Built Environment and Population Health in Small-Town America

Built Environment and Population Health in Small-Town America

Learning from Small Cities of Kansas

MAHBUB RASHID

Johns Hopkins University Press

Baltimore

2 4 6 8 9 7 5 3 1

Johns Hopkins University Press
2715 North Charles Street
Baltimore, Maryland 21218
www.press.jhu.edu

Library of Congress Cataloging-in-Publication Data is available.

A catalog record for this book is available from the British Library.

ISBN 978-1-4214-4799-5 (hardcover)
ISBN 978-1-4214-4800-8 (ebook)

Special discounts are available for bulk purchases of this book. For more information, please contact Special Sales at specialsales@jh.edu.

To my students and teachers

CONTENTS

List of Figures and Tables   ix

Preface   xi

Acknowledgments   xxv

1 Introduction to Population Health: *From Theory to Practice*   1

PART I   SMALL-TOWN AMERICA AND ITS
POPULATION HEALTH CONTEXTS

2 Rural and Small-Town America: *Definitions*   37

3 The Rural Contexts of Population Health in Small-Town America:
Consequences of Ongoing Changes   49

PART II   STORIES OF SMALL CITIES OF KANSAS

4 Small Cities of Kansas: *Stories of Recent Changes*   75

5 Health in Small Cities of Kansas: *Stories of Recent Concerns*   94

PART III   APPROACHES, METHODS, AND STUDY SAMPLE

6 Approaches and Methods: *How to Study Spatial Associations
of Population Health in Small-Town America*   119

7 The Study Sample: *A Description of Its Spatial,
Lifestyle, and Health Data*   152

PART IV   RURALITY, SPATIAL FACTORS,
AND LIFESTYLE IN SMALL CITIES OF KANSAS

8   Spatial Associations of Lifestyle in Small Cities of Kansas:
Correlational Analyses   171

9   Rurality and Spatial Associations of Lifestyle in Small Cities of Kansas:
Comparative Correlational Analyses   195

PART V   RURALITY, SPATIAL FACTORS, AND
HEALTH STATUS IN SMALL CITIES OF KANSAS

10   Spatial Associations of Health in Small Cities of Kansas:
Correlational Analyses   229

11   Rurality and Spatial Associations of Health in Small Cities of Kansas:
Comparative Correlational Analyses   251

PART VI   PROBLEMS AND PROSPECTS OF SPATIAL
PLANNING AND DESIGN FOR POPULATION HEALTH
IN SMALL-TOWN AMERICA

12   Built Environment and Population Health in Small Cities of Kansas:
Study Limitations, Findings, and Implications   285

13   Health Promotion in Small-Town America: *Traditional and
Participatory Approaches and Some General Principles*   314

References   355
Index   421

FIGURES

1.1. A high-level depiction of the socio-ecological approach
to health   6

1.2. Interactions among different spatial scales and
organizational levels of health   20

1.3. Potential pathways through which spatial design and
planning factors may influence health and health-
related behaviors   23

6.1. Potential pathways through which spatial design and
planning factors may influence health and health-
related behaviors, highlighting the pathways studied
in this book   127

7.1. Locations of the small cities in the study sample   154

TABLES

5.1. Health rankings for Johnson and Wyandotte Counties,
Kansas   109

5.2. Measures for different health outcomes and factors for
Johnson and Wyandotte Counties, Kansas   110

7.1. Population and land area of the sample cities   153

7.2. Descriptive statistics for different measures of the
spatial factors in the sample cities   159

7.3. Descriptive statistics for different measures of lifestyle
in the sample cities   161

7.4. Descriptive statistics for different measures of health
in the sample cities   164

*8.1.   Correlations between lifestyle and city size, density, availability of key destinations and facilities, and land use types and mix

*8.2.   Correlations between different lifestyle behaviors and street properties

9.1.   Significant correlations between spatial factors and work-related travel behaviors   203

9.2.   Significant correlations between spatial factors and food-shopping and eating behaviors   210

9.3.   Significant correlations between spatial factors and physical and sedentary activities   218

9.4.   Ranking of significant correlations between spatial factors and lifestyle   222

*10.1.   Correlations between different health indicators and city size, density, availability of key destinations and facilities, and land use types and mix

*10.2.   Correlations between different health indicators and street properties

11.1.   Significant correlations between spatial factors and mortality and morbidity indicators   257

11.2.   Significant correlations between spatial factors and physical health indicators   262

11.3.   Significant correlations between spatial factors and mental health indicators   267

11.4.   Significant correlations between spatial factors and social health indicators   275

11.5.   Ranking of significant correlations between spatial factors and health outcomes and indicators   278

Problem and Purpose

Places of living—buildings, neighborhoods, cities—help contextualize health and population health by uniquely combining physical, social, and natural features. On the one hand, they protect and promote health and healthy behaviors. On the other hand, they contribute to health risks [1–3]. Health status, health care access, health service use, health service deficits, and adequacy of health care are all dependent on places of living [4–13]. As the need to address avoidable health-related inequities continues to grow [14, 15], it is important to recognize that an extensive body of public and population health–related research already shows place of living as a significant factor for health disparities. According to this literature, everything else remaining constant, health inequities vary for people living in different places.

Even though literature in social epidemiology [1] and population health [16] has only recently recognized the importance of rurality—a concept that defines the status of a place based on its lack of urbanity—it already includes enough evidence suggesting that population health disparities may exist within and between urban and rural areas [14, 17]. Despite the debate surrounding various methods of classifying what constitutes a rural or urban area [18], studies continue to find that differences in health between rural and urban populations are real [19–22] and that living in a rural area brings higher risk of substantial health disadvantages, in some cases alarmingly so, in comparison to urban areas [23, 24]. In rural areas, the population at large experiences avoidable "differences in the incidence, prevalence, mortality, and burden of diseases and other adverse health conditions" [25]. This knowledge indicates a serious need for addressing rural health to improve the quality of life. Does such a need exist in small towns and cities? Is population health there any different from rural areas?

A lack of evidence prevents us from suggesting that small-town populations suffer place-based health disparities similar to those of rural populations. One important misconception has been that small-town America is indistinguishable from rural America and, therefore, the population health of small-town America is no different from that of rural America. In this book, I aim to clarify this misconception. For political, administrative, and census reasons, small-town America is often considered a part of rural America. As a geographical and sociological unit, however, small-town America is very different from the rest of rural America, and so are its population health concerns. These population health concerns are also different from those of urban America due to many differences in environmental context and scale, social and cultural norms, economic and lifestyle opportunities, and demographic composition of urban and small-town America.

The purpose of this book is to describe the population health concerns of small-town America and to learn how these concerns are affected by their unique characteristics, with a focus on the built environment. I use the isolated small cities of the state of Kansas in the United States as case studies. Dictated by a socio-ecological approach, in these studies I use various spatial design and planning factors describing the *built environment* at the city or community level; lifestyle, morbidity and mortality, and physical, mental, and social health risk factors and outcomes describing *population health*; and population size and density, change in population due to daytime travel, distance from the nearest city with 50,000 or more people, and commuting time describing *rurality*.

First, I introduce the sample of small cities from Kansas using spatial, lifestyle, and health data. Following this, I explore spatial associations of lifestyle and health for the whole sample as well as for different subsamples of small cities, defined based on rurality. Using the findings of these studies and those reported in the literature, I then provide spatial design and planning guidelines, policies, and strategies to promote health in small-town America toward the end of the book.

Why Small Cities of Kansas?

Kansas is a predominantly rural state with numerous isolated small cities. The physical, political, social, and economic geographies of these small cities are constantly shifting. Although agriculture is still the economic backbone of these small cities, their continued existence heavily depends on big cities with supermarkets, hospitals, schools, churches, courts, restaurants, retail stores, and shopping centers. As in most states, small cities in Kansas face many health-related challenges. These challenges include shrinking population, poverty and isolation, limited access to health care, increasing prevalence of obesity and chronic diseases, and limited job and food availability.

Some simple facts about the state may help put things in perspective. According to the 2020 data from the Kansas Department of Health and Environment, on average there are 99 live births every day in Kansas. The number includes 36 births to unwed mothers and 6 to teenagers, 7 births with low birthweight, and some infant deaths. Clearly, several births daily in Kansas are occurring in unfavorable conditions. Corollary to that, there are 76 deaths every day in Kansas. Several of these deaths are probably preventable and untimely [26]. Put simply, Kansas as a state does poorly in terms of many basic health indicators.

The poor population health conditions of many rural states like Kansas remained largely unnoticed until the recent tragedies caused by the SARS-CoV-2 global pandemic brought them to the forefront. According to Google's COVID-19 Open Data on May 30, 2021, the total number of reported COVID-19 cases in Kansas was 312,997. The number of cases per 1 million people in the state was 107,437, which is higher than the national number of 100,858 cases per 1 million people. The data provided by Google also reported the number of cases per million people for 36 counties out of 105 counties of the state. Out of these 36 counties, 23 had a higher number of cases per million than the national number, and 18 had a higher number than the state number. Out of 105 counties in Kanas, 79 counties had a death rate per 10,000 people due to COVID higher than the state rate of 161.57; 70 counties had a death rate higher than the national rate of 178.77; and 54 counties had a death rate higher than the world rate of 207.92. At least 99 of these counties had over 100 deaths per 10,000 people, which is a much higher death rate than the combined death rate per 10,000 for the 10 leading causes of death in the United States.

COVID-19 was able to wreak such havoc in Kansas because there are high rates of *diabetes*, *obesity*, *depression*, and *anxiety* in Kansas, along with many other chronic health conditions [27, 28]. The percentage of adults 65 and older is also high in many places in Kansas. COVID-19 has been particularly deadly for older people and for people with comorbidity.

COVID-19 has also been deadly among people who have household incomes at or below the poverty level. According to a report by ABC News [29], the death rate was 1.6 times higher in counties where the median household income was below $35,000 than in counties where household income was higher than $75,000. The death rate was 2.5 times higher in the very poorest counties, where a quarter of residents are below the poverty line, than it was in the richest counties. In Kansas, 11.4% of the total population lives in poverty. Of this, 15.5% are 65 and older. The 2015–2019 median household income (in 2019 dollars) was only $59,597 in Kansas, indicating that a large percentage of its population may be close to poverty.

Along with poor health and poverty, a lack of hospitals with intensive care unit (ICU) beds is notable in many Kansas counties and was a contributing factor for high COVID-19 deaths in the state. Most Kansas counties have critical access hospitals, which offer 24-hour emergency care services 7 days a week. These hospitals do not have more than 25 beds and cannot keep patients over 4 days for inpatient care. Traditionally, they relied on partner hospitals for patients who needed ICU care. During the COVID-19 pandemic, most partner hospitals ran out of ICU beds, causing delays in transferring patients from critical access hospitals—which proved deadly in many cases.

Making matters worse, local health departments in Kansas and around the country had already faced significant obstacles over the past decade. In addition to an 18% drop in national spending for local health departments since 2010, at least 38,000 state and local public health jobs have been eliminated since the 2008 recession, leaving behind a skeletal workforce, according to an investigation by Kaiser Health News and the Associated Press [30]. A lack of health care workers has been particularly severe in poor rural places in several states, including Kansas, for several years now. These are the places where one does not wish to live during a global pandemic.

Regarding the spread of COVID-19 in rural communities of Kansas and other midwestern states, the most harmful element might have been the sense of independence and freedom these communities had developed over many generations. "I think early on people just thought, 'Well, we're either going to get it or we're not going to get it,' or 'I'm not ever going to wear a mask,'" said one resident. Another resident observed, "An oasis in the desert, where we can do what we want . . . because this is still America, and we still have our freedoms, and we don't like to give them up much." When the governor of Kansas issued an executive order in early July 2020 requiring masks in public places, many Kansas counties opted out of a mandate. A county police chief noted on Facebook, "It has come to our attention that some are concerned that we are not enforcing laws to protect our communities. . . . The Governor's order is NOT a law. It has not been passed by our state legislature and therefore, not a criminal law that we can, nor will, enforce" [31].

Put simply, the status of the population health of Kansas is poor, with many contributing factors, which became clear during the COVID-19 global pandemic. Improving the health status of the state will require significant changes in many areas. This book does not cover all these different areas related to population health. Rather, it explores ways to improve the population health status of small-town residents of the state through changes in the built environment only.

Relevance for Small-Town America

One might ask why a book written on the built environment and population health of small cities in Kansas should be relevant to the other parts of small-town America. After all, small-town America shows significant differences within its vast territories. The rural high plains have had a history of population loss for over a century, something that has not occurred in many other parts of rural or small-town America. Will someone working on the population health of a small city in Florida, Alabama, or Georgia find this book useful? How about someone working on that of small towns and cities of Maine or California?

A similarly conceived book on another part of small-town America may produce results different from what I present in this book. While these differences matter, the built environment of small towns and cities has not yet been studied in relation to population health. Therefore, we must start somewhere. It matters less if a study is confined to one state only. The analogical use of studies done in one context to another is common in the literature. For example, health effects of the built environment are likely to be different in different metropolitan areas. Yet we continue to study these effects in different metropolitan areas for generalizable findings with the hope that generalizability depends less on *what* we study and more on *how* we study.

Besides giving us a glimpse of how the built environment of small cities in Kansas is related to population health, the significance of this book also rests on the fact that spatial design and planning dynamics generally are more consistent across small-town America than they are across metropolitan or urban America. The basic job requirements of small-town design and planning professionals, the planning provisions in small towns, the need to plan for preserving natural resources and enhancing economic opportunities in small towns, and a general lack of proper zoning ordinances, subdivision regulations and public infrastructure in small towns are among many things that seem to remain similar across small-town America, from Florida to Washington and from California to Maine. In this sense, small-town design and planning professionals across different regions may be able to learn relevant lessons based on studies of small cities and towns in any US region despite specific regional differences in population health and built environments.

Relevance for Urban America

A reader interested in the population health of urban America may find this book less interesting, but there are several points to be made in this regard. These points, as described below, indicate that the significance of small-town design and planning for population health should continue to grow for both urban and rural America.

First, this book should make the reader aware that the contrasts between small-town America and urban America are great. These contrasts should make the reader think differently about how built environments are associated with population health. For example, some neighborhood qualities may not have similar associations with population health in urban and small-town America.

Second, the problems of population health are often geographically determined, but their effects are not always geographically confined. While the associations between the built environment and population health in urban and rural America may be different, these differences are less important than health disparities that arise due to these differential associations. Anyone interested in rural-urban population health disparities must find this book on the population health of small-town America as relevant as any book on the population health of urban America.

Third, since the time it was founded as a discipline, public health has remained focused on urban health problems. Now, it is time to shift its focus away from more urbanized metropolitan areas to less urbanized rural areas before some of these less urbanized areas become heavily urbanized or become an extended part of a metropolitan area. In this regard, we should note that population health problems in small towns and cities are difficult to solve, but they remain more manageable than the problems we find in large cities. It is true that steps to mitigate population health problems in rural and small-town areas are long overdue, but the significance of these problems has never been clear in our urban consciousness. Thanks to COVID-19, now it has become clear.

Lessons to Be Learned

The extent of population health problems in small-town America is alarming. Still, no book that considers the built environment of small-town America in relation to its population health problems has been written to dispel the myth that small-town America is generally healthier than urban America.

There is nothing homogeneous about small-town America. The built environment and population health of small cities and towns of this country and its states vary significantly based on their rurality. Their social, economic, and political structures providing the context for spatial design and planning are complex. They provide very little support for spatial design and planning services and activities promoting health. Conventional urban design and planning approaches and techniques are inadequate to deal with spatial design and planning problems related to population health in small-town America.

There is no easy way to solve spatial design and planning problems related to population health in small-town America. The nature of these problems varies depending on how one looks at them. For example, there is no single way to define the rurality of small towns and cities. The status of a small city or town may change based on how one defines rurality, which then changes the way spatial design and planning factors are considered in relation to population health problems. Notably, rurality is just one of many factors that can affect spatial associations of population health in small-town America. Therefore, finding ways to define and characterize the differences between small towns and cities is important for health promotion through appropriate and effective spatial design and planning strategies.

Spatial design and planning strategies are not enough for health promotion in small cities and towns, however. Most small cities and towns generally lack the tools, provisions, and resources necessary to implement effective spatial planning and design strategies promoting population health. Small-town design and planning professionals must participate in a constant struggle for improving the health of a population who may know very little about what these professionals do. Therefore, they must consider community participation and empowerment along with spatial design and planning for health promotion in small towns and cities of the county.

Key Points

This book makes six key points. First, rural America, urban America, and their relationships are changing. These changes are having indelible effects on small-town America, giving rise to significant population health problems. Second, the population health problems of small-town America are as severe as the problems of some of the most deprived parts in urban America. These problems are related to lifestyle and to physical, mental, and social health and well-being. The nature of these problems, however, is different in small-town America from urban America. Third, the built environment of small-town America presents population health threats, as does the built environment of urban America, but the nature of these threats is different in small-town America. Fourth, there are far fewer studies on the effects of built environments on population health in small-town America than in urban America. Fifth, many features of the built environment that show significant health effects on urban population, such as zoning, subdivision regulations, and public transportation systems, either do not exist in small towns or do not work in the same way as they do in urban America. Many other features of the built environment that show significant health effects on urban populations show either dissimilar health effects or different mechanisms for similar health effects on small-town populations. Finally, spatial planning and design approaches for improving population health must consider the differences and similarities between small-town America and urban America, acknowledging that small-town planning and design are different from urban planning and design.

Other Books on the Subject

Sociological and social science studies on rural America focusing on the changing structure of agriculture, natural resources and the environment, economy, demography, migration and immigration, diversity, and life in rural communities are extensive. They span over a century. Among the recently published books, some are broad in scope [32–40]. Others are narrow in scope, covering such topics as housing in rural America [41]; rural aging in the 21st century [42] in relation to economy, race, ethnicity, migration, and other social structures and patterns [43]; rural poverty [44, 45]; race and identity [46]; mental health [47] and other critical health issues [48]; and rural health care services and delivery [47, 49–52].

Books looking at the relationships between population health and the built environment of small towns and cities in rural areas, however, have not yet been written. This contrasts with the fact that quite a few books have looked at the relationships between health and the built environment in large cities [53–59]. Focusing on large cities, many books have covered topics such as urban poverty, race, and environmental injustice [60]; the social determinants of health in the urban context and the role of local government [61]; the effects of sprawling urban development [62]; the effects of active transportation and air pollution exposure [63]; and the US food system and its interrelationships with public health, the environment, equity, and society [64]. Existing books have also covered various research approaches [65], design strategies [66, 67], and decision-making frameworks [68].

By comprehensively looking at the relationships between population health and the built environment of small towns and cities in rural America, this book will help fill in the gap that currently exists in the literature.

Outline of the Book

There are thirteen chapters in the book, twelve of which are divided into six parts. In chapter 1, health is described as a broad concept that includes physical, mental, and social health and well-being. Following this, the key principles of population health are described as a new approach to health promotion. A multidimensional socio-ecological model is provided that describes potential links between population health and social, built, and natural environments. Next, various pathways of influences are identified that show how spatial factors of the built environment may affect population health. The final two sections of the chapter describe the projects and programs of Healthy Cities and Communities. Sponsored by the World Health Organization, these projects and programs in different countries use a socio-ecological approach to health promotion. The basic concepts and processes of these projects and programs are described and their limitations are identified.

Part I considers small-town America and its population health contexts. In chapter 2, the definitions of rural and small-town America are discussed. Many would agree that one important difficulty in examining population health in small-town America is a lack of consistent definitions for small towns and cities. Without proper definitions, doubts may arise about the validity and utility of research studies presented in this book. Therefore, an attempt is made to define small towns and cities. The consequences of many ongoing changes in the rural contexts of small-town America are discussed in chapter 3.

In part II, I tell the stories of small cities of Kansas. Chapter 4 provides an account of recent economic, demographic, and environmental changes in small cities of Kansas using stories published in local and national news sources or in scholarly publications when available. Chapter 5 offers an account of population health in small cities of Kansas focusing on a few factors and indicators of population health for which the state ranks poorly.

Chapters 6 and 7 constitute part III. In chapter 6, I describe the general approach to research, the specific pathways of influence, the study variables, and the general principles of statistical analyses used in the studies of the book. Among other things, a scale- and place-based approach to understanding the effects of the built environment on population health in small towns and cities is emphasized. In chapter 7, I explain the selection of the sample of small cities of Kansas for the studies of the book, beginning with why and how they were selected. Following this, I describe the sources of socio-economic, demographic, crime, health, and spatial data used in the studies as well as the built environments and the lifestyles and the health status of the people of these cities.

Part IV includes chapters 8 and 9. In chapter 8, the associations of spatial (planning and design) factors with lifestyles in small cities of Kansas are explored using correlational analyses. This is accompanied by a review of the literature reporting these associations. In chapter 9, the effects of rurality on the associations between spatial factors and lifestyles in small cities of Kansas are explored, taking into account various factors of rurality.

In chapter 10 of part V, I use correlational analyses to explore the associations of spatial factors with health outcomes and indicators in small cities of Kansas. This is also accompanied by a review of the literature reporting these associations. In chapter 11, the effects of rurality on the associations between spatial factors and health outcomes and indicators in small cities of Kansas are explored, taking into account various factors of rurality.

In chapter 12 of part VI, the limitations of the studies presented in this book are discussed, focusing on the definitions of small towns and cities, the socio-ecological model of population health, the lifestyles and health outcomes and indicators, the study sample and the study data, and the analysis of data. Following this, I present the findings of the studies and their implications for small-town design and planning from a population health perspective.

Finally, in chapter 13, two different but complementary approaches to health promotion are described. They are the traditional spatial design and planning approach and the somewhat nontraditional participatory design and planning approach. First, I explain the various contextual complexities and constraints faced by small-town design and planning professionals. Then, I go on to describe the participatory design and planning approach to health promotion, highlighting its limitations, advantages, and status in rural areas and small towns and cities. The description borrows from the community participation approaches of Healthy Cities and Communities presented in the introductory chapter of the book. Finally, in the third part of the chapter, I present a set of general principles for small-town design and planning professionals to follow as they try to fulfill their mission in the intellectual and professional vacuum of small towns and cities. Following this, a separate set of general principles for participatory design and planning is provided for small towns and cities focusing on, among other things, health in all policies, empowerment, and health equality.

Intended Audience

The book explores the relationships between the built environment and population health in small-town America. It also explores the effects of rurality on these relationships. Being exploratory in nature, the book should be appropriate for both undergraduate and graduate students seeking to learn about these topics. The chapters are interconnected; however, they are also written as stand-alone parts, each with its own introduction and conclusions. Therefore, these chapters can potentially be short readings for a wide range of courses in different academic disciplines, including community planning and development, urban design and planning, rural planning and development, public and population health, and public policy and administration.

Overall, this book is for anyone who wants to know how spatial factors of the built environment may be associated with population health in small-town America, and how small-town communities can manage these associations through both a traditional spatial design and planning approach and a nontraditional participatory design and planning approach to promoting population health.

NOTES

1. Berke, "Geographic Information Systems (GIS)."
2. Koh, Graham, and Glied, "Reducing Racial and Ethnic Disparities."
3. Cummins et al., "Understanding and Representing 'Place' in Health Research."
4. Beyer et al., "Explaining Place-Based Colorectal Cancer Health Disparities."
5. Singh, "Rural-Urban Trends and Patterns."

6. Krishna, Gillespie, and McBride, "Diabetes Burden and Access to Preventive Care."

7. Lutfiyya et al., "Are There Disparities in Diabetes Care?"

8. Lutfiyya et al., "Is Rural Residency a Risk Factor?"

9. Lutfiyya, Chang, and Lipsky, "A Cross-Sectional Study of US Rural Adults' Consumption of Fruits and Vegetables."

10. Lutfiyya et al., "Adolescent Daily Cigarette Smoking."

11. Lutfiyya, McCullough, and Lipsky, "A Population-Based Study of Health Service Deficits."

12. Lutfiyya et al., "Adequacy of Diabetes Care for Older US Rural Adults."

13. Lutfiyya et al., "A Comparison of Quality of Care Indicators."

14. Bellamy, Bolin, and Gamm, "Rural Healthy People 2010, 2020, and Beyond."

15. Bolin et al., "Rural Healthy People 2020."

16. Hartley, "Rural Health Disparities, Population Health, and Rural Culture."

17. Lutfiyya et al., "Rurality as a Root or Fundamental Social Determinant of Health."

18. Hart, Larson, and Lishner, "Rural Definitions for Health Policy and Research."

19. Johnson et al., "Rural-Urban Health Care Provider Disparities."

20. Joynt et al., "Quality of Care and Patient Outcomes in Critical Access Rural Hospitals."

21. Ingram and Franco, *2013 NCHS Urban-Rural Classification Scheme for Counties.*

22. National Center for Health Statistics, *Health, United States, 2013.*

23. Erwin et al., "Health Disparities in Rural Areas."

24. Braveman, "AOTA's Statement on Health Disparities."

25. US Congress, "Minority Health and Health Disparities."

26. Norman, *2020: The State of the Health of Kansans.*

27. Bureau of Epidemiology and Public Health Informatics, *Kansas: Annual Summary of Vital Statistics, 2019.*

28. United Health Foundation, *America's Health Rankings: Annual Report 2020.*

29. Schumaker and Nichols, "An American Tragedy."

30. Weber et al., "Hollowed-Out Public Health System Faces More Cuts Amid Virus."

31. Maxouris, "For Months, a Rural Kansas Community Watched the COVID-19 Pandemic Unfold from Afar."

32. Bailey, Jensen, and Ransom, eds. *Rural America in a Globalizing World.*

33. Brown, and Swanson, *Challenges for Rural America in the Twenty-First Century.*

34. Flora, Flora, and Gasteyer, *Rural Communities.*

35. Fuguitt, Brown, and Beale, *Rural and Small Town America.*

36. Hicks, Powers, and Broderick, *Small Town.*

37. Kley and Paul, *Rural America.*

38. Moore, *The Hidden America.*

39. Riney-Kehrberg, *The Routledge History of Rural America.*

40. Wuthnow, *Small-Town America.*

41. Belden and Wiener, *Housing in Rural America.*

42. Youmans, *Older Rural Americans.*

43. Glasgow, Berry, and Edmund, *Rural Aging in 21st Century America.*

44. Dáil, *Hard Living in America's Heartland.*

45. Tickamyer, Sherman, and Warlick, *Rural Poverty in the United States.*

46. Lensmire, *White Folks.*

47. Smalley, Warren, and Rainer, *Rural Mental Health.*

48. Crosby et al., *Rural Populations and Health.*

49. Fitzpatrick and Merwin, *Focus on Rural Health.*

50. Gesler and Ricketts, *Health in Rural North America.*

51. Ricketts, *Rural Health in the United States.*

52. Stamm, *Rural Behavioral Health Care.*
53. Barton et al., *The Routledge Handbook of Planning for Health and Well-Being.*
54. Freudenberg, Galea, and Vlahov, *Cities and the Health of the Public.*
55. Freudenberg, Klitzman, and Saegert, *Urban Health and Society.*
56. Gatrell and Elliott, *Geographies of Health.*
57. Hynes and Lopez, *Urban Health.*
58. Nieuwenhuijsen and Khreis, *Integrating Human Health into Urban and Transport Planning.*
59. Lopez, *The Built Environment and Public Health.*
60. Fitzpatrick and LaGory, *Unhealthy Cities.*
61. WHO Commission on Social Determinants of Health, *Addressing the Social Determinants of Health.*
62. Frumkin, Frank, and Jackson, *Urban Sprawl and Public Health.*
63. Frank et al., "Many Pathways from Land Use to Health."
64. Neff, *Introduction to the US Food System.*
65. Sarkar, Webster, and Gallacher, *Healthy Cities.*
66. Gaston and Kreyling, *Shaping the Healthy Community.*
67. Jackson and Sinclair, *Designing Healthy Communities.*
68. Corburn, *Toward the Healthy City.*

ACKNOWLEDGMENTS

I would like to thank the students of my seminar classes, who helped me conceive the book. I would also like to thank Bushra Obeidat, Lingling Li, Bushra Nayeem, and Monalipa Dash for helping me collect the data for the book. Additionally, I would like to thank Johns Hopkins University Press for taking up my book project for publication. Finally, I would like to thank my parents and my siblings and their children, who never lost faith in my abilities, and my wife and children for their love and patience.

Built Environment and Population Health in Small-Town America

CHAPTER ONE

Introduction to Population Health

From Theory to Practice

That the built environment can affect health and health-related behaviors has been known since the dawn of human civilization. Our earliest cities were designed with various positive health outcomes in mind: the orientation of a city was based on sunlight availability and wind directions; unwanted land uses were placed away from the main areas of the city; fortifications were designed to protect and save lives; and so on [1–4]. More recently, modern city and urban planning fields were created to protect and improve public health and safety in our early industrial cities. Construed based on normative knowledge, in all these and other early spatial design and planning efforts, health remained narrowly defined as a disease-free state of human body, and the effects of the built environment on health and health-related behaviors were rarely considered empirically and systematically.

Today, due to progress made in public and population health, there has been a noticeable shift away from the traditional concept of health as a disease-free state of human body and the built environment as an undefinable factor of health and health-related behaviors. Highlighting that the narrowly defined traditional concepts had underestimated the scope of health and the role of the built environment as an active agent of individual and population health, the broad contemporary concepts have redefined health as a positive state, not just a disease-free state, and have stressed the importance of built, natural, and social environments as agents determining, shaping, and moderating health and health-related behaviors.

The purpose of this introductory chapter is to describe the broad contemporary concepts of health to guide research linking population health and environments. First, focusing on its physiological, mental, and social dimensions, the concept of health is described as something more than a disease-free state of human body [5]. Next, an attempt to define the concept of population health is made. A socio-ecological framework of population health is presented, where health is considered in relation to different spatial scales and organizational levels of its environmental contexts. Concerning the framework, first the contexts of population health are described, which include built, social, and natural environments. Then, the spatial scales and the organizational levels of these environments, as well as the interactions across these spatial scales and organizational levels, are described. Based on the socio-ecological framework, pathways of influence are also identified, showing how spatial (design and planning) factors may affect health and population health.

In recent years, spatial design and planning professionals have been among many who have embraced the population health concept as an approach to building healthy cities and communities in many countries around the world, sometimes with support from the World Health Organization (WHO). In the final sections of this chapter, this professional approach to health promotion is discussed, highlighting its lack of research-based evidence. This lack of evidence is particularly noticeable for small towns and cities in the United States and other countries. As a remarkably understudied area of research and practice, health promotion in small towns and cities requires serious attention not only from spatial design and planning researchers and professionals but also from public and population health experts and policymakers.

Health: An Evolving Concept

Health is more than a disease-free state of human body. The WHO's definition of health, formulated in 1948, was an early attempt to consider health more broadly beyond a disease-free physical state. It described health as "a state of complete physical, mental and social well-being and not merely the absence of disease or infirmity" [6]. In this definition, physical or physiological health is the presence or absence of infectious, chronic, or life-threatening diseases or physical disabilities. Mental health, on the other hand, is believed to concern the prevalence of common psychiatric disorders, including depression, anxiety, and cognitive impairment. More broadly, mental health refers to subjective well-being, perceived self-efficacy, autonomy, and competence. It is about enhancing competencies of individuals and communities and enabling them to achieve their self-determined goals. Finally, social health is essentially governed by social interactions affecting health, social support promoting a sense of community necessary to help each other, and social well-being promoting, among other things, a sense of safety, satisfaction, and happiness within groups and communities [7].

By emphasizing mental health and well-being along with physical health, the WHO made mental health a concern for all of us, rather than for only those who suffer from a mental disorder, at a time when its significance generally was ignored. Mental health problems affect society, and not just a small, isolated segment. Depression, for example, has been a leading contributor to the global burden of disease [8]. No group is immune to mental disorders, but the risk is higher among people who live in poverty, people without housing, people who are unemployed, people with low education, victims of violence, migrants and refugees, Indigenous populations, children and adolescents, abused women, and the neglected elderly. Still today, more than six decades after the WHO provided its definition of health, mental health is not accorded anywhere near the same degree of importance as physical health in most parts of the world. Rather, it is largely ignored or neglected.

By emphasizing social health and well-being, the WHO's definition recognized that individual health and well-being cannot be separated from social health; that social realities defined based on beliefs, customs, tradition, culture, religion, and social class are important for individual and social health; and that the unequal distribution of health-damaging experiences is not in any sense a "natural" phenomenon but is the result of a combination of poor spatial design and planning, poor social and environmental policies, unfair economic arrangements, and other inflexible realities of a society [9, 10]. Though it was not acknowledged as important at the time the WHO provided its definition, it is now acknowledged that good social health can enhance government performance, improve social justice and democracy [11], prevent crime and delinquency, and promote population health [12].

Social health has individual as well as collective dimensions [13]. The individual dimensions of social health include an individual's well-being that concerns how she gets along with other people, how other people react to her, and how she interacts with social institutions and societal mores [14]. These individual dimensions often dictate individual behaviors, including alcohol consumption, tobacco use, and sexual activity [11, 15, 16]. Better social health as it pertains to individuals is often associated with significant decreases in mental health problems and lower rates of homicide, suicide, and alcohol and drug abuse [11, 17]. The collective dimensions of social health include trust and cohesion; willingness to act for the community's benefit; community engagement, such as voting or volunteering; behavior norms; and gender norms. They are evident in the fact that when people come together for the common good, communities are better able to use their resources and efforts to reduce levels of crime and violence [11, 18] and improve food access [11, 19].

Groundbreaking in its breadth and ambition, the WHO's definition provided, and still provides, an understanding that health encompasses physical, mental, and social well-being, as well as their interactions. Though it was not known clearly at the time the WHO formulated its definition, now we know that mental disorders (e.g., depression, anxiety, and substance abuse) occur in people suffering from both noncommunicable and communicable diseases more often than would be expected by chance. And people suffering from chronic physical conditions have a greater probability of developing mental disorders such as depression. The rate of suicide is higher among people with physical disorders than among people without these disorders. Social isolation and loneliness can lead to mental and physical health problems.

Today, the WHO has taken an even broader view of health. According to its Ottawa Charter, health is understood as "a resource for everyday life," which allows an individual or group "to identify and to realize aspirations, to satisfy needs, and to change or cope with the environment," whereas health promotion has been defined as "the process of enabling people to increase control over, and to improve, their health" [20]. In this regard, the concept of population health becomes relevant because it considers the WHO's broad definition of health and health promotion.

Population Health: A New Approach to Health Promotion
The Concept of Population Health

As early as 1990, Evans and Stoddart described population health as a framework characterized by a broad definition of health. This framework recognized health determinants that exist outside health care systems and explicitly acknowledged trade-offs between investing in health care and investing in other social goods [21, 22]. Later, Kindig and Stoddart defined population health as "the health outcomes of a group of individuals, including the distribution of such outcomes within the group" [23]. Subsequent definitions have proposed refinements [24], but their primary focus has remained on the aggregate or population dimension, as distinct from the health of an individual.

In its more recent use, population health signifies a conceptual approach to understanding the drivers of health and consequently the strategies most useful to improving health. This approach is consistent with broad definitions of public health as a field of study with a purpose to understand the drivers of the health of the public, encompassing both distal and proximal factors [25], as well as a field of actions that a society defines and undertakes collectively to ensure conditions for people to remain physically, mentally, and socially healthy [26].

One of the three key principles of population health is that it embraces the WHO's positive concept of health. According to this principle, there is a need to integrate physical, mental, and social health in the promotion of population health. The second key principle is that "Health for All"—a concept requiring health be brought within reach of everyone—cannot be attained without taking a socio-ecological viewpoint. Discussed more thoroughly in the next few sections of this chapter, the socio-ecological viewpoint of population health recognizes that the determinants of health include various aspects of the natural, physical, and social environments extending from the individual level to that of our culture and the global ecosystem. Clearly, Health for All embraces a broad range of strategies, including public policies at the national and local levels. The third key principle is that it is not possible to substantially improve the health of a population without addressing health inequities it suffers. Simply put, the determinants of health inequities generally are the determinants of population health. Therefore, population health must be explicitly concerned with health equity [27].

The Socio-Ecological Model of Health

Figure 1.1 provides a high-level depiction of the socio-ecological model of health. As shown in the figure and as described below, the contexts of health include built, social, and natural environments. Each of these environments can directly influence health. Each can also indirectly influence health through its influence on the relationships between health and the other environments. For those familiar with public health literature, the conceptual framework has obvious and intentional antecedents: Barton and Grant's settlement health map [28]; Hancock's "mandala of health" linking health and the human ecosystem [29]; and more specifically, Dahlgren and Whitehead's model of the social determinants of health [30].

The socio-ecological model considers health at different organizational levels, such as individual, group, and community. It also considers environments at different spatial scales, such as micro, meso, and macro scales. In the model, the health of an individual, a group, or a community can be affected differently by different environmental factors of different scales, giving rise to nu-

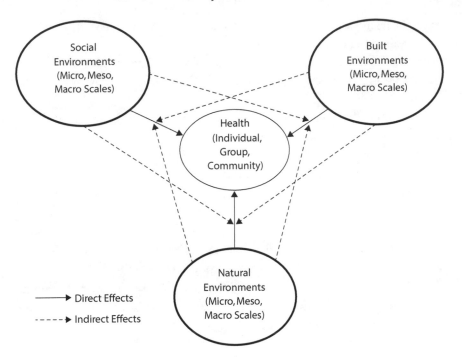

Figure 1.1. A high-level depiction of the socio-ecological approach to health. When considering human health, we must link the built, social, and natural environments.

merous pathways of health influence. According to the model, spatial design and planning factors of the built environment are important because they can directly affect health, or they can indirectly affect health by moderating or mediating the relationships between the natural or social environments and health. The model suggests that healthy spatial design and planning require interventions that should be guided by considerations for each environment at different scales.

CONTEXTS OF HEALTH

According to a socio-ecological model of health, the contexts of health must include all relevant distal and proximal factors of the natural, built, and social environments of a population. These contextual factors frequently interact and cannot be disassociated when trying to understand and improve health inequities [31, 32]. Access to food, natural and social resources, inclusive transportation systems and other public infrastructure, affordable housing, safe neighborhoods, and many other things play a crucial role in shaping social equity and inclusion and, therefore, population health outcomes [33].

Natural Environments. Natural environments (the natural world or simply *nature*) include natural resources, such as land, air, forests, mountains, rivers, seas, minerals, water, and climate, as well as different forms of energy. Humans are fundamentally dependent on nature [34, 35]. All systems and goods that support health and well-being can ultimately be traced back to nature [36]. Yet human activities continue to cause many harmful changes to natural environments. These changes increase the frequency of extreme events, threaten ecological balance, and affect food systems. They also increase conflicts and displacement of people, with consequent health impacts. Environmental changes have, and will increasingly have, an enormous impact on human health.

We can use increased air pollution as an example to illustrate how anthropogenic activities might have caused significant changes to natural environments during the last century or so. In the first half of the twentieth century, air pollution in the developed world increased steadily as industrialization progressed, industries and homes used coal for power and heat, and automobiles proliferated. As a result, cities had the worst pollution [37]. In the second half of the century, however, and especially in the last few decades, many forms of pollution decreased in urban areas as coal was phased out, manufacturing plants moved to the suburbs or to the developing world, lead was banned from gasoline, and the automobile industry was forced to build cleaner cars.

Despite many advances, the global disease burden attributed to air pollution from all sources did not change [38]. In modern cities, air pollution continues to cause asthma and wheezing [39, 40], impair lung function [41], restrict physical activity [41], and increase hospital admissions [41]. It also increases cardiovascular mortality and morbidity [41, 42] and all-cause mortality [40, 41]. As late as the mid-1990s, researchers estimated that urban air pollution contributed to 30,000–60,000 deaths per year in the United States [43, 44]. Likewise, in Britain, it is estimated that poor air quality is responsible for 29,000 premature deaths, 5% of the total every year, with an average reduction in life span of 11 years [45]. Many developing nations face similar or worse urban pollution problems as they industrialize.

Health inequities due to anthropogenic changes in natural environments are stark, and concerns are growing. While people who are wealthy tend to be primarily responsible for the creation of anthropogenic pollutants, those who live in poverty tend to suffer the most from these pollutants [46]. In low- and middle-income countries, increasing population concentrations, industrial pollution and burning of solid fuels, and the unprecedented rise in motor vehicle ownership have become significant health risk factors [47, 48]. Every year, more than 2.1 million people die prematurely in Asia from poor air quality. Air pollution in 180 Indian cities is more than six times higher than WHO's accepted standards and is the country's fifth-biggest killer [49].

Besides global disparities, health disparities due to anthropogenic changes to nature are also found at the national, regional, and local levels. Nationally, anthropogenic changes to nature follow different pathways of health influence in urban versus rural areas and in different geographically distinct regions such as coastal regions versus inland areas. Regionally, they show differences between metropolitan regions and their peripheral nonmetropolitan regions. Locally, they show differences among city cores, suburbs, and rural areas within metropolitan regions. Reported studies rarely look at these differences in a systematic manner.

While nature and anthropogenic changes to nature can present health risks, unspoiled, functioning, and resilient nature can help mitigate extreme events and effects of natural disasters. Nature can be salutogenic by limiting human exposure to pathogens. Modified or not, nature can affect the ways communities sustain themselves. It can shape the culture of a place. It can influence the rate of development and growth of the place. The presence of natural elements, such as green spaces, woods, rivers, and lakes, in built environments can reduce air pollution and mitigate greenhouse effects. Built environments rich in natural features can increase physical activity and improve mental well-being among all, but particularly among low-income groups [50].

Growing understanding of how natural environments support, protect, and threaten health underlines the importance of the links between population health policy and practice regarding nature [51]. The vastness of nature and its enormous abilities to affect human health often require that natural environments be managed by governmental agencies under a multiple-use mandate. Generally, the mandate has been to ensure a balanced mix of benefits to society ranging from traditional "hard" economic resources, such as minerals, timber, and livestock forage, to the more recent "amenity" resources such as clean air and water, outdoor recreation, wilderness experience, and natural scenic beauty. The problem, of course, is how to provide adequate amounts of any of these resources without undue damage or waste. A precondition is to have some means of knowing how much of each resource is available and how various policies and actions will affect the amount and quality of each.

Research has taken many different approaches when focusing on natural environments' benefits to human health. Two among these approaches are particularly notable. The first approach considers *natural environments as important ecological resources*, something that requires protection and preservation for human benefits. Therefore, studies on soil preservation, landscape preservation, preservation of wildlife habitat, reduction of air and water pollution, and so on are needed. The second approach focuses on *the perceived qualities of the natural environment*, which include natural scenic beauty, wilderness experience, outdoor recreation opportunity, and visibility values. These environmental aspects generally do not lend themselves well to traditional physical or biological assessments because they all have a central element that is fundamentally psychological in nature. This creates an important opportunity, and perhaps a responsibility, for psychologists and related social scientists to play an increased role in environmental policy, planning, and management, as evident in some work [52–54].

Built Environments. Modifying natural environments, humans create built environments for different purposes. Extents of their modifications can vary significantly, ranging from extremely urbanized places with high levels of human interventions to extremely rural places with low levels of interventions. Research evidence suggests that the built environment can affect health in many direct and indirect ways at different spatial scales and organizational levels. Among the spatial design and planning factors of the built environment, buildings, exterior spaces and places, streets, utilities, and parks and playgrounds can be important for human health. Among the ambient factors of the built environment, outdoor noise levels, air pollution, and urban heat sinks can be important. Among the factors of housing and workplaces, layouts of buildings, lighting, furniture and finishes, noise, and air quality can be important for human health.

The literature on the relationships between built environments and health is quite extensive. The studies reported in the literature extend from individual spaces to residences to neighborhoods to cities. They involve individuals, groups, and communities. They concern lifestyle and physical, mental, and social health. They include different socioeconomic, sociocultural, and sociodemographic groups or classes. They involve local, regional, and global contexts. Many studies will be reviewed selectively throughout this book, but here I will provide examples of many others that will not be reviewed elsewhere in the book.

Earlier, it was noted how anthropogenic activities affect natural environments, with a focus on air pollution. That is because the effects of air pollution are rarely limited to a place. In contrast, noise decays quickly. Hence, its effects are often limited to a place. Chronic outdoor and indoor noise exposure has implications for physical and mental health through annoyance, sleep disturbance, and chronic stress pathways [55]. Road traffic noise is the most important source of outdoor noise exposure worldwide [55–57]. It has been associated with cardiovascular disease and hypertension [57–60]. Airport noise has been associated with reduced quality of life, impaired cognitive development in children [58], and reduced psychological well-being [61]. A recent meta-analysis concluded that traffic noise in Europe caused between 400 and 1,500 disability-adjusted life years (DALYs) per one million people [62].

Besides air pollution and noise, many other anthropogenic activities can affect human health, demonstrating the importance of interactions between built and natural environments. Highways and streets can pollute water through runoff. They can destroy nature. They can affect air pollution through motor vehicle use. They can contribute to urban heat sink by absorbing heat that can increase the temperature in cities by several degrees. As power, water, drainage, and sewer systems age in a period of declining municipal resources, breakdowns may increase and cause health problems [63, 64]. Aging systems can become vulnerable to natural or human-made disasters. Other examples of anthropogenic activities affecting health include hazardous landfills, often located in or near urban areas, which have been associated with risks of low birth weight, birth defects, and cancers through their effects on water, air, and food [65].

Many psychological, psychosocial, and physical design aspects of the built environment are important for human health, demonstrating close interactions among built and social environments. For example, *privacy* from external and internal noise and visual intrusion can be compromised by the way the environment is designed, which can lead to social withdrawal or tension and conflicts among coworkers, neighbors, or family members, thus creating stress. *Attachment and belonging* can be affected by the character of neighborhoods, including those related to local traditions and styles, and are generally important for mental well-being, particularly for children as they grow up. *Competency* is related to the fact that environments can help us learn new skills and stretch our abilities. For example, children can develop physical prowess climbing stairs, and people can learn spatial skills exploring cities. *Autonomy and independence* are related to the fact that environments can help or hinder people's ability to manage everyday life, which becomes important as people age. *Controllability* differs in terms of how much environments can be altered and controlled by people, or how far they allow people to pursue their individual goals [8]. It has been known for quite some time that the design of built environments can influence *crime* and *violence* [18, 66]. *Disabilities* are important when one considers the interactions among built and social environments in terms of health. Our built environments are rarely designed for people with disabilities. Another way to put this is that we have created disabilities due to our failures to construct environments that can accommodate people with disabilities. In this sense, if designed properly, the built environment can play an important role to de-medicalize disabilities. Similar observations can be made concerning how the built environment can promote health through social justice and equity.

Social Environments. Within a socio-ecological model of health, social environments refer to socioeconomic status; demographic characteristics; social support, relations, and networks; social, cultural, and economic activities; and different social institutions related to governance, public policy, public administration, and educational opportunities and interventions. Put simply, social environments extend beyond socioeconomic factors to include a broader array of factors that constitute the social determinants of population health [67–69]. They include various life-enhancing resources and services, the distribution of which across populations effectively determines the quality of life, and a lack of these is often considered an important cause of health disparities.

Social environments influence health through a variety of pathways. They can support or discourage individual or group behaviors affecting health (e.g., smoking, diet, exercise, sexual behavior) [70]. They can buffer the impact of stressors. They can affect access to goods and services that influence health (e.g., housing, food, informal health care). Limited social support may predispose persons to poor coping skills and health. High levels of social stressors, such as social isolation and violence, can adversely affect health. Stress from a lack of social ties and support can contribute to low birth weight, which increases risk of infant death, slow cognitive development, hyperactivity, breathing problems, becoming overweight, and heart disease [31]. Social support buffers stressful situations, prevents isolation, contributes to self-esteem, and reduces the risk of early death [71]. Crime affects safety and perceived safety. If a neighborhood is not considered safe, physical activity decreases, which negatively affects health. Lack of neighborhood safety has also been associated with parental anxiety, in turn affecting children's physical activity [72, 73].

Perhaps the most well-researched aspects of the social environment are the influences of economic status or class on health and well-being. Studies show a clear relationship between income and health. Except the wealthiest members of a society, everyone is likely to experience slightly worse health than those who are marginally better off [74]. This is known as the "social gradient" in health and is observable in most countries. According to the WHO European review of social determinants of health and the health divide [75], people living in poverty often lack control over where they live, which exposes them to a variety of adverse conditions of daily living that increase risks to their health. These conditions include biological and chemical contamination; air pollution; flooding; poor sanitation and water scarcity; noise pollution; road traffic; hazardous waste sites; places that feel unsafe, unwelcoming, and uncongenial; scarcity of green space; unsafe transport; food deserts; and fewer opportunities for healthy activities.

The cumulative health impact of adverse social conditions on people living in poverty is significant, resulting in shorter and less healthy lives [75]. One 2016 study [76] found a gap in life expectancy of about 15 years for men and 10 years for women when comparing the most affluent 1% of individuals with the poorest 1%. To put this into perspective, a lifetime of smoking reduces life expectancy by 10 years for women. Interestingly, several studies show that the detrimental effects of individual poverty on health are reduced when people with lower incomes live in a socially mixed neighborhood with more affluent and educated people [77, 78]. While debate continues on whether absolute or relative poverty matters more for health, there is agreement that being living in poverty anywhere increases one's likelihood of a range of health risks across the life course, from infant mortality and low birth weight to stunted physical and cognitive development to early onset chronic illnesses and higher rates of infections [75].

Among other social determinants, racial/ethnic diversity has the potential to enhance health (e.g., broaden social support) or to damage it (e.g., a breakdown in traditional values). Racial diversity at the scale of a city may simply mask increased racial segregation at the scale of neighborhoods, which has been associated with poor health outcomes [79, 80]. Between 1980 and 2000, segregation of African Americans in the US declined, but levels were still highest for Black people. However, several measures of the segregation of Hispanic and Asian populations did increase during the same period [81].

It is well documented that health disparities are generally severe among racial and ethnic minorities [82, 83]. Each population faces specific challenges, but many indicators of health, access to care, and health care quality are worse for racial/ethnic minorities than for white people. For example, African Americans die earlier than white Americans. Life expectancy for African American males is almost seven years less than white males. The difference of five years for African American versus white women is smaller, but still alarming. Non-Hispanic black Americans have the highest prevalence of obesity among all racial and ethnic groups (37.7%), while Asian Americans have the lowest obesity prevalence (10.2%) [84].

The influences of education on health and well-being are well-researched aspects of the social environment. Although the average health of the US population improved over the past decades [85, 86], the gains largely went to the most educated groups. Health and longevity are deteriorating among those with less education [87–90]. Empirically, hundreds of studies have documented "the gradient" whereby more schooling is linked with better health and longer life. Since the 1970s, nearly all health outcomes were strongly patterned by education [91–96]. Less educated adults report worse general health [97, 98], more chronic conditions [99, 100], and more functional limitations and disability than do more educated adults [90, 101–103]. Objective measures of health, such as biological risk levels, are similarly correlated with educational attainment [104, 105], showing that the gradient is not a function of differential reporting or knowledge.

Effects of disability, gender orientation, and cultural norms are no less important for population health. For instance, the degree of isolation in rural areas / small towns likely has various effects on marginalized populations. So, even if there are high levels of social support, social integration, or religious participation, this may be exclusive to certain groups and less available to marginalized populations (e.g., LGBTQ individuals, racial minorities, or new immigrants). Likewise, rural areas are often characterized by risk behaviors—smoking, drinking, lack of preventive care, and so forth—because of normative and learned behaviors linked to masculinity, agriculture, poverty, or lack of alternative options. Other social issues affecting health include collective efficacy, powerlessness, discrimination, social contagion, and politics [106–108].

The economic opportunities of a place also affect health. Neighborhood grocery stores support nutritious diets. Local financial institutions help families create and maintain wealth that can affect health. Local businesses can act as sources for employment and culturally appropriate food and other services. Displacement of local businesses can adversely affect health by altering the availability and affordability of essential goods and services and the type of local employment possibilities. Business displacement can also contribute to physical blight, which is all too common in poor neighborhoods where widespread property abandonment has taken hold. Property abandonment can adversely influence health by increasing the likelihood of illegal dumping of garbage and hazardous wastes. Neighborhoods with high concentrations of property abandonment raise safety concerns and discourage active living.

There are differences in the social determinants of population health in urban and rural communities. Out-migration of younger individuals from rural communities can leave behind older populations. Higher rates of chronic conditions among older populations can place a heavy strain on rural health resources [109]. Many rural communities also have large concentrations of minority populations, leading to pronounced health disparities [110]. In one study on rural health disparities due to social factors, Murray and colleagues divided the US population into "eight Americas" based on such factors as race, income, and place of residence (by county). These different Americas have distinctly diverse mortality rates, highlighting huge disparities among different subpopulations such as southern, low-income Black people; low-income white populations in Appalachia and the Mississippi Valley; western Native Americans; and northland low-income rural white people [111].

SPATIAL SCALES OF HEALTH CONTEXTS

The environmental factors of health described above can be considered at micro, meso, and macro spatial scales. At different scales, these factors can affect health differently.

Micro-Spatial Scale: Residential and Work Environments. The micro-spatial level of health includes spaces of individual actions. Sanitation, indoor air quality, noise, lighting, dampness, sunlight hours, floor space size and shape, and heating are among the factors defining these spaces [112]. The associations between micro-spatial factors and health outcomes are complex, as these associations are often mediated and moderated by social factors.

The most common micro-spatial environments are residential or housing environments. They define the immediate environment where individuals spend most of their time [113] and will spend even more time in the coming decades as commuting is being discouraged for reduced carbon footprints. The importance of quality and quantity of housing for urban health has been emphasized by the United Nations Human Settlement Program (UN-Habitat), which holistically defines adequate housing as:

> more than a roof over one's head. It also means adequate privacy; adequate space; physical accessibility; adequate security; security of tenure; structural stability and durability; adequate lighting, heating and ventilation; adequate basic infrastructure, such as water-supply, sanitation and waste-management facilities; suitable environmental quality and health-related factors; and adequate and accessible location with regard to work and basic facilities: all of which should be available at an affordable cost. Adequacy should be determined together with the people concerned, bearing in mind the prospect for gradual development. Adequacy often varies from country to country, since it depends on specific cultural, social, environmental and economic factors. Gender-specific and age-specific factors, such as the exposure of children and women to toxic substances, should be considered in this context. [114]

Residential environments are often composed of many residential units. Each of these units consists of various health-influencing biochemical factors. Each unit has a different ability to shield individuals from exposure to adverse climatic conditions, vector-borne pathogens, and pollutants. Each unit has a unique set of personal and household hygiene-related attributes such as dampness, lighting, indoor pollution, supply of potable water, sanitation, waste disposal, storage, space and methods of food storage and preparation, and so on [115]. Residential units provide an environment for the household economic activities. These activities carry various types of health risks that are mitigated or enhanced by the configuration of internal and external spaces. Residential units also provide private and non-private spaces for relaxation and interaction for a family and its guests. The arrangements of residential units can foster social bonds, support specific living arrangements, and alleviate psychological stress processes.

Research already indicates connections between different microenvironments and the physical and mental health of individuals [7]. The micro-spatial factors assume particular importance in high-density and impoverished households [116]. Poverty is more likely to be associated with cold and damp houses infested with spores of fungi [117–119]. Several individual members of a family living in poverty may occupy a single room, often lacking proper ventilation and sanitary facilities. Harmful microenvironmental factors in impoverished households may exacerbate chronic asthma [120]. Household overcrowding may make individuals more prone to infectious diseases [121,

122] and to the stress of forced involuntary social interactions. Contrasting these risks, increased interpersonal contacts in dense housing may result in enhanced social capital and support [61, 123, 124].

Micro-spatial factors affecting health, however, are not confined to only residential environments. These factors are found in every environmental setting of individual actions, including offices, learning environments, recreational settings, health care settings, and factories. Occupational health hazards often originate from agents of air, water, noise, thermal, and radioactive pollution and interpersonal contacts in places of employment. In places of employment with poor air quality, poor lighting conditions, high levels of noise, high density, or with other environmental stressors, workers may also suffer from work-related anxiety, cardiovascular disease, and other work-related chronic disorders [125–127].

Meso-Spatial Scale: Neighborhoods and Campuses. The meso-spatial scale of health is the scale of a neighborhood or a campus. Housing should not be considered in isolation but as part of a neighborhood. When appropriate, workplaces should be considered as part of a campus or a larger environment within which they are found. At this level, environments are rarely homogeneous. In a neighborhood, we commonly find workplaces, recreational facilities, parks, and learning environments along with places of residence. Likewise, a campus is often composed of many interconnected buildings serving many different functions. At the meso-spatial level, density, location, and externalities from proximate land uses have an indirect influence on the health of one or more user groups.

People residing in houses located in a spatially well-integrated, prosperous neighborhood may enjoy the benefits of an optimized density of health-promoting resources; an optimized mix of land uses; a street configuration conducive to walkability; denser social networks and levels of social capital; and greater density of accessible welfare-enhancing destinations. Conversely, a neighborhood may discourage active living if its spaces and units are not spatially well integrated; if it lacks density, diversity, and design promoting healthy living; if it lacks safety and access to healthy food and health-promoting resources; and so on [128–134].

Neighborhood safety is a foundational element of health in urban areas, or "urban health." When residents worry about neighborhood safety, they curtail their outdoor activities, reducing the extent of their physical activities and interactions with others. Indirect effects of neighborhood violence and crime include fear, stress, anxiety and unhealthy coping behaviors, overeating, smoking and alcohol/drug abuse. In poor neighborhoods, fear of crime can force children to stay indoors, increasing exposure to toxic indoor air and allergens and limiting physical activity outside [18, 135–140].

Macro-Spatial Scale: Communities and Cities. At the macro-spatial level, health factors may include those associated with the overall quality of the built, social, and natural environments, such as ethnicity; socioeconomic classes; air, water, and noise pollution; proximity to waste disposal sites; density; street network; accessibility to services; land use mix; and food environments. Residents living close to major roads may be prone to the negative health effects of poor air quality and elevated noise levels from traffic flows [141–144], while residents living in the vicinity of major industrial sites may have a higher rate of chronic diseases due to higher levels of air and water pollution [145, 146]. At the macro-spatial level, other health-defining factors include access to nature and natural amenities [147–149], manmade electromagnetic fields [150, 151], urban heat island effects [152, 153], smog, deforestation, and climate change [154–161].

Often, cultural, socioeconomic, and political factors can help determine how macro-spatial factors are related to health [33, 75, 162]. One major example of a spatial factor defined by social and political factors in cities is spatial segregation. Many cities worldwide are highly segregated with discrimination against certain racial, ethnic, caste, or tribal groups. Spatial segregation can have harmful effects. A community when spatially segregated may show homogeneity and lack social resources. People who live in segregated, low-income communities often have disproportionate exposure, susceptibility, and response to economic and social deprivation, toxic substances, and hazardous conditions [31, 71].

ORGANIZATIONAL LEVELS OF HEALTH

In a socio-ecological model, health is considered at different organizational levels. These levels range from individuals to groups to communities. At higher levels, organizations show differences in density, complexity, diversity, and administrative apparatus with different implications for health.

Individuals. Population health does not consider individual health and factors affecting individual health. Instead, it focuses on those factors that affect group and community health described below. There is rarely any one-to-one correspondence between individual and aggregate health. A group or community may never be exposed to the same set of health determinants as individuals. Nevertheless, individuals remain a concern for population health.

They are essential units of health and health-related theories, research, and practice. Individuals consist of many inherent unique factors that govern the nature and degree to which they react to the surrounding environment. Population health is interested in these factors to the extent they help categorize individuals into population groups based on the degree of risk or proneness of individuals to a particular health issue. Such factors may include age, gender, ethnicity, color, and socioeconomic status. These may also include such attributes as beliefs, expectations, motives, values, perceptions, and other cognitive elements.

Groups. The next higher organizational level of health study and interventions is a *group*. At this level, interpersonal relations, networks, and communication are important. There are different pathways through which interpersonal networks and relations can influence health and well-being. They can provide intimacy and companionship, resources to cope with illness, and new information and resources to buffer oneself from stress. Interpersonal networks and relations can play a positive or negative role in determining health—a point worth remembering when considering health and health-related behaviors.

Communities. At an even higher level of health study and interventions, we have *communities*. A community may include many different groups of individuals. A community may also include groups representing specific demographic or behavioral types such as older adults, children, smokers, and so on that may extend beyond any geographical limits. *Composition* [32] refers to the socioeconomic and demographic characteristics of a community. It can have profound influence on population health.

It is at this level of study that various aspects of social structure (social capital and support) and culture (distinct sets of attitudes, beliefs, values, knowledge systems, and behavioral habits) are generally expressed. Characterized by specific built and natural environments, and social and cultural preference structures, communities are rarely homogeneous. Within a community, diverse group susceptibilities and exposures, as determined by composition, are interlinked, producing overall population-level risk factors [7]. The disadvantages that minorities so often experience in the United States are partly due to composition and are often compounded by the disadvantages created by the lack of socioeconomic opportunities as well as historical policies. It is no wonder that minorities in the rural parts of the United States have been referred to as a forgotten population [110].

Significance of Organizational Levels. A proper understanding of the interdependence of different organizational levels is vital to health promotion and enhancement. Designing initiatives to change health behavior and environment for communities and targeted groups, not just single individuals, is at the heart of a population health approach. Experts have explicitly recommended that policy and design interventions for environmental and behavioral factors related to health should consider interconnected levels of influence, extending from individuals to groups to communities [163–165].

The above recommendation is based on the limited reach and staying power of individual health behavior interventions for health promotion. By the late 1980s, it was clear that an exclusive reliance on individually oriented interventions would be inadequate to achieve pressing population health and health care goals; and that the targets of effective health interventions and promotion are not individuals but the broader contexts in which they live and work. This shift in paradigm fueled the rise of socio-ecological models of health. Whereas experts once might have seen their roles as working at a particular level of intervention (such as changing organizational or individual health behaviors) or employing a specific type of behavior change strategy (such as group interventions or individual counseling), they now realize that multiple interventions at multiple levels are often needed to initiate and sustain behavior change effectively [165].

INTERACTIONS BETWEEN SPATIAL SCALES
AND ORGANIZATIONAL LEVELS

As different spatial scales and organizational levels of health are important, so are the interactions occurring within and across these scales and levels, both in upward and downward directions. Downwardly, factors at a higher spatial scale can affect those at the lower scales. Therefore, factors at the macro-spatial scale of cities can affect those at the meso-spatial scale of neighborhoods and micro-spatial scale of environments. Similarly, factors at the meso-spatial scale of neighborhood can affect those at the micro-spatial scale of environments. Similar downward interaction processes occur within different organizational levels—communities can affect groups and individuals; and groups, in turn, can affect individuals.

Upwardly, factors at the micro-spatial scale of environments can affect those at the meso-spatial scale of neighborhoods; and factors at the meso-spatial scale of neighborhoods can affect those at the macro-spatial scale of cities. Likewise, individuals can affect groups, and groups can affect communities.

More interestingly, factors at different spatial scales and organizational

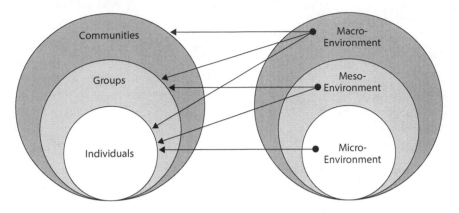

Figure 1.2. Interactions among different spatial scales and organizational levels of health.

levels also interact. As shown in figure 1.2, factors of the macro-spatial scale of cities can affect communities, groups, and individuals; those of the meso-spatial scale of neighborhoods can affect groups and individuals; and those at the micro-spatial scale of environments can affect individuals and, maybe, some small groups. These cross-domain interactions can help define the scope of population health studies involving the built environment. These studies can focus on the effects of the macro-spatial factors on health in communities, groups, and/or individuals, and on the effects of the meso-spatial factors on health in groups and/or individuals. Studies on the effects of the micro-spatial factors on individual health, however, are less interesting from a population health perspective. Since it seems impossible for a study to focus on all these effects at the same time, researchers generally focus on a select set of effects in population health studies.

Pathways of Influence

At a granular level, a socio-ecological model of health can be complicated. Interactions among various components of the model are generally fluid, nonlinear, and scale dependent. In this model, the pathways of influence of a health factor can be many. To illustrate this, we can use education as an example. There are many pathways for education to influence health. The most prominent among these pathways can be grouped into four categories: economic, health-behavioral, social-psychological, and access to health care. Education leads to better, more stable jobs that pay higher incomes and allow families to accumulate wealth that can be used to improve health [166]. In this sense, the economic factors are an important link between schooling and health, estimated to account for about 30% of the correlation [167]. Health behaviors are undoubtedly an important proximal determinant of health, but they explain only a part of the effect of education on health: adults with less education are more likely to smoke, have unhealthy diets, and lack exercise [168–171]. Social-psychological pathways include successful long-term marriages and other sources of social support that people gain through education to help cope with stressors and daily hassles [172, 173]. Access to health care, while important to individual and population health overall, has a modest role in explaining health inequalities by education [174–176], highlighting the need to look upstream beyond the health care system toward social factors that underlie social disparities in health. Beyond these four groups of mechanisms or pathways, the literature explores several other pathways involving stress, cognitive and noncognitive skills, or environmental exposures for education to influence health [116, 166, 167, 177–179].

Like the pathways for education to influence health, the potential pathways for the built environment to influence health are likely to be complex. The studies of this book will consider some of these potential pathways for spatial design and planning factors of the built environment to influence health. Inspired by Giles-Corti et al. [180], figure 1.3 is a detailed illustration of the potential direct and indirect pathways through which spatial design and planning factors (column 1) might be associated with lifestyle behaviors (column 3), health risk factors (column 4), and health outcomes (column 5). In column 1, spatial design and planning factors include macro-, meso-, and micro-scale elements. In column 3, lifestyle behaviors include work-related travel behaviors, employment and living conditions, use of health care services, use of food outlets and eating behaviors, participation in social activities, use of parks and recreational facilities, and active living. In column 4, health risk factors include traffic incidents, environmental pollution, urban heat island effects, greenhouse effects, social isolation, safety and crime, physical inactivity, prolonged sitting, obesity and overweight, unhealthy diet, substance abuse, drinking, and smoking. In column 5, health outcomes include mortality and morbidity factors and different physical, mental, and social health outcomes.

Moving from left to right, the figure shows how spatial design and planning factors of different scales (column 1) may be associated with lifestyle behaviors (column 3), health risk factors (column 4), and health outcomes (column 5) and how any such associations may be influenced by various actors, user attitudes and preferences, social and cultural norms, levels of rurality or urbanicity of a place, demographics, socioeconomic status, and health care services (column 2). For example, destination accessibility (column1) may be associated with work-related travel behaviors (column 3), but the strength of such associations may depend on socioeconomic factors (column 2).

The figure also shows how spatial design and planning factors (column 1) may have indirect associations with health risk factors (column 4) and health outcomes (column 5) due to their direct associations with lifestyle (column 3). Again, it should be noted that any direct associations between spatial design and planning factors (column 1) and lifestyle (column 3) could still be influenced by the factors in column 2. For example, influenced by socioeconomic factors (column 2), spatial design and planning factors (column 1) may encourage sedentary activities (column 3) that lead to obesity (column 4), which is a risk factor for cardiovascular diseases (column 5).

Additionally, the figure shows how health risk factors (column 4) may affect each other and health outcomes (column 5), which ultimately determine the quality of life, as well as health, social, and environmental equity. For example, traffic incidents may determine road trauma; increased environmental pollution may determine greenhouse effects, particulate matter emissions, and climate change, leading to respiratory diseases, heat stress, infectious diseases, and mental illnesses; social isolation may result in mental illnesses, increased crime, and diminished safety; and physical inactivity, prolonged sitting, and unhealthy diet may cause obesity, overweight, and cardio-metabolic risk factors leading to type 2 diabetes, cancer, and cardiovascular diseases. While some direct connections between health risk factors and outcomes are shown using arrows, many others are not shown in the figure. For example, traffic incidents are linked to trauma, but trauma may be linked to other health outcomes, including mental illnesses, which are not shown in the figure. Any relationships within and between health risk factors and outcomes, however, generally fall under the purview of health professionals; therefore, they are less important for spatial design and planning research and practice.

In general, as shown in figure 1.3, spatial design and planning factors can potentially affect mental, physical, and social health in many ways, connecting different factors of different environments at different spatial scales and organizational levels. A great deal of research evidence already exists supporting some of these pathways [181]. Presented throughout this book, most existing research deals with only urban areas. As a result, we do not know if these pathways of health influence also apply to small towns and rural areas, which are often significantly different from urban areas in terms of health and

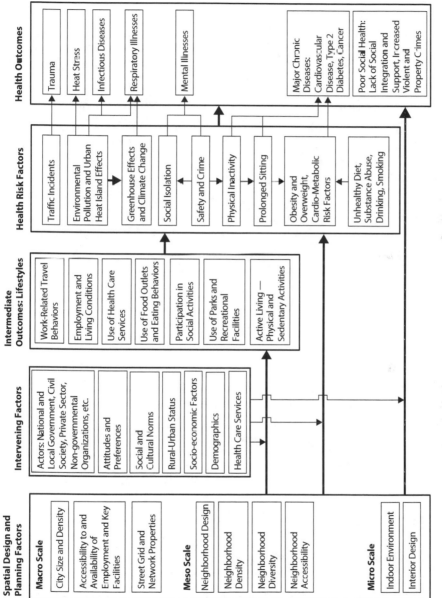

Figure 1.3. Potential pathways through which spatial design and planning factors may influence health and health-related behaviors.

its determinants. To improve our understanding about this less-studied area of population health, this book presents studies unraveling the pathways for spatial factors to influence health in small towns of rural America. The relevance of these studies is presented in the next two sections of this chapter using the examples of Healthy Cities and Communities.

Healthy Cities and Communities: A Population Health Approach to Health Promotion

Since the mid-1980s, Healthy Cities and Communities have been designed by numerous local or city governments in Europe [182, 183], the United States [184, 185], and elsewhere [186, 187], sometimes with help from the WHO, to promote health and to reduce health inequalities using a population health–based approach [188]. These projects and programs help develop healthy public policies and spatial design and planning strategies at the local level through a multisectoral approach and increased community participation [189–194] with goals to empower people to control and improve their health, as was envisioned in the definition of "health promotion" provided by the Ottawa Charter for Health Promotion [20].

Conceived as a major vehicle for health promotion through community empowerment, healthy cities and communities aim to achieve "Health for All." It is, however, difficult to generalize or to draw clear differences between many projects and programs around the world that could be termed as healthy cities or communities. Nevertheless, European projects and programs show more similarities, most likely because of the extensive technical support provided by the WHO European Regional Office. In the United States and elsewhere, these projects and programs show significant dissimilarities because they are often initiated independently with different focuses or emphases and with different sponsoring organizations and funding [195].

Regardless of similarities and differences, all healthy cities and communities are generally conceived around a broad concept of health and a set of strategies to achieve it. As discussed, this broad concept of health focuses on a positive model of health that emphasizes social and personal resources as well as physical capacities, an ecological model of health, and a concern with health inequalities [5]. In response to this concept, the strategies of healthy cities and communities emphasize processes, public policies, and community empowerment [5]. The *processes* of healthy cities and communities generally involve establishing a broad-based structure for projects and programs, encouraging community participation, assessing community needs, establishing priorities and strategic plans, soliciting political support, taking local action, and evaluating progress [196, 197]. In the strategies of healthy cities and communities, the essential environmental dictum has been "think globally and act locally."

Health-related *public policies* generally supported by various healthy cities and communities involve such issues as promoting equity, altering lifestyles, improving political environment for a health agenda, and reorienting health services toward prevention and health promotion [198–201]. The European projects and programs generally follow four common approaches to policy change: First, they adopt position statements and advocate for city council resolutions. Second, they facilitate adoption of policies on health issues, population groups, geographic areas, or services. Third, they support the formulation and adoption of comprehensive city health plans. Finally, they advocate for assessments of the impact of city policies on health and the use of assessments by decision makers [195].

Aligning with the Ottawa Charter for Health Promotion [20], healthy cities and communities put great emphasis on *community empowerment*. In simple words, healthy cities and communities suggest a restructuring of the health decision-making process, shifting power to the local level. Successful community empowerment generally includes the processes that promote advocacy, enablement, and mediation; the processes that seek to strengthen community action, develop personal skills, and reorient health services; and the processes that seek to identify and learn from multisector coalitions with demonstrated success addressing the social determinants of health. Most projects and programs of healthy cities and communities are intended to build health into the decision-making processes of local governments, community organizations, and businesses to develop a broad range of strategies to address the social, environmental, and economic determinants of health and to change the community culture by incorporating health [188].

Characteristics of successful healthy cities and communities, as have been reported based on experiences in Europe and North America [202–204], include effective leadership; a multisectoral committee or steering group that directs the project; strong economy; community participation; information used in citywide planning; obtaining needed technical support; being viewed as a credible resource for health in the community; and effective networking [195].

Concerns about Healthy Cities and Communities

While the projects and programs related to healthy cities and communities provide useful examples illustrating how to promote population health, they present many concerns. The primary concern arises from the fact that they are conceived, organized, or created at the local level by community activists, politicians, government officials, or community members. These people are interested in action rather than research. Therefore, it is not surprising that academic involvement has not been a central part of health promotion in the projects and programs of healthy cities and communities [5]. These projects and programs provide challenges to the dominant health and public health paradigms in the United States and other countries for their emphasis on community participation and empowerment.

The concern about the positive model of health used in the projects and programs of healthy cities and communities is that the health of a city and of its citizens need to be assessed in terms of their physical, mental, and social well-being or fitness as much as, if not more than, their mortality, morbidity, or hospitalization rates. Unfortunately, there is so far no widespread agreement among international, national, and local organizations on these measures. The data do not, for the most part, exist (and certainly not at the local level); and simple, cheap, and effective methodologies for assessing physical, mental, and social well-being and fitness at the local level are not readily available. The studies of this book will focus on such concerns using data on lifestyle, mortality and morbidity, and physical, mental, and social health of the population of small cities of Kansas, made available primarily through the US Census Bureau and the state and local governments working with the Centers for Disease Control and Prevention (CDC).

The concern about a socio-ecological model of health used in the projects and programs of healthy cities and communities is how to replace pathogenic epidemiology (a disease-based approach) with salutogenic epidemiology (an approach focused on the causation of good health) in population health [5]. Antonovsky [205–207] used the term "salutogenesis" as the opposite of "pathogenesis" to explain why it was that some populations survive or remain relatively well-off in situations where others do not. Clearly, there are many salutogens, but equally clearly, some are likely to be more fundamental than others in terms of positive health benefits. The most fundamental salutogens generally include food, shelter, clean water, a safe environment, and peace. Sadly, they are lacking for large groups of population, particularly in small towns and rural areas, in the United States and other countries. It is hoped that the studies of this book will help identify the salutogenic (positive) effects of spatial design and planning factors on health in small towns and cities, which can then be used to build healthy small cities and communities in rural areas.

The concern for the projects and programs of healthy cities and communities is also that socio-ecological research is interdisciplinary in nature. Clearly, research limited to any one area does not provide necessary knowledge to address population health issues. Using theories, methods, and data from different areas related to population health, the studies in the book will provide examples illustrating how to mitigate this concern in the projects and programs of healthy small cities and communities in rural areas of the United States and other countries.

Arguably, dealing with inequality is among the most important concerns in the projects and programs of healthy cities and communities. It requires us to figure out the most important determinants of health and health inequalities. It also requires us to develop reliable, cheap, and easy-to-apply methods of assessing health status and health determinants in cities of different sizes. This is so that inequalities in health and inequities in access to health can be documented and monitored at all levels, and comparisons can be made between and within different groups of cities. Finally, research is needed on the impact of steps taken to reduce inequity in access to basic determinants of health; and the results in terms of physical, mental, and social well-being need to be documented, preferably over short, medium, and long terms [5]. It is hoped that the studies of this book will provide some examples showing reliable, cheap, and easy-to-apply methods of assessing health determinants in small cities to help achieve health equity through projects and programs in small cities in the United States and other countries.

Conclusions

Population health is a function of interactions among multiple environmental factors working at multiple spatial and organizational scales. Studies exploring the effects of built environments on population health have increasingly pointed to many conceptual and methodological challenges [208, 209]. The risk factors operating at multiple spatial scales and organizational levels of population health are often interdependent, and it is highly unlikely that causality in population health studies is unidirectional and continuous in nature. The simple fact that people select where to live, work, and play based on personal preference, socioeconomic constraints, perceived degree of satisfaction, safety, and so on makes any causal inferences based on statistical associations between population health and built environments difficult. Additionally, any health effects of risk factors are cumulative in nature. People adapt their behaviors according to the characteristics of their social and economic classes and environments, following one or more pathways of influence. Similarly, people and their built environment configure one another, each adapting in response to the other.

In order to address many constraints and concerns, therefore, a socio-ecological approach to population health studies is needed, as many have argued [181, 210]. This approach acknowledges that various health-defining factors and processes take place at multiple spatial and organizational scales and that interactions of these factors and processes are nonlinear, acting along highly differentiated and specific pathways, for many of which there are no well-defined theories. Nevertheless, the pathways described in this chapter are important as they may help explain how spatial design and planning factors might produce population health inequalities. According to these pathways, population health inequalities may be produced by the differences in the associations between spatial design and planning factors and health and health-related behaviors and by the influence of actors, user attitude and preferences, social and cultural norms, mobility needs, rural-urban status, and demographic and socioeconomic factors on such associations. Improving health and reducing inequalities, therefore, requires effective spatial design and planning interventions, primarily for people living in poverty, who generally have disproportionate exposure and susceptibility to economic and social deprivations, extreme rurality, negative attitudes and preferences, and restrictive social and cultural norms [31, 211].

Based on the concept of population health and the socio-ecological model of population health, cities and communities around the world have been investing in projects and programs to promote health and to reduce health inequalities. Though they have seen successes, they have also seen barriers, primarily due to a lack of research-based evidence promoting health. On the one hand, it has been difficult to get action-oriented community activists excited about research. On the other hand, it has been difficult to get academics interested in projects and programs that thrive on community participation and empowerment and that do not fall within the traditional research paradigms of health and population health.

Even though exceptional in relation to the dominant paradigms of health and population health research, the studies of this book endorse the socio-ecological perspective of population health. They explore how spatial design and planning factors affect lifestyle and health outcomes in a sample of small cities in Kansas. Regarding spatial scales, these studies do not involve the meso-spatial scale of neighborhoods and micro-spatial scale of housing units and workplaces as shown in the pathways of influence diagram (figure 1.3). Concerning organizational levels, these studies deal with population health described using aggregate data. These and other dimensions of study design are discussed thoroughly in part III.

Before that, chapter 2 of part I of the book attempts to define small-town America. Following that, chapter 3 discusses the ongoing changes affecting population health in small-town America. Chapter 4 of part II then presents the stories of recent changes in small cities of Kansas, and chapter 5 reports the stories of health concerns in these small cities. The purpose of parts I and II together is to provide the reader with background on small-town America and small cities of Kansas before the methods, the study sample, and the studies exploring spatial associations of lifestyle and health are presented in parts III, IV, and V.

NOTES

1. Alberti, *On the Art of Building in Ten Books.*
2. Vitruvius, *Vitruvius: The Ten Books on Architecture.*
3. Aristotle, *Politics.* Book 2, section 1267b.
4. Aristotle, *Politics.* Book 7, section 1330b.
5. Hancock, *The Healthy City from Concept to Application.*
6. World Health Organization, *Constitution of the World Health Organization.*
7. Sarkar, Webster, and Gallacher, *Healthy Cities.*
8. Burton, "Mental Well-Being and the Influence of Place."
9. Marmot et al., "Building of the Global Movement for Health Equity."
10. Marmot et al., "Closing the Gap in a Generation."
11. Putnam, *Bowling Alone.*
12. Kawachi et al., "Social Capital, Income Inequality, and Mortality."
13. McDowell and Newell, *Measuring Health.*
14. Larson, "The Conceptualization of Health."
15. Perry, "Preadolescent and Adolescent Influences on Health."
16. Curry et al., "Assessment of Community-Level Influences."
17. Wandersman and Nation, "Urban Neighborhoods and Mental Health."
18. Sampson, Raudenbush, and Earls, "Neighborhoods and Violent Crime."
19. Pothukuchi, "Attracting Grocery Retail Investment to Inner-City Neighborhoods."
20. World Health Organization, *The Ottawa Charter for Health Promotion.*
21. Evans and Stoddart, "Producing Health, Consuming Health Care."
22. Evans and Stoddart, "Consuming Health Care, Producing Health."

23. Kindig and Stoddart, "What Is Population Health?," 380.
24. Jacobson and Teutsch. *An Environmental Scan of Integrated Approaches.*
25. Goldberg, "In Support of a Broad Model of Public Health."
26. Institute of Medicine, Committee for the Study of the Future of Public Health, and Remington, *The Future of Public Health*, 2.
27. Diez-Roux, "On the Distinction—or Lack of Distinction—between Population Health and Public Health."
28. Barton and Grant, "A Health Map for the Local Human Habitat."
29. Hancock and Perkins, "The Mandala of Health."
30. Dahlgren and Whitehead, *Policies and Strategies to Promote Social Equity in Health*, 1–69.
31. Corburn, "Urban Inequities, Population Health and Spatial Planning."
32. Phillips and McLeroy, "Health in Rural America."
33. Marmot, *Status Syndrome.*
34. World Health Organization, *Nature, Biodiversity and Health.*
35. United Nations, *Global Environment Outlook—GEO-6.*
36. United Nations, *Preventing the Next Pandemic.*
37. McNeill, *Something New Under the Sun.*
38. Lim et al., "*A Comparative Risk Assessment of Burden of Disease and Injury.*"
39. Gasana et al., "Motor Vehicle Air Pollution and Asthma in Children."
40. Yang and Omaye, "Air Pollutants, Oxidative Stress and Human Health."
41. Samet and Krewski, "Health Effects Associated with Exposure to Ambient Air Pollution."
42. Shah et al., "Global Association of Air Pollution and Heart Failure."
43. Dockery et al., "An Association between Air Pollution and Mortality."
44. Sarnat, Schwartz, and Suh, "Fine Particulate Air Pollution and Mortality."
45. Committee on the Medical Effects of Air Pollutants, *The Mortality Effects of Long-Term Exposure.*
46. Jephcote and Chen, "Environmental Injustices of Children's Exposure to Air Pollution."
47. Samet, "Community Design and Air Quality."
48. Cervero, "Linking Urban Transport and Land Use in Developing Countries."
49. Intergovernmental Panel on Climate Change, *Climate Change 2014.*
50. Mitchell and Popham, "Effect of Exposure to Natural Environment on Health Inequalities."
51. ten Brink et al., *The Health and Social Benefits of Nature and Biodiversity Protection.*
52. Kaplan, "Aesthetics, Affect, and Cognition."
53. Ulrich et al., "Stress Recovery during Exposure to Natural and Urban Environments."
54. Daniel, "Measuring the Quality of the Natural Environment."
55. Ising and Kruppa, "Health Effects Caused by Noise."
56. Tobías et al., "Health Impact Assessment of Traffic Noise."
57. Moudon, "Real Noise from the Urban Environment."
58. Clark and Stansfeld, "The Effect of Transportation Noise on Health and Cognitive Development."
59. Van Kempen et al., "The Association between Noise Exposure and Blood Pressure."
60. Babisch, "Road Traffic Noise and Cardiovascular Risk."
61. Evans, "The Built Environment and Mental Health."
62. Hänninen et al., "Environmental Burden of Disease in Europe."
63. Melosi, *The Sanitary City.*
64. Garrett, *Betrayal of Trust.*

65. Vrijheid, "Health Effects of Residence near Hazardous Waste Landfill Sites."
66. Newman, *Defensible Space: Crime Prevention through Urban Design.*
67. Kawachi and Kennedy, "Socioeconomic Determinants of Health."
68. WHO Commission on Social Determinants of Health, *Addressing the Social Determinants of Health.*
69. Wilkinson and Marmot, *Social Determinants of Health.*
70. King et al., "Smoking in Cape Town."
71. Corburn, *Toward the Healthy City.*
72. Carver, Timperio, and Crawford, "Playing It Safe."
73. Weir, Etelson, and Brand, "Parents' Perceptions of Neighborhood Safety."
74. Allen and Allen, "Health Inequalities and the Role of the Physical and Social Environment."
75. Marmot "WHO European Review of Social Determinants."
76. Chetty et al., "The Association between Income and Life Expectancy."
77. Wen, Browning, and Cagney, "Poverty, Affluence, and Income Inequality."
78. Ellaway et al., " 'Getting Sicker Quicker.' "
79. Acevedo-Garcia et al., "Future Directions in Residential Segregation and Health Research."
80. Williams, "*Race, Socioeconomic Status, and Health.*"
81. Iceland, Weinberg, and Steinmetz, *Racial and Ethnic Residential Segregation.*
82. Centers for Disease Control and Prevention, "CDC Health Disparities and Inequalities Report."
83. US Department of Health Human Services, "Agency for Healthcare Research and Quality."
84. Cohen et al., "A Closer Look at Rural-Urban Health Disparities."
85. Jemal et al., "Trends in the Leading Causes of Death."
86. Martin, Schoeni, and Andreski, "Trends in Health of Older Adults in the United States."
87. Meara, Richards, and Cutler, "The Gap Gets Bigger."
88. Montez and Zajacova, "Trends in Mortality Risk."
89. Shiels et al., "Trends in Premature Mortality."
90. Zajacova and Montez, "Physical Functioning Trends."
91. Christenson and Johnson, "Educational Inequality in Adult Mortality."
92. Elo and Preston, "Educational Differentials in Mortality."
93. Feldman et al., "National Trends in Educational Differentials in Mortality."
94. Kitagawa and Hauser, *Differential Mortality in the United States.*
95. Rogot, Sorlie, and Johnson, "Life Expectancy by Employment Status, Income, and Education."
96. Sorlie, Backlund, and Keller, "US Mortality by Economic, Demographic, and Social Characteristics."
97. Mirowsky and Ross, "Education and Self-Rated Health."
98. Zajacova, Hummer, and Rogers, "Education and Health among US Working-Age Adults."
99. Johnson-Lawrence, Zajacova, and Sneed, "Education, Race/Ethnicity, and Multimorbidity."
100. Quiñones, Markwardt, and Botoseneanu, "Multimorbidity Combinations and Disability in Older Adults."
101. Schoeni, Freedman, and Wallace, "Persistent, Consistent, Widespread, and Robust?"
102. Schoeni et al., "Persistent and Growing Socioeconomic Disparities."
103. Tsai, "Education and Disability Trends of Older Americans."

104. Crimmins, Kim, and Vasunilashorn, "Biodemography."
105. Zajacova, Dowd, and Aiello, "Socioeconomic and Race/Ethnic Patterns."
106. Mayer and Jencks, "War on Poverty."
107. Macintyre and Ellaway, "Neighborhoods and Health."
108. Macintyre and Ellaway, "Ecological Approaches."
109. Corrigan et al., *Quality through Collaboration.*
110. Probst et al., "Person and Place."
111. Murray et al., "Eight Americas."
112. Howden-Chapman, "*Housing Standards.*"
113. Leech et al., "*It's About Time.*"
114. United Nations Commission on Human Settlements, "Report of the United Nations Conference on Human Settlements (Habitat II)," 34.
115. World Health Organization, *Indoor Environment.*
116. Evans and Kantrowitz, "Socioeconomic Status and Health."
117. Burr, St Leger, and Yarnell, "Wheezing, Dampness, and Coal Fires."
118. Billings and Howard, "Damp Housing and Asthma."
119. Martin, Platt, and Hunt, "Housing Conditions and Ill Health."
120. Sandel and Wright, "When Home Is Where the Stress Is."
121. Fonseca et al., "Risk Factors for Childhood Pneumonia."
122. Kellett, "Crowding and Mortality in London Boroughs."
123. Evans and Lepore, "Household Crowding and Social Support."
124. Evans et al., "Residential Density and Psychological Health."
125. Landsbergis et al., "The Workplace and Cardiovascular Disease."
126. Belkic et al., "Is Job Strain a Major Source of Cardiovascular Disease Risk?"
127. Lang, Fouriaud, and Jacquinet-Salord, "Length of Occupational Noise Exposure and Blood Pressure."
128. Cohen et al., "Neighborhood Physical Conditions and Health."
129. Flowerdew, Manley, and Sabel, "Neighbourhood Effects on Health."
130. Frank et al., "Many Pathways from Land Use to Health."
131. Kaczynski, Johnson, and Saelens, "Neighborhood Land Use Diversity."
132. Orstad et al., "A Systematic Review of Agreement."
133. Sallis et al., "Neighborhood Environments and Physical Activity among Adults."
134. Sallis et al., "Neighborhood Built Environment and Socioeconomic Status."
135. Newman, *Defensible Space.*
136. Perkins, Meeks, and Taylor, "The Physical Environment of Street Blocks."
137. Perkins et al., "The Physical Environment of Street Crime."
138. Rand, "*Crime and Environment.*"
139. Taylor and Harrell, *Physical Environment and Crime.*
140. Foster, Giles-Corti, and Knuiman, "Neighbourhood Design and Fear of Crime."
141. Stansfeld, Haines, and Brown, "Noise and Health in the Urban Environment."
142. Stansfeld and Matheson, "Noise Pollution."
143. Künzli et al., "Public-Health Impact of Outdoor and Traffic-Related Air Pollution."
144. Brauer et al., "Air Pollution from Traffic."
145. Ginns and Gatrell, "Respiratory Health Effects of Industrial Air Pollution."
146. Elliott et al., "The Power of Perception."
147. De Vries et al., "Natural Environments—Healthy Environments?"
148. Lachowycz and Jones, "Greenspace and Obesity."
149. Beil and Hanes, "The Influence of Urban Natural and Built Environments."
150. Knave, "*Electric and Magnetic Fields and Health Outcomes.*"
151. Röösli, "Radiofrequency Electromagnetic Field Exposure."

152. Heaviside, Macintyre, and Vardoulakis, "The Urban Heat Island."
153. Tan et al., "The Urban Heat Island and Its Impact."
154. Patz and Norris, "Land Use Change and Human Health."
155. Butler, *Climate Change and Global Health.*
156. Costello et al., "Managing the Health Effects of Climate Change."
157. Epstein, "Climate Change and Human Health."
158. Haines et al., "Climate Change and Human Health."
159. Haines and Patz, "Health Effects of Climate Change."
160. McMichael, Woodruff, and Hales, "Climate Change and Human Health."
161. Patz et al., "Impact of Regional Climate Change on Human Health."
162. Schüle and Bolte, "Interactive and Independent Associations."
163. Committee on Capitalizing on Social Science and Behavioral Research to Improve the Public's Health, Division of Health Promotion Disease Prevention, and Institute of Medicine, "Promoting Health."
164. McLeroy et al., "An Ecological Perspective on Health Promotion Programs."
165. Glanz, Rimer, and Viswanath, *Health Behavior and Health Education.*
166. Mirowsky and Ross, *Education, Social Status, and Health.*
167. Cutler and Lleras-Muney, "Education and Health."
168. Cutler and Lleras-Muney, "Understanding Differences in Health Behaviors by Education."
169. Lawrence, "Why Do College Graduates Behave More Healthfully."
170. Pampel, Krueger, and Denney, "Socioeconomic Disparities in Health Behaviors."
171. Schoenborn, Adams, and Peregoy, "Health Behaviors of Adults."
172. Taylor and Seeman, "Psychosocial Resources and the SES-Health Relationship."
173. Waite and Gallagher, *The Case for Marriage.*
174. Hoffmann, *Socioeconomic Differences in Old Age Mortality.*
175. Ross and Wu, "The Links between Education and Health."
176. Williams, "Socioeconomic Differentials in Health."
177. Adler and Ostrove, "Socioeconomic Status and Health."
178. Baum, Garofalo, and Yali, "Socioeconomic Status and Chronic Stress."
179. Hummer and Lariscy, "Educational Attainment and Adult Mortality."
180. Giles-Corti et al., "City Planning and Population Health."
181. International Council for Science, *Report of the ICSU Planning Group.*
182. Davies and Kelly, *Healthy Cities.*
183. Tsouros, "City Leadership for Health and Sustainable Development."
184. Flynn, "*Healthy Cities within the American Context.*"
185. Easterling, Conner, and Larson, "Creating a Healthy Civic Infrastructure."
186. Werna et al., *Healthy City Projects in Developing Countries.*
187. de Leeuw and Simos, "Healthy Cities Move to Maturity."
188. Hancock, "The Evolution, Impact and Significance of the Healthy Cities/Healthy Communities Movement."
189. Ashton, *Healthy Cities*, 235.
190. Kickbusch, "Healthy Cities."
191. Tsouros, "The WHO Healthy Cities Project."
192. Ashton, Grey, and Barnard, "Healthy Cities—WHO's New Public Health Initiative."
193. Barton and Grant, "Urban Planning for Healthy Cities."
194. Tsouros, "Healthy Cities: A Political Movement."
195. Flynn, "Healthy Cities: Toward Worldwide Health Promotion."
196. Duhl, "The Healthy City."
197. World Health Organization, *Twenty Steps for Developing a Healthy Cities Project.*

198. Draper et al., *WHO Healthy Cities Project.*
199. Evers, Farrant, and Trojan, *Healthy Public Policy at the Local Level.*
200. Kickbusch, *Good Planets Are Hard to Find.*
201. Milio, "Healthy Cities."
202. Ziglio, Hagard, and Griffiths, "Health Promotion Development in Europe."
203. Tsouros, "Healthy Cities: A Political Project."
204. de Leeuw, "Evaluating WHO Healthy Cities in Europe."
205. Antonovsky, "The Salutogenic Model as a Theory to Guide Health Promotion."
206. Antonovsky, *Unraveling the Mystery of Health.*
207. Antonovsky, "The Structure and Properties of the Sense of Coherence Scale."
208. Auchincloss and Diez-Roux, "A New Tool for Epidemiology."
209. Galea, Riddle, and Kaplan, "Causal Thinking and Complex System Approaches in Epidemiology."
210. Rydin et al., "Shaping Cities for Health."
211. Gordon-Larsen et al., "Inequality in the Built Environment Underlies Key Health Disparities."

PART ONE

SMALL-TOWN AMERICA
AND ITS POPULATION
HEALTH CONTEXTS

CHAPTER TWO

Rural and Small-Town America

Definitions

In 2010, nearly one-fifth of the US population lived in mostly rural nonmetro statistical areas covering over three-quarters of all counties of the country [1, 2]. A vast majority of this population lived in small towns and cities (also called *small-town America*) in these rural counties. Often geographically isolated from one another and from other larger cities by mountains, deserts, rivers, forests, prairies, rangeland, unused land, or land used for agricultural production and processing, mining, and recreation [3], these small towns and cities generally serve similar functions as the urban core of a metropolitan area but at a much smaller scale. As settlement types, they are important because they facilitate many different forms of social, technological, and economic exchanges and interactions necessary to bridge the divide between urban and rural areas.

Today, many isolated small towns and cities in the United States face existential threats. With neglected and abandoned houses, poorly maintained roads and bridges, dilapidated and dangerous parks and open spaces, food deserts, dysfunctional traffic systems, and failing health care facilities, the built environments of these small towns and cities raise profound population health and social justice concerns. These concerns are distinct and different from those of big cities and suburbs, and from the rural counties where these small cities and towns are located. In densely built big cities, traffic exposure, air pollution, noise, and urban heat island effects are important population health concerns, but not in these small towns and cities. In small towns and cities—as in many deprived urban areas with poor populations—mental health, inactive lifestyles, obesity, crime, social isolation, drug use, traffic fatalities, work-related injuries, suicides, and high mortality and morbidity are significant population health concerns. Despite having many population health concerns, a general focus on urban, suburban, and rural areas in population and public health literature has left small towns and cities poorly studied, without much understanding of the unique characteristics of these communities and their environmental conditions affecting population health.

While examining population health in small-town America, it is important to notice the lack of a consistent definition for small towns and cities. Defining a small town or city, however, is not easy. The phrase "rural America" has often been used as a synonym of "small-town America" even though they are not the same. The oft-used phrase "rural and small-town America" not only undermines the distinctions between them, but it also tends to put more emphasis on rural America over small-town America. It assumes that small-town America is contained in rural America. When using the phrase, researchers therefore find it acceptable to consider small-town America as an indistinguishable part of rural America or to avoid acknowledging it as different for all things related to rural America. If, for any reason, they are unable to consider or to ignore small-town America in their studies on rural America, they make it an anomaly in the otherwise "homogeneous" landscape of rural America.

Nowadays, many prefer to downplay the homogeneity of rural America, emphasizing that it is more diverse than it was ever before. In this regard, national and regional perspectives can be helpful. Geographically, rural America was and is diverse at the national level. With almost 80% of the total US land area, rural America encompasses the vast agricultural heartland of the Great Plains of the Midwest; the desert lands and mountains of the Southwest; the deep, mountainous forests of the Pacific Northwest; the isolated, hilly terrain of the Appalachian Mountains; the rocky shorelines and working forests of New England; and the flat and humid coastal plains of the Southeast.

In contrast, rural America has not been as diverse racially and ethnically as the nation overall. The 2010 Census reports that approximately 78% of the rural population is white and non-Hispanic, compared to 64% of the population of the nation. The location and concentration of minorities in rural areas vary across regions, however, adding notable diversity to the social landscape of rural America. For example, nearly 90% of rural African Americans reside in the southern region of the United States. The southern "Black Belt" communities of Alabama, Georgia, Mississippi, North Carolina, South Carolina, and Virginia as well as the Lower Mississippi Delta states of Arkansas, Mississippi, and Louisiana have even larger portions of African American population. The Midwest plains, the Southwest, and Alaska have the most rural Native Americans residing on or near Native American reservations and trust lands. Texas, California, New Mexico, and Arizona are home to more than half of all rural Hispanics in the country. In fact, just under one quarter of all rural Hispanics live in Texas alone [4].

Even though rural America is geographically and socially diverse across regions within the United States, diversity within an otherwise rural region or locality can be complex. Some parts of many rural regions are quite homogeneous, even as other parts become increasingly diverse. In most cases, diversity is increasing in small towns and cities as it is decreasing in rural hinterlands. This is evident in that the built environment of small towns and cities generally remains significantly diverse in size, shape, and form. This is also evident in that many small towns and cities have been demographically diverse since the time they were founded and that they continue to remain relatively diverse because most demographic, economic, social, and physical changes within rural regions occur here. While it is true that many small towns and cities are losing population due to out-migration to more urbanized areas, many others are also seeing a rise in population as they become bedroom communities within sprawling metropolitan regions or destinations for amenity seekers.

Another less noted but important fact related to population change is in-migration to small towns and cities from their own rural hinterlands. Poor rural hinterlands often have more problems than small towns and cities. As a result, these hinterlands are losing population to nearby small towns and cities and becoming socially and demographically more homogeneous. Against these common trends, however, some rural areas have observed increasing retail, recreational, manufacturing, and food processing activities in recent years. Many small towns and cities, therefore, are adapting to or wrestling with racial and ethnic changes caused by immigrants, who are taking low-paying jobs in these facilities [5]. In many cases, these changes are seen as indicators of success and a healthy economy. Reversing a trend of depopulation, immigrants are repopulating several of these small towns and cities with new life and vigor [6, 7]. In contrast, in many other cases immigrants make it difficult for communities to meet their fiscal, social, environmental, and public health goals, giving rise to ethnic/racial tensions [8].

Put simply, it is difficult to generalize if rural America is becoming either more or less diverse. Within rural regions, it may be wise to treat small towns and cities differently from their rural hinterlands because they show significant differences in terms of physical, social, and economic contexts and demographic compositions. Yet small-town America rarely finds a place in many disciplinary studies that include population health. This is primarily because small towns do not serve as important administrative and political units of the state or federal government. In the United States, generally counties are the primary administrative units of local government. They have programmatic importance at the federal and state levels, and their boundaries are relatively stable [9]. Another important geographical unit is the census tract, which is a relatively stable geographic unit for the collection and presentation of statistical data by the US Census Bureau. The spatial size of census tracts can vary widely depending on the density of settlements. Therefore, the number of census tracts of a county may not correlate with the size of the county. A geographically small county with high population density can have more census tracts than a geographically large county with low population density. Most population and public health studies on rural areas generally use counties or census tracts as the geographical units of analysis because most data collected by federal and state entities are readily available for these units. These studies, however, are less relevant to the population health concerns of small towns and cities because as geographical units they are often different from rural counties or census tracts.

A book exploring the relationships between the built environment and population health in small-town America needs a proper definition for small towns or cities to enhance the validity and utility of its research. Such a definition must recognize that, despite differences, a small town or city is a rural phenomenon. Yet it is not completely rural. Nor is it a small version of urban America.

Defining Rurality

The term "rural" is easily taken for granted, but it is difficult to define given that rurality is associated with the geography, demography, economy, and culture of a place. Multiple definitions of rurality exist for both research and policy purposes in the United States [1, 10–13]. Even federal organizations do not use consistent criteria to define "rural," which is not without reasons. Most definitions are designed to target assistance to a specific problem that occurs in some rural communities but not in all. Rural communities face many problems, such as getting a school or a hospital, recruiting teachers and doctors, getting affordable housing and broadband access, providing transportation services to seniors who cannot drive anymore, protecting farmers from disastrous losses, or maintaining roads and repairing bridges. In many cases, the survival of a small town depends on receiving state or federal help with some of these problems.

Since not all rural areas face all these problems, thoughtful, targeted definitions are needed to make government assistance programs most helpful to those who need them most. A simpler definition is not always better, nor is it more efficient. Different government programs have different purposes and therefore need different parameters. One program may be targeted for small cities with 10,000 to 25,000 people. Another may be targeted for small cities with fewer than 2,500 people. Both are often considered rural, but the programs need to define "rural" specifically so they can hit the right target. Over the past few decades, the patterns of development have changed and so have the definitions of urban and rural. The problem is that by the time an agency decides to switch to a new definition or classification system, it already has legacy programs based on the old definition or classification. As a result, it is not easy to replace an old definition with a new one.

In general, a simple definition of "rural" is either so inclusive that many better-off communities may not need the help being offered by a federal entity (but would take it anyway), or so restrictive that some struggling communities may not be able to get the help they need from the same entity. Still, most common definitions generally assume a simplistic rural-urban dichotomy, where one is defined by the absence of or in relation to the other. Rigorous criteria are rarely applied to assess such a dichotomous relation. Recent studies have cautioned against such oversimplification of rurality based on the argument that dichotomous definitions assume that these two categories are homogeneous and mutually exclusive [14–17]. The assumption is problematic because similarities and differences are common within and between rural and urban areas.

Some other common ways to define rural areas in policy analysis and research come from the federal government's Office of Management and Budget (OMB), the US Census Bureau, and the US Department of Agriculture (USDA) Economic Research Service [18, 19]. Interestingly, the definitions put forth by these agencies do not actually strive to define rurality. The US Census Bureau and OMB typically define urban and metropolitan, with "rural" being functionally defined as any area that is not urban or metropolitan [19]. In contrast, the USDA defines geographical areas on a continuum where none—rural or urban—is defined with any certainty.

From 1910 to 1950, "rural" included all people outside incorporated places with a population of more than 2,500 residents, with those living in such incorporated places constituting the urban sector [20]. Since 1950, the definition has been modified to reflect increasingly decentralized settlements. In 2000, the US Census Bureau defined rural as consisting of all territory, population, and housing units outside of an urbanized area of 50,000 or more people and outside urban clusters with at least 2,500 people. Since the Census Bureau uses census tracts and blocks, the new definition is difficult to apply and can lead to seeming "islands" of urbanicity within otherwise rural areas or of rurality within otherwise urban areas [21].

In contrast, the OMB uses the terms "metropolitan" and "nonmetropolitan" instead of "rural" and "urban." A nonmetropolitan area is outside of a metro area and has no cities with more than 50,000 residents. This is useful as a clear-cut, mostly objective definition that can be easily applied (thus its widespread use); however, it focuses only on population size, ignoring the many other factors of rurality. It also does not take into account wide variations that can occur within a single county, particularly counties with large geographical areas [21]. Therefore, a person living in a nonmetropolitan county as defined by the OMB may live in an urban area of greater than 2,500 using the census definition.

As used in the definitions provided by the US Census Bureau and OMB, rural and nonmetropolitan, however, are far from synonymous. Noted earlier, according to these definitions, nonmetropolitan areas can include urban population, and there can be considerable rural population inside metropolitan areas. Consequently, the Census Bureau classifies 61.7 million (25%) of the total population as rural, OMB classifies 55.9 million (23%) of the total population as nonmetropolitan [21]; and, based on these definitions, only 13% of the urban population is nonmetropolitan, whereas 39% of the rural population is metropolitan [20]. Therefore, both a rural-urban and a metropolitan-nonmetropolitan distinction are important because the rural and urban components of metropolitan areas may be expected to differ considerably from those in nonmetropolitan areas.

Different from the defining criteria used by the US Census Bureau and OMB, the USDA has five different ways of classifying rural and urban areas, many of which measure rurality and urbanicity on a continuum. The two most-used USDA classifications include the Rural-Urban Continuum Codes (RUCCs) and the Rural-Urban Community Areas (RUCAs). The USDA RUCCs classify counties according to a continuum defined based on population size, level of urbanization (metro vs. nonmetro), and proximity to metropolitan areas (adjacent vs. nonadjacent) [19]. In contrast, the USDA RUCA codes classify census tracts using a scale based on population density, level of urbanization, and the degree to which residents of the area commute to more urbanized areas. The classification codes are important from a policy perspective because they are used in combination with the county-level census definition to define eligibility for rural-specific funding administered by the Health Resources and Services Administration (HRSA), but they are complex and difficult to both apply and interpret since even areas with the same code generally have many differences [19].

An emphasis on proximity to metropolitan areas and the degree to which residents of the area commute to more urbanized areas in the USDA's definitions of rurality are important, however. They are related to remoteness or isolation in rurality, which helps define rural residents as independent and self-sufficient individuals. The norms of self-reliance among rural residents in remote areas often affect health through an individual's or a group's willingness to seek care. For mental health in particular, resistance to therapeutic techniques and unwillingness to reveal mental illnesses to friends and families are often amplified in rural settings.

In addition to separating rural communities from other communities, geographic remoteness or isolation also contributes to the potentially life-threatening distance to many essential medical and mental health care services. A potentially life-threatening distance from rural areas to emergency and routine medical care [22, 23], again, fosters a notion of self-reliance among rural populations concerning health [24, 25]. Isolated rural residents likely perceive seeking health care as an inconvenience and a burden to friends and family because of increased travel distance [26]. For health care providers, this can lead to a perception of noncompliance that is dictated less by choice than by circumstance.

Other measures of rurality, such as population size and density, are important and easy to define but not easy to apply. For example, the rural parts of Montgomery County, Maryland (population over 1 million and population density close to 2,000 persons per square mile) are not like those of Kent County, Maryland (population less than 20,000 and population density close to 73 persons per square mile). Likewise, the state of Alaska, with its vast swaths of wilderness, has an average population density of 1.25 persons per square mile. If we take out Anchorage, the density goes down to 0.7 persons per square mile. Therefore, rurality in terms of density in Alaska cannot be compared to that in Maryland. Likewise, many metropolitan areas often contain census tracts with lower population density than many census tracts in nonmetropolitan rural areas.

A comprehensive examination of the strengths and weaknesses of the OMB, Census Bureau, and USDA classifications can be found in a 2005 article published by Hart, Larson, and Lishner [1] in the *American Journal of Public Health*. Additional definitions and typologies of rural, such as frontier rural, are also found in the literature. Frontier communities represent the extreme of rurality, with definitions ranging from population densities less than or equal to six persons per square mile [27] to complex scoring methods that take into account travel time to market centers and medical care [28].

Regardless of how accurately various geographical dimensions of rurality are described, rurality can be neither dichotomous nor one-dimensional. As a multidimensional construct, it can affect not only the potential health care needs of rural populations but also the ways in which rural populations will seek out assistance and care (or avoid them) and will lead their everyday lives. The dimensions of rurality must be considered carefully in the planning, execution, and even the evaluation of rural health to ensure the success of any population health efforts. The problem, however, is how to capture and analyze the dimensions of rurality consistently.

Defining Small-Town America

Even though small-town America is often considered a part of rural America, they have significant differences. Writing about small-town America almost a century ago, sociologist H. Paul Douglass noted that there was something perennially distinctive about these places. It mattered that they were incorporated and were places in which people worked and lived, not apart from one another as they did in the countryside, but together on a small scale. The togetherness was what mattered [29]. Writing about them a hundred years later, sociologist Robert Wuthnow evokes a similar sentiment:

> To be sure, friends and neighbors are crucial to people who live in small towns. But so is the fact that they live in a community. The town has an identity as a community. Its meanings are inscribed in particular places and the tangible aspects of these places. . . . The town's identity is reinforced in festivals and ball

games, small acts of kindness, recovering from a disaster, and the stories that are repeated about these events, and by the local cultural leaders who keep the stories alive. Towns are defined as well by that which they are not—cities, unfamiliar places, and big government. The stories and symbolic markers of difference define a place as a community [30].

According to these and other sociologists, it is quite clear that small-town America is very different not only from rural America but also from cities, as emphasized previously. They are characterized by unique physical settings, social structures, economic imperatives, and cultural and religious practices and perspectives, which cannot be generalized over rural America.

Another sociologist, Suzanne Keller [31], identified ten building blocks of a small town based on her ethnographic research, qualitative interviews, and survey of a small-town community. These building blocks include territory, membership criteria, an institutional framework, cultural values, a belief system, myths, rituals and celebrations, leadership structure, social networks, and the spirit of community—all specific to the place itself. While there is a need to define each one of Keller's building blocks for small-town America separately from rural America, a physical and/or population-based territorial definition for a small town seems more pressing for a book that explores the relationships of the built environment with population health in small-town America. For Keller, *territory* or turf is figuratively, if not also literally, the bedrock of community, serving as the bounded site in which it exists and providing it with a spatial signature, physical identity, and perhaps sense of security and closure. However, a physical or a population-based definition of such a territory for a small town is not immediately found.

In the absence of a general definition, for the purposes of this book, a small town or city is defined as *an incorporated town or a civil township that falls in the category of urban clusters (UCs) with US Census Bureau population between 2,500 and 49,999 and that is formed under the general laws of a US state or under a charter adopted by the local voters.* According to the US Census Bureau, places with fewer than 2,500 people are rural areas; and places with 50,000 or more people are urban areas (UAs) of the OMB's metropolitan category. In 2010, the United States had 486 UAs with 71.2% or 219.9 million of the nation's population; 3,087 UCs with 9.5% or 29.3 million of the nation's population; and rural areas (any area outside UAs and UCs) with 19.3% or 59.9 million of the nation's population [32].

Though the debate over an appropriate population size threshold between rural and urban clusters is ongoing, it seems reasonable to assume that any place with fewer than 2,500 people might not be able to maintain the levels and diversity of employment, goods, and services necessary for its own governance. Keeping the upper threshold at 49,999 people ensures that the education and income levels of the populations of these places are somewhat closer to those of the general US population since most of the country's population lives in UAs. Keeping the upper threshold at 49,999 people also aligns with the 2002 farm bill, which includes areas outside census places of 50,000 or more and their adjacent areas for several USDA funding programs. Additionally, it ensures that small towns include OMB's micropolitan areas with populations between 10,000 and 49,999, greatly increasing the flexibility in tailoring rural programs to different target populations [33]. In contrast, lowering the upper threshold from 49,999 to 25,000 or to 10,000 may decrease the size of qualifying population who live in small cities and towns significantly. For example, lowering the threshold to 10,000 may decrease the population from 17% to 7%, leaving out a significant chunk of small-town population that consistently shows lower education and income levels than the overall US population.

Notably, keeping the upper threshold at 49,999 people also allows the two nonmetropolitan levels, micropolitan (10,000–49,999) and noncore (2,500–9,999), of the six urbanization levels of the National Center for Health Statistics (NCHS) Urban-Rural Classification Scheme for Counties to remain within small-town categories. The other four metro levels are large central metro, large fringe metro, medium metro, and small metro. An alignment of a small-town definition with the NCHS classification scheme is important because application of the scheme to National Vital Statistics System (NVSS) and National Health Interview Survey (NHIS) data has demonstrated that these six categories are useful for assessing and monitoring health differences among communities across the full urbanization spectrum [9].

Following the USDA classification systems, population density, proximity to metropolitan areas (adjacent and nonadjacent), and commute to more urbanized areas [34] are used in addition to population size in this book to measure the rurality of a small town or city. Taken together, these measurements of rurality should help enhance the definition of small towns and cities in the studies of the book on the effects of rurality on spatial associations of population health in small-town America. It should be noted, however, that the qualitative dimensions described by Keller [31] will not be used here to limit the scope of these studies and to align them with previous studies on spatial associations of population health reported in the literature.   .

Conclusions

Primarily a rural phenomenon, small-town America is not quite rural. Even though it serves some urban functions, small-town America is not urban either. It is different from both rural and urban America. In the United States, rurality has been defined differently over time by different institutions to serve different purposes. Among them, institutional definitions that use simple spatial and population terms have continued to serve important functions. In contrast, definitions that must use complex economic, social, and cultural terms have remained difficult to operationalize.

This chapter provides a definition for small towns and cities for use in the studies of the book exploring how rurality affects spatial associations of lifestyles and health indicators and outcomes in small towns and cities. Though defined based on population size, the definition will be enhanced by population density, commute time, and proximity to urban areas following the USDA's rurality (or urbanicity) classification. The complex social, economic, and cultural factors will not be used in defining small towns and cities.

In the next chapter, the population health contexts of small towns and cities in the United States will be described as background to what follows in part II. In the two chapters (chapters 4 and 5) of part II, the stories of recent changes and health concerns in rural Kansas will be described relative to the US contexts described in chapter 3.

NOTES

1. Hart, Larson, and Lishner, "Rural Definitions."
2. US Census Bureau. "Explore Census Data."
3. Dalbey, "Implementing Smart Growth Strategies."
4. Housing Assistance Council. "Race and Ethnicity in Rural America."
5. Fennelly, "Prejudice toward Immigrants in the Midwest."
6. Kandel and Cromartie, *New Patterns of Hispanic Settlement in Rural America.*
7. McConnell and Miraftab, "Sundown Town to 'Little Mexico.'"
8. Muro and Puentes, *Investing in a Better Future.*
9. Ingram and Franco, *2013 NCHS Urban-Rural Classification Scheme,* 1–73.
10. US Office of Management and Budget, "2010 Standards for Delineating Metropolitan and Micropolitan Statistical Areas."
11. Isserman, "In the National Interest."
12. Woods, "Rural Geography."

13. Hall, Kaufman, and Ricketts, "Defining Urban and Rural Areas."
14. Cutler and Coward, "Residence Differences."
15. Krout, "Rural versus Urban Differences."
16. Miller and Luloff, *Who Is Rural?*
17. Rowles, *What's Rural About Rural Aging?*
18. Ricketts, Johnson-Webb, and Taylor, *Definitions of Rural.*
19. Warren and Smalley, *What Is Rural?*
20. Fuguitt, Brown, and Beale, *Rural and Small Town America.*
21. Smalley and Warren, *Rural Public Health.*
22. Connor, Kralewski, and Hillson, "Measuring Geographic Access to Health Care."
23. Weinert and Boik, "MSU Rurality Index."
24. Long and Weinert, "Rural Nursing."
25. Weinert and Long, "Understanding the Health Care Needs of Rural Families."
26. Mohatt et al., *Mental Health and Rural America.*
27. Hewitt, *Defining "Rural" Areas.*
28. Frontier Education Center, *Frontier.*
29. Douglass, *The Little Town.*
30. Wuthnow, *Small-Town America*, 3.
31. Keller, *Community.*
32. US Census Bureau, "Growth in Urban Population Outpaces Rest of Nation."
33. Cromartie and Bucholtz, "Defining the 'Rural' in Rural America."
34. Crosby et al., *Rural Populations and Health.*

CHAPTER THREE

The Rural Contexts of Population Health in Small-Town America

Consequences of Ongoing Changes

The United States had been a predominantly rural society until at least the end of the nineteenth century. The people of this rural society settled sparsely, with enough land to grow sufficient food and other agricultural products to survive and prosper. Nearby small towns and cities worked as economic hubs, where people could buy and sell everyday products. These towns were also the places where agricultural surpluses were collected and stored for trading with the world outside and where social and cultural identities of a frontier society were produced and reproduced.

Things have been changing quite significantly in rural and small-town America since the late 19th century. Through urbanization and concomitant deconcentration, urban and metropolitan influences have already penetrated deeply into what formerly were entirely rural areas. As a result, the relationships between rural and urban America have become complicated, with the former often exploited by the latter. In the process, many small towns and cities in America have lost their traditional significance as economic, social, and cultural hubs while many others have continued to thrive and flourish through many changes [1].

Today, both rural and small-town America face many economic, social, environmental, and population health challenges that they have not known before. For various reasons, however, these challenges affect small-town America differently from rural America. In geographical terms, small towns and cities occupy small segments of rural counties of the United States, but they contain almost one-half of the population living outside metropolitan areas [1]. They generally have higher population densities; denser and more diverse built environments; more public and private institutions; more economic functions and opportunities; and better and more health, utility, and transport facilities and infrastructures than the rest of the rural counties within which they are located. Yet like most other things, the population health issues of small-town America remain intrinsically related to rural America. Therefore, to understand the population health issues of small-town America, we must first consider rural America and its changing trends.

Changing Trends in Rural America
Relative Shrinking of Rural Population

Throughout the 20th century, the absolute size of rural US population has remained relatively stable, between 51 and 65 million people [1], while its relative size with respect to urban population has decreased significantly. In 1900, the urban share of US population was 39.5%. By 1950, the percentage increased to 64%. In 2000, 79% of the US population was urban [2], and in 2010, that percentage increased to 83%. Put simply, by 2010, the 65% of US counties classified as rural were home to only 17% of the population (about 52 million people) [3].

Among many other things, rural out-migration has been an important factor for the relative shrinkage of rural population. In general, for much of the 20th century, most rural communities experienced out-migration and population loss as millions left rural areas for booming cities. The volume of rural out-migration varied from decade to decade, but the direction of flows did not. Even today, more people consistently leave rural areas than come to them [4]. Within this overall relative shrinking trend, however, some rural counties continue to grow. As the economies of scale and geographic proximity that long provided a significant competitive advantage for locations in urban cores keep eroding by congestion, high housing costs and densities, land shortages, and high labor costs, more people and businesses are migrating to rural areas than they did previously in search of cheaper, quieter, and healthier lifestyles. Such selective urban to rural migration, however, has not been able to reverse the trend of shrinking rural America.

To understand why rural America is shrinking, natural increase (the excess of births over deaths) and decrease (the excess of deaths over births) must be considered along with out-migration. Historically, high rural fertility contributed to the greater levels of natural increase. Farm families and small-town residents had more children than their urban counterparts, and enough babies were born to offset the steady departure of working-age people. But over the last few decades, rural women have been bearing fewer children. Though they still marry earlier and have children earlier than their urban counterparts, these differences are diminishing. Fertility levels among the two groups are now virtually indistinguishable [6, 7]. The incidence of natural decrease in rural America is now higher than at any point in history. Over 40% of America's rural counties have experienced natural decrease since 2000. These 850 counties are concentrated in agricultural regions of the Great Plains and Corn Belt and in parts of the upper Great Lakes, the Ozarks, and Appalachia. Because most counties with natural decrease are also experiencing net out-migration, the prospects for future population gains in these rural counties are limited at best [5].

The shrinking patterns of rural America are often complex and subtle, but their impacts on population health in rural and small-town America are not. We see it in persistent poverty and diminished community capacity, strained infrastructure and institutions, poor housing conditions, and poor population health. The study of geographic differences presented in the 2001 urban and rural health chartbook [8] showed that rural areas in general ranked poorly on 21 of 23 selected population health indicators, including health behaviors, mortality, morbidity, and maternal and child health.

Diminishing Demand for Labor and Age-Selective Rural Migration

The past few decades have brought an unprecedented ebb and flow of migration between urban and rural areas and between metropolitan and nonmetropolitan areas. These changing migration patterns can be misleading, but the relative rates of out-migration from rural areas have always been higher than from urban areas [9]. A smaller rural population has been exporting a larger share of its population to urban areas. In contrast, a larger urban population has been exporting a smaller share of its population to rural areas.

Another interesting fact is that rural out-migration has always been age selective [10–12]. Even though the magnitude of rural out-migration has varied, age-selective out-migration has remained strikingly consistent in rural areas over the years. Its incidence rate has been the highest among young adults, who are attracted to a metro area's economic advantages, especially given the diminishing demand for labor in farming and mining and low wages in many rural industries [13]. Since the out-migration of young adults increases the overall age and decreases the overall earnings of rural population, it also increases traditional rural-urban health, income, and spatial inequalities.

As rural America continues to lose its young, best, and brightest to metropolitan areas, the least educated and least skilled are left behind. Low economic returns on education generally motivate out-migration of the most educated or those with high educational and occupational aspirations among young adults. For the least educated residents, however, urban-rural wage differentials are often small. As a result, they have no good reason to leave rural areas. Their decisions to stay or leave are generally affected by the relative importance of other factors (such as family and friends) [14, 15]. The effects of an uneven but persistent out-migration of a productive, young population are often substantial on small rural communities, even though the magnitude is small in relation to the overall population of the country [16, 17]. It reinforces cultural homogeneity and common social values among older adults who are left behind.

In contrast, rural heterogeneity and change come mostly from the in-migration of older urban residents seeking recreational and leisurely activities in rural areas. Not surprisingly, in-migration often leads to cultural clashes between urban newcomers and longtime rural residents [18]. In many instances, urban newcomers seek to halt new growth lest the community lose the special appeal that first attracted them. Urban and rural values often collide in the form of contentious local politics, leading to conflicts at the cost of community health.

In recent years, the percentage of rural elderly has grown significantly [19]. Many rural areas have seen a growth in their elderly population due to the out-migration of young adults. Fewer other areas have seen the same due to aging in place. Still fewer have seen the elderly population grow due to in-migration of urban retirees. Growth in the elderly population greatly influences the health status and health care needs of a rural community, where the resources necessary to take care of older citizens are generally limited. This is seen in that the risk of serious illness and death is high among elderly populations (aged 65 and older) in rural counties [20]. A lack of rural health care resources is worsened by the fact that most rural elderly populations in the United States are generally living in poverty due to high medical expenses. In 2002, populations aged 65 and up were responsible for 36% of total personal health care expenditures but constituted only 13% of the US population [21]. In 2010, Medicare—the federal health insurance entitlement program for people who are 65 and older—was the payment source for almost one-third of all hospital care expenditures [22]. In many parts of rural America, population health continues to decline as poverty continues to rise due, in part, to the increased elderly population.

Increasing Diversity

A common image of rural America is one of racial and ethnic homogeneity— that is, rural places are mostly where white people live. While this is true for much of rural America, there are substantial African American concentrations in the Southeast, Hispanic concentrations in the Southwest, and Native American concentrations in the northern Great Plains and upper Great Lakes [5]. In addition, a surprising number of recent immigrants, especially from Mexico and Latin America, are now settling in many rural destination communities [23–25].

Though racial diversity is growing locally across rural America, it is not always noticeable in all rural communities due to lower numbers of non-white population. In many counties, the foreign-born populations exceeded 5% of the total population for the first time in 2000. Some of these counties are nonmetropolitan, and they cluster on the peripheries of existing regions with large concentrations of foreign-born people. Some cluster in the isolated counties of the rural Midwest to work in meatpacking and food processing plants [25]. Recent evidence suggests that many new immigrants—those who arrived in the past 5 to 10 years—are bypassing the gateway cities and regions (or residing there only briefly) for more geographically dispersed rural locations [26].

Despite increasing diversity, many racial and ethnic groups remain underrepresented in rural and nonmetropolitan areas. Only American Indians are predominantly nonmetropolitan, while the proportion of Black, Hispanic, and Asian and Pacific Islander residents living in nonmetropolitan areas is much smaller than proportion of the total US population. These four groups combined account for a much smaller segment of the nonmetropolitan population compared with the same groups as a segment of the metropolitan population [1].

In addition to being underrepresented, many racial and ethnic groups are unevenly distributed across rural and nonmetropolitan areas. In most of the South, for example, Black citizens still account for large fractions and even majorities of the rural and small-town population. In contrast, they are almost totally absent in rural and nonmetropolitan areas outside of this region. This situation is worsened by the fact that racial and ethnic minorities tend to be concentrated in rural and nonmetropolitan areas that are socially disadvantaged and are experiencing slow economic growth or decline.

It is important to note that while immigrants are a small percentage of the rural population, they have accounted for a disproportionate share of the nonmetropolitan growth since 1990 [5]. For example, during the first decade of the 21st century, Hispanics and other minorities accounted for only 21% of the rural population, but they contributed to 83% of overall rural population growth [27]. Immigrants tend to be young, so they bring the vigor and energy of youth to rural communities that have been losing much of their young adult population for decades. Young immigrants also tend to have higher fertility than native-born residents, so they bring the potential for a new generation to many rural areas that have been experiencing minimal natural increase or outright natural decrease. Current high rates of immigrant fertility, combined with overall low fertility and aging among the white population, also mean that rural ethno-racial heterogeneity will continue to grow in the coming years.

Increasing rural diversity due to new immigration clearly is linked to the changing global economy. New immigrants today, compared with those of the 1960s, are less fluent in English, less educated and skilled, and more likely to be undocumented [28]. Not surprisingly, the presence of new immigrants has sometimes created racial and ethnic tensions within many rural communities. Longtime white rural residents are generally unaccustomed to living with minorities who speak different languages and bring unfamiliar customs to the community [29–31]. They also fear that immigrants will change the fundamental character of their communities, spur new tax increases to pay for social services and special education programs, and raise local crime rates [32]. Consequently, supporting their longtime residents, many small communities have imposed new anti-immigrant ordinances in hopes of discouraging foreign-born newcomers, especially undocumented workers [33].

Sociological concerns raised by new rural immigration, however, are many [34, 35]. Hispanic-white segregation levels are higher in many new rural destination communities than they are in traditional gateway cities. Small rural communities are now experiencing "white flight"—a phenomenon usually associated with the movement of white residents to suburbs due to racial changes in inner-city neighborhoods—because of increasing new immigration. Ethnic enclaves are forming in some of these small communities. All these spatial changes are likely to have population health implications, which have not yet been studied thoroughly [36].

Changing Agriculture

Rural areas and farming remain inextricably but often mistakenly linked in the public mind. This is despite industrialization and globalization of US agricultural production having reshaped rural America in profound ways over the past century while also introducing new environmental and population health problems. Federal policies and tax laws, trade liberalization, and market rules regulating international agricultural trade have often favored corporate actors over smaller farm operations. As a result, the concentration of production of internationally traded commodities continues to grow among fewer and larger farming units [37] at the cost of more numerous and diversified smaller farming units.

In general, the past century was marked by a massive shift away from labor-intensive, small, diversified farms (producing different crops and animals) that served nearby communities and surrounding regions to an agricultural sector that is increasingly dominated by large, specialized farms [38]. These large farms employ only a tiny fraction of the workforce that previously served smaller farms and often produce crops that local communities and surrounding regions do not use or need. Between 1900 and 2000, the share of the workforce employed in agriculture declined from 41% to 2%. With the exception of 403 rural counties where farming still dominates the local economy and another 113 counties where mining (which includes oil and gas extraction) remains a major economic enterprise, most rural areas employ significantly fewer farmworkers than they did in the past [39]. Rural areas have a long history of slow population growth or outright decline and have experienced significant net out-migration for decades [10, 11, 40]. They continue to shed jobs and consolidate. In many rural areas, only a few young adults remain, and births no longer offset deaths.

A dramatic decline in the overall farm population, however, did not change the absolute size of the total US rural population in the 20th century. Instead, population shifted from farms to rural towns and communities, with the resulting decrease in farm population generally offset by an increase in small-town population. The movement of people from farms to rural towns began in earnest circa World War II. Labor shortages associated with war efforts encouraged farm mechanization, freeing many farmworkers for off-farm jobs after the war ended. Many joined what was then an expanding farm service sector—businesses that were selling new, technologically superior tools to farmers, tools that caused a sharp rise in farm output, creating surplus supplies and lowering farm prices. Nationally, the massive migration of people from farms to small towns was hardly noticeable. The enormity of rural America, with its thousands of small towns, allowed a few dozen farm families to migrate in each county each year almost imperceptibly. The movement process was spread out over several decades, further softening its impact and lessening its visibility [41].

With the migration obscured by space and softened by time, most Americans remained more impressed with the stability of rural America than with its ongoing changes. Rural stability was reflected in the perceived serenity of small towns and in the perceived unchanging nature of farmsteads even as science continued revolutionizing agricultural production and supplies through all types of economic adversity. Farmers and farm output seemed almost insulated from these macro cycles, capable of meeting almost any challenge—a reassuring image to most Americans wary of change [41].

Behind the facade of rural stability was an onslaught of new technology that imposed constant change on farm families. Like the fact that the nation's rapid economic development in the 19th century eventually came under question, the successful adoption of new agricultural technology has run into economic, social, and environmental limitations in the 20th century. The replacement of family farms with corporate agriculture has seemingly eroded many of the most salient aspects of rural and small-town community life in America [41]. Groundwater contamination, pesticide residues, pollution of waterways, erosion of fragile cropland, and food-safety questions relating to the use of growth hormones in livestock farming have all become national concerns.

The rise of corporate agriculture, which rapidly displaced family farms and caused economic dislocations in family farm–dependent communities, also occurred in concert with the growth of so-called food deserts in rural areas. Fewer rural people grow their own food, while the introduction of large regional retailers such as Walmart has forced many locally owned groceries out of business. Residents in remote rural places now must travel long distances to shop for fresh and nutritious food in urban commercial centers, but they lack the necessary transportation [42]. Not surprisingly, rural food deserts have been linked to poverty, food insecurity, and obesity [43, 44].

As the rise of corporate agriculture frees up a major segment of the rural labor force, rural industries become diversified with clothing manufacturers, meatpacking plants, auto parts makers, and computer equipment manufacturers taking advantage of cheap labor. The proportion of the rural labor force employed in manufacturing in 2003 was 12.4%, substantially higher than the

8.4% figure in metropolitan areas. The transition from heavy reliance on employment in an extractive economy to a more diversified economy has not, however, fulfilled the promise of increased employment and better incomes for rural residents in the most recent period. Instead, rural residents have experienced increased rates of unemployment and declining incomes compared with their urban and metropolitan counterparts. During the last few decades, the increased globalization of manufacturing has cost many traditional rural manufacturing jobs. The low-technology, low-wage labor that traditional rural manufacturing and processing plants specialized in is now shifting offshore. The impact of these trends is clearly reflected in the dramatically reduced levels of population growth and modest net migration gains in manufacturing counties since 2000 [45]. It does not appear that rural industries will come to rescue many poor parts of rural America.

Overall, rural residents face substantial disadvantages in terms of economic opportunities. The level of labor force participation in rural areas continues to be lower than in urban and metropolitan areas. This persistent gap is associated with older age among the rural labor force. It is also associated with a greater prevalence of work-limiting disability, which is a continuing legacy of agriculture, mining, and other types of goods-producing industries that are concentrated in rural economies. The dramatic industrial transformation of nonmetropolitan economies along with their smaller labor markets and greater level of specialization are also more vulnerable to cyclical changes [1]. As a result, rural areas experience a disproportionate share of employment declines, and because goods production is now concentrated in rural areas, they recover more slowly from any economic recession. Urban economies, in contrast, are larger and more diversified and depend more on services for employment. Unsurprisingly, urban and suburban areas have returned to their pre-recession employment rates since the national economic downturn and recession of 2008, but rural areas have not fully recovered or seen overall net employment growth [46].

Increasing Rural Consumption

Throughout history, the well-being of rural America has remained connected to its natural resources, including scenic mountains, lakes, rivers, and seashores, but the nature of these connections has changed over time. Today, rural America represents a new twist on long-dominant patterns of Americans exploiting their natural resources. Originally, the exploitation occurred through extractive industries; but in contemporary rural America, bountiful natural and recreational amenities offer new opportunities for growth and de-velopment through recreation, tourism, and retirement. The counties offering such opportunities are commonly found in the mountain and coastal re-gions of the West, in the upper Great Lakes, in the coastal and scenic areas of New England and Upstate New York, in the foothills of the Appalachians and Ozarks, and in coastal regions from Virginia to Florida [5]. Between 1970 and 1996, average population growth in rural counties rich in natural amenities was significant compared with essentially no growth among rural counties lacking amenities. Among such counties, retirement counties grew by more than 2.6% annually in the 1990s, with growth continuing after 2000. And rec-reational and amenity counties grew at a slightly slower rate of 2.1% annually during the 1990s. Even though growth slowed after 2000, gains still far ex-ceeded those in rural counties generally [47, 48].

As demands for recreation, tourism, and retirement grow, many parts of rural America with beaches or mountains, cultural or historic sites, or na-tional parks and recreational areas have become places of consumption, pro-viding spatial arenas for interaction between rural natives and urban visitors. They provide goods and services directed toward, and consumed dispropor-tionately by, people with strong ties to urban and big-city populations. The effects of such consumption are never straightforward. Recreation and tour-ism often generate such positive income multiplier effects on the local rural economy that annual median family income can be more than $3,000 higher in counties high in recreation and tourism than in otherwise similar rural counties [49]. However, tourist-related development may disregard the in-terests of local residents who want to preserve traditional livelihoods in favor of the interests of developers and other community residents seeking to cre-ate new jobs in the community [50].

Like the effects of tourism and recreation, the effects of increasing second-home ownership in rural America are not straightforward. Between 1980 and 2000, second homes increased from 1.9% to 3.4% of all housing units in the United States, and they were much more prevalent in rural than in urban communities [51]. Many urban dwellers who own second homes in rural areas are older adults who find the outdoor and cultural amenities of rural areas attractive. Described as "gray gold" [52], these older adults are gradually dis-engaging themselves from the labor force with good pensions and social se-curity income. In some cases, the numbers of older urban adults retiring are high enough that they turn rural communities into retirement communities. Again, benefits come with costs. For example, older in-migrants often strengthen the real estate market, but this may inflate prices and displace local service workers. They enhance local institutions through leadership and volunteering, but they may impose their own values and preferences on natives. Many older in-migrants are retired professionals. They are eager to offer free technical assistance to local governments, but this can undermine the demand for such services by local professionals. They thwart the natural increase of population, but their wealth may help create permanent job opportunities for younger residents, who can boost the natural increase of population, creating additional demand for facilities that support raising children.

Besides older adults, other second-home owners in rural areas are seasonal working-age urban migrants (consultants, contract employees, freelancers), for whom new communications technologies and changes in the organization of work allow more flexibility in choosing a rural place of residence. As the amount of time they spend at their second homes increases, many eventually consider retiring to the area. As part-time residents, these younger second-home owners make significant contributions to the local economy [53]. To meet their growing demands, new jobs and opportunities are created in construction, retail, health care, and education, benefiting local residents [12]. So, young adults who previously had to migrate to urban areas for employment are now able to stay. Like any other growing rural areas, however, as the number of second homes rises, property values and taxes also rise, forcing many local long-term residents to relocate elsewhere at the cost of local communities.

Regardless of types and services, rural places of consumption are often vulnerable to swings in the national business cycle. They often face seasonal variability in demand. They see conflicts between seasonal homeowners and year-round residents. The limits on community carrying capacity and the provision of social services of these places are put to the test during peak seasons. For some communities, tourism and recreational development pose new environmental risks to water quality and marine ecosystems, forest fragmentation, and biodiversity. Not only second homes but also any urban-related growth of rural areas may inflate local property values and taxes, displace longtime residents who can no longer afford to live in the community, and undermine community attachment and solidarity.

While the economic effects of retirees and amenity migrants are easily recognized for remote rural areas rich in natural resources, the secondary effects of their presence in terms of social, cultural, and health costs remain less recognized. In the deep and enduring relationships of dominance, dependency, and unequal power between rural areas and their urban counterparts, rural counterparts have always operated from a disadvantageous position. To say the least, the core of these relationships has been defined based on the exploitation of rural resources in various forms. Retirement and recreation are just two among many forms of exploitation. More recently, America's increasing energy problems have brought the nation's rural resources to the center. Most solutions to these energy problems reside in rural areas. These include new plant-based feedstocks (e.g., switchgrass) for ethanol; wind generation of electricity; and the use of new technologies, such as hydraulic fracturing (fracking), to extract gas from rock formations deep underground. Each brings different economic and community interests into potential conflict. As in the past, new energy technologies infuse capital into rural economies from metropolitan and global sources. Yet the environmental and population health effects of these energy technologies on rural populations will remain unknown for years to come, highlighting persistent rural-urban imbalances in political and economic power and control [54].

Growing Rural-Urban Interdependency

Rural-urban spatial interdependencies are not new [55]. New ideas, technology, and public opinion have always spread outward from cities to the countryside [56]. What is different now is the accelerated pace of changing spatial and social boundaries due to technological innovations in production, transportation, and communication. Past technological innovations (e.g., railroads, interstate highways, and air transportation) had large spatial impacts by virtue of improving the movement of products and people. In contrast, today's innovations have greatly facilitated the rapid (and relatively costless) movement of information and capital (e.g., internet, cable and satellite TV, broadband, mobile banking). They have stitched together America's rural and urban communities as never before and linked rural people and communities directly to the global economy [13].

Though isolation remains a factor for many rural communities, rural America is generally much less isolated than before. This is true not just socially and spatially but also economically. Arising out of the interdependence between rural and urban America, the putative negative effects of corporate farming on rural community well-being [57, 58], the economic and social implications of transnational corporate investments (e.g., Walmart or Conagra) for small towns [59, 60], the breakdown of small-town values and community attachment [61, 62], and the definition and meaning of rural and rurality in relation to modern urban societies [63–66] are all significant concerns for rural America today. Evidence for many negative impacts of increasing rural-urban dependency can be found in the way growth in urban areas takes advantage of proximity to rural areas and vice versa; in lifestyle changes at the rural-urban fringe; in the many instances of environmental injustice; and in the changing patterns of agriculture, consumption, and poverty.

Notably, as rural-urban dependencies increase, traditional stereotypes of rural America are breaking down [13], often to the detriment of rural America. Americans' perceptions of rural areas show a mismatch between rural stereotypes and reality, and they are dominated by images of "the family farm, crops and pastures" [67]. Most Americans believe that rural residents have stronger families and kinship networks than people in cities and their suburbs. The reality is that rural family life looks remarkably similar to urban areas today, if measured by shares of single-parent families and rates of nonmarital fertility, cohabitation, and divorce [68, 69].

Often characterized as urban sprawl, population deconcentration has been one of the most visible and impactful spatial manifestations of rural-urban dependencies in recent decades. Even though sprawl affects rural areas more than urban areas, most current discussions of sprawl are dominated by city and suburban interests. Many rural and small-town governments are not fully prepared to meet the serious challenges posed by a rapid influx of people and businesses due to sprawl. Besides land grabbing and conversion, sprawl accelerates the demand for new schools, roads, sewers, emergency and health care services, and a myriad of other services. The substantial upfront cost of all these improvements often exceeds any revenue gains. As a result, many rural and small-town governments face serious fiscal stress [70].

Evolving Forms at the Rural-Urban Fringe

The rural-urban fringe includes places outside the city in rural areas. Growth at the fringe occurs as proximate urban areas grow outward, and population eventually spills over urban boundaries into surrounding rural areas in different forms. Often generically identified as urban sprawl, growth at the fringe includes suburbs, exurbs, edge cities, and bedroom communities. They blur the line that traditionally separated urban from rural or metropolitan from nonmetropolitan areas [71, 72].

The social, economic, and cultural connections linking rural and urban areas at the fringe are enormous and ever growing [64, 71]. These areas are close enough to give people access to the urban labor market, amenities, and services. Many businesses see advantages to locating in such areas because of lower land costs, less congestion, and access to a high-quality labor force. At the same time, many people view rural counties adjacent to metropolitan areas to be an excellent compromise between rural and urban life. Opinion polls consistently show a preference among many Americans to live in smaller places that are proximate to urban areas rather than in urban cores [73].

The fringe, however, puts enormous pressure on rural land use patterns, including the conversion of agricultural land for residential and commercial use [74, 75]. Between 1980 and 2003, the developed land area of the United States increased by more than 30 million acres, with projections published in 2009 suggesting an additional 57 million acres converted by 2030 [76]. Land conversion may be troubling, but it does not represent a large share of the nation's total land base, nor does it threaten the nation's agricultural industry [13]. Though the expansion of urban settlements into rural fringe destroys natural land and resources, in some cases it can bring people into closer contact with animals (e.g., livestock and wildlife) and natural ecosystems. From a public health perspective, however, urban development into rural areas raises a specter of health concerns [77]. It can increase commute time and environmental pollution and can destroy preexisting rural communities and their ways of living, which affects physical, mental, and social health. Similarly, the development of former wildlands creates new costs and challenges for managing wildfires, water use and quality, wildlife resources (e.g., fish, game), and so forth [78].

Growth at or beyond the fringe comes with some obvious externalities, especially for rural communities. So-called bedroom communities, which often develop in small towns and cities closer to larger urban areas, may lack the usual ingredients that characterize socially cohesive and civically engaged communities. As commuting to and from work consumes more time, money, and energy, it also reduces the same from other productive community activities, including volunteerism [79]. As a result, long commutes often diminish social good. Still, the Americans who generally fare best on the health indicators are the residents of the fringe counties of large metro areas. Nationally, people living in fringe counties have the lowest levels of premature mortality. Teens in fringe counties have the lowest levels of teenage childbearing. The percent of the population with no health insurance and no dental visits in the past year also is the lowest in fringe counties [3]. According to a 2001 urban and rural health chartbook [8], the healthier, wealthier residents of "large fringe" counties—those who live in large metropolitan areas that do not include any part of the largest central city—were better off on nearly every indicator than any of the other residential categories used in the report (urban core, small urban, rural with a city of ≥10,000 residents, and rural without a city of ≥10,000 residents). Growth at and beyond the fringe, therefore, has given rise to a profound contradiction between social good and individual health in the United States.

Rising Social and Environmental Justice Concerns

Despite its somewhat negative effects, in relative terms, urban sprawl still is a better spatial outcome of the rural-urban dependency in the United States compared to other spatial outcomes of the dependency. Due to better transportation and communication systems, more prisons, slaughterhouses, feedlots, landfills, and hazardous and toxic waste sites are being built in rural areas, raising serious social and environmental concerns. The siting of these locally undesirable land uses (LULUs), planned for by urban elites, typically preys on relatively powerless and lower-income people, especially minorities in rural areas [80, 81]. Despite the promise of economic growth, new health concerns often cause rural residents to leave communities with hazardous waste sites, large landfills, or prisons. Therefore, it is unclear whether LULUs create new economic growth or crowd out other jobs by creating new environmental disamenities.

How LULUs find their places in rural areas is a bit convoluted. For example, efforts to attract prisons reflect the common belief that they will spur local economic development and prosperity [82]. Many economically depressed communities actively engage in bidding wars for prisons, offering tax breaks, infrastructure (such as roads and sewers), and land at below-market prices [83]. Interestingly, prisons rarely deliver their supposed benefits to rural communities. Rural prisons typically import prisoners from metropolitan areas. They seemingly benefit largely white rural communities at the expense of incarcerated minority prisoners and the urban communities from which they come [84]. While one study found that prison towns benefited from greater job and wage growth, retail sales, housing occupancy rates, and housing values [85], others found quite the opposite. One study reported that prison construction actually impeded economic growth in many lagging rural counties [86]. Another recorded no evidence of positive impacts of state-run prisons on county economic and population growth [83]. Yet another showed that prisons drive away or crowd out other types of local economic development [84].

The restructuring of meat production and processing also promises to bring positive change to rural America. To meet the nation's demand for meat and processed food, giant commercial feedlots, slaughterhouses, and food processing plants are often built in rural areas. These facilities create economic opportunities, but they also expose rural residents to noxious fumes, potential health hazards, and water pollution (e.g., wastewater runoff and contamination). The negative effects of these establishments often extend beyond their operating life. When a meatpacking or food-processing plant relocates or goes out of business, a rural community can take a downturn economically as well as environmentally. This was the case when Conagra closed its plant in Garden City, Kansas [87]. In essence, once rural communities fall into the trap of urban corporate profitability, rarely can they escape negative population health consequences.

The Alarming State of Rural Poverty

In the United States, rural areas have a disproportionate share of poverty [88]. More than 386 rural counties—almost 20%—have had poverty rates of 20% or more since 1970 [89, 90]; and approximately 28% of people living in completely rural counties were also residing in persistently poor counties [91]. This is alarming because a county's economic well-being in general, and the share of its population living below the poverty threshold in particular, greatly influences its health and health care needs [92].

Poverty in rural areas is not simply a result of the lack of economic growth, income, or employment. It is also the result of inequality in the distribution of income, employment, and resources within communities and regions [93, 94]. Rural areas are often dominated by low-wage employment in agriculture, service, and manufacturing sectors. The industries that pay relatively high wages, such as mining and other resource extraction, tend to be hazardous and volatile [95]. Many other jobs are part-time and seasonal, such as in agriculture and construction. As a result, underemployment is a chronic condition for the working rural poor [88, 96, 97]. While many combine off-farm employment with farm labor to raise income, many others are still unable to earn enough to escape poverty [98–100].

Although there are compositional differences between the rural and urban poor (the rural poor are more likely to be white, elderly, or in two-parent households with at least one worker), those who are most vulnerable in the central cities—Black people, children, and those in female-headed households—are even more likely to be poor if they live in rural areas. Rural counties with large Black populations are more likely to suffer plant and employment losses

[101]. Large gaps between white and Black workers in rural areas persist in all economic sectors [102]. Southern rural Black Americans are particularly vulnerable to underemployment, with rates 39% higher than for urban Black Americans in the same region [97]. Women have limited employment opportunities, flat earnings curves, and high poverty rates in rural counties and labor market areas dominated by agriculture and mining [103, 104]. Rural child poverty rates are higher than urban child poverty rates in every racial and ethnic group; and the highest poverty rates are in the most rural places [105]. In all, 48 of the 50 counties with the highest child poverty rates are in rural America, and the gap between urban and rural child poverty has widened since the late 1990s [5, 106].

The movement of people with lower and higher incomes between rural and urban areas has historically contributed to higher rates of poverty in rural areas [13]. Since the scarcity of work and the inadequacy of wages are generally serious for young people in rural areas, poverty for young rural adults increases faster than for older workers [107]. Young adults seek every opportunity to migrate out of their own places. In many cases, they move to counties that are poorer than the counties they leave behind [108], therefore making their destination counties even poorer. At the same time, as young people migrate out, many rural areas are left with more elderly poor [109, 110].

Poverty has both behavioral and spatial components. Many recent empirical studies emphasize the maladaptive behaviors and values of the urban underclass living in poor and racially segregated neighborhoods or ethnic enclaves [13]. The extent and social implications of concentrated poverty in the United States, especially in inner-city neighborhoods of major metropolitan cities, have been well-documented [111, 112]. In contrast, America's so-called rural ghettos have received much less systematic attention than their urban counterparts [113–115]. The physical and social isolation associated with rural poverty creates problems different from those in densely settled urban areas. Due to a lack of transportation and the considerable distances to be traveled, people living in impoverished rural areas often lack access to government services and the help they need to navigate the intricacies of the social services system.

Similarly, while issues of access to quality health care are relevant in both urban and rural areas, there are important differences. In urban areas, questions of access to care often revolve around whether all segments of the population have access to the full range of specialized medical centers serving the metropolitan area. In rural areas, the issue is often whether there are any health care facilities and providers to access at all. Large metropolitan counties have nearly four times as many physicians per 100,000 residents as do rural counties with only small towns. Access to specialized medical care in rural areas is even more problematic. Small rural counties have only one-sixth as many specialists per 100,000 residents as do large metropolitan areas. The relative dearth of health care professionals and hospitals in rural areas is worsened by the distances rural residents must travel to get to them. The consequences can be particularly dire when time is critical, as with accidents involving severe trauma or life-threatening illnesses. The higher fatality rates in rural areas for infants, young adults, middle-aged adults, and victims of motor vehicle crashes are a sober reminder that where you reside sometimes determines whether you would survive after a tragic event has happened [116].

Conclusions

Rural America has been undergoing significant changes. In general, the population of rural America is shrinking relative to urban population. Young rural adults on balance favor migrating out to urban areas. In contrast, older rural adults favor staying in rural areas. Within this overall trend, however, some rural areas continue to show significant population growth. These areas generally are close to metro areas or are rich in natural and recreational amenities. They attract mostly wealthy, retiring-age populations with the potential to affect local demography, economy, culture, society, and the built environment.

Dominant secular trends, such as persistent low fertility, the aging of large baby boom cohorts, and increased longevity, have shaped age composition in both urban and rural areas in recent years, but the rural population has aged more than the metropolitan population because of aging in place and net in-migration of elderly persons. The rural elderly population still is generally poorer than the urban elderly population despite an increasing rate of elderly in-migration from urban to rural areas.

Rural America continues to be socioculturally conducive to earlier and greater childbearing in a way that is not true of metropolitan society. This is despite underrepresentation of Black and Hispanic Americans, two of the groups with the highest propensity for early childbearing, in the rural and nonmetropolitan population. Rural America also continues to be characterized by a more traditional household structure. A high proportion of rural and small-town family households contain a married couple, and a small proportion comprise single parents. Generally, elderly persons, not young adults, live alone in rural areas and small towns because of the out-migration of young adults.

Rural economies have observed significant changes during the past few decades. Agriculture has ceased to be the major component in the economies of many rural areas. Many rural areas have observed significant growth in manufacturing and service industries. The use of rural areas for recreation and retirement purposes has also increased due to an elevated importance of quality-of-life considerations in migration decisions. As a result, the rural-urban economic dependency has become stronger by the years, but at the cost of the rural counterpart. Issues of poverty, consumption, and environmental justice come up often in discussions related to rural America.

Rural and urban people living in poverty clearly have different social and demographic characteristics. People living under the poverty line in rural and nonmetropolitan areas are more likely to be elderly and white. Rural workers are often less educated and less skilled than urban workers. Therefore, they earn less and are poorer than urban workers. Even worse, rural workers generally receive lower payoff for each year of higher education than urban workers. They also receive lower wages than urban workers with jobs in the same industrial categories [1]. Unsurprisingly, in recent years rural America's poverty has become more concentrated among youth, who lack both education and skills.

Changes in rural America are having indelible effects on small-town America. With changing economies and declining populations, the older economic and social structures of small-town America are falling apart along with their facilities and infrastructure. As population declines, local institutions with traditional local jobs shut down, increasing unemployment. With increasing unemployment, social and behavioral problems such as crime, alcohol abuse, and domestic violence increase as resources to deal with these problems decrease [117]. In many small towns and cities, as traditional local jobs vanish, new jobs become available in food processing and packing plants, manufacturing and chemical plants, and construction and service industries. Oriented to national and international markets, these jobs attract immigrants to small towns and cities. Immigrants bring strong work ethic, family values, and religious beliefs. They help boost the natural increase rate of an otherwise decreasing local population. As a result, some small towns and cities experience rapid shifts in their racial, ethnic, and cultural makeup. Even though several of these shifts are usually important for small-town America, the differences in culture, language, and race that immigrants introduce are not. These differences put significant stress on already dwindling local resources.

As some towns and cities grow due to immigration, others observe a sizeable out-migration that can reduce population base to a point where public financing for essential institutions becomes difficult. This is particularly true for K-12 education and health care. As local schools lose their base of support and consolidate, many are forced to shut down. As a result, educational opportunities for children diminish; families with school-age children move out. A community cannot maintain good health when it lacks children and basic educational opportunities. Likewise, as the population decreases, local hospitals shut their doors, often putting both the health and the economy of these towns and cities in peril. Additionally, it is difficult to attract teachers and health care workers to a small town or city that has been on a path of decline for some time.

The church is another significant institution in small-town America. Many small towns usually had several churches [118, 119], but with more personal transportation, the residents of small towns and rural areas now often seek alternatives in the form of bigger, out-of-town churches. Decreasing church attendance reduces church income. Church closings and consolidations reflect further community decline in small-town America [118].

Everywhere, small towns and cities are undercut by big changes in American life—automobiles and interstate highways, supermarkets and malls, big hospitals, schools and recreational centers, the mechanization of farming, and more recently, internet—so that the prospect of a prosperous life in small towns has become almost impossible. As wages in big cities skyrocket, the small-town garage, hardware store, or general store cannot compete. Social institutions and entertainment spots, sports events, movies, and cafes start to decline because of declining profits. As population and institutions decline, many small towns and cities struggle to survive. Community functions and services come to depend on government subsidies, and so does agriculture. With government subsidies also come government regulations. The more these towns and cities come to depend on and be regulated by state or federal government, the less they need or use their local community resources. As small towns and cities turn more to sources outside their communities, the cohesion of the community becomes strained, and older and disadvantaged citizens suffer for a lack of assistance and care.

It should be noted here that population decline does not always need to be associated with business or institution decline in small-town America. To some extent, the belief that small towns are dying is based on the decline of their businesses and institutions more than the decline of their population. While it is true that the rural population in the United States is declining in relative terms, this is often not the case for many small towns and cities. Rural out-migration often contributes to the growth of population in many small towns and cities. For example, between 1950 and 1970, small towns of fewer than 2,500 people had an average decline of nearly one-third in the number of consumer business establishments with a visible negative impact on the physical fabric of towns. Yet some of these towns actually gained population during the same period [120], indicating that business and/or economic decline does not preclude population gain. This is not surprising considering that the nation's elderly population is leaving large cities for smaller, quieter places and that a significant part of the nation's population lives in one place and works, shops, or plays in another. The separations between young and old and between places of living and working have their own predicaments in terms of the physical, mental, and social health of small towns and cities, regardless of whether they have economic benefits or not.

Simply put, alongside rural America, small-town America has been undergoing drastic changes over the last several decades, with potentially significant impacts on its population health. Yet changes in individual towns and cities are not all the same, as they are not in rural areas across the country. Small towns and cities vary in terms of geographical regions, proximity to urban areas, economic opportunities, demographic trends, and many other socio-ecological factors. As a result, health concerns in these small towns and cities are likely to be different from one another.

Part II will describe small Kansas cities, focusing on their recent changes and health concerns. This description will provide the much-needed background for analytic studies and health promotion strategies presented in the latter parts of the book.

NOTES

1. Fuguitt, Brown, and Beale, *Rural and Small Town America.*
2. Suchan et al., "Population Distribution."
3. Meit et al., *The 2014 Update of the Rural-Urban Chartbook.*
4. US Census Bureau, "Nation's Urban and Rural Populations Shift."
5. Johnson, *Demographic Trends.*
6. Heaton, Lichter, and Amoateng, "The Timing of Family Formation."
7. Long and Nucci, "Accounting for Two Population Turnarounds."

8. Eberhardt et al., *Health, United States, 2001.*
9. Economic Research Service, "Rural America at a Glance."
10. Fuguitt and Heaton, "The Impact of Migration."
11. Johnson and Fuguitt, "Continuity and Change."
12. Johnson et al., *"Temporal and Spatial Variation."*
13. Lichter and Brown, "Rural America in an Urban Society."
14. Lichter, McLaughlin, and Cornwell, "Migration and the Loss of Human Resources."
15. Carr and Kefalas, *Hollowing Out the Middle.*
16. Domina, "What Clean Break?"
17. Weber et al., "Education's Effect on Poverty."
18. Salamon, *Newcomers to Old Towns.*
19. Jones, Kandel, and Parker, *Population Dynamics Are Changing the Profile.*
20. Murphy, Xu, and Kochanek, "Deaths."
21. Stanton, "The High Concentration of U.S. Health Care Expenditures."
22. National Center for Health Statistics, "Health, United States, 2012."
23. Johnson and Lichter, "Natural Increase."
24. Nelson, Lee, and Nelson, "Linking Baby Boomer and Hispanic Migration Streams."
25. Kandel and *New Patterns of Hispanic Settlement in Rural America.*
26. Lichter and Johnson, "Emerging Rural Settlement Patterns."
27. Bailey, Jensen, and Ransom, *Rural America in a Globalizing World.*
28. Farmer and Moon, "An Empirical Examination of Characteristics."
29. Chavez, "Community, Ethnicity, and Class."
30. Oropesa and Jensen, "Dominican Immigrants and Discrimination."
31. Fennelly, "Prejudice toward Immigrants in the Midwest."
32. Crowley and Lichter, "Social Disorganization in New Latino Destinations?"
33. O'Neil, "Hazelton and Beyond."
34. McConnell and Miraftab, "Sundown Town to 'Little Mexico.'"
35. Pfeffer and Parra, "Strong Ties, Weak Ties."
36. Lichter et al., "Residential Segregation in New Hispanic Destinations."
37. McMichael, "The Impact of Global Economic Practices."
38. Dimitri, Effland, and Conklin, *The 20th Century Transformation.*
39. Jackson-Smith and Jensen, "Finding Farms."
40. Johnson, "Recent Population Redistribution Trends."
41. Mayer, "Agricultural Change and Rural America."
42. Ver Ploeg et al. *Access to Affordable and Nutritious Food.*
43. Morton et al., "Solving the Problems of Iowa Food Deserts."
44. Schafft, Jensen, and Hinrichs, "Food Deserts and Overweight Schoolchildren."
45. Johnson and Cromartie, "The Rural Rebound and Its Aftermath."
46. Bolin et al., "Rural Healthy People 2020."
47. Johnson and Beale, "Nonmetro Recreation Counties."
48. McGranahan, *Natural Amenities Drive Rural Population Change.*
49. Krannich and Petrzelka, "Tourism and Natural Amenity Development."
50. Petrzelka, Krannich, and Brehm, "Identification with Resource-Based Occupations and Desire for Tourism."
51. Stedman, Goetz, and Weagraff, "Does Second Home Development Adversely Affect Rural Life?"
52. Brown and Glasgow, *Rural Retirement Migration.*
53. Johnson and Stewart, "Amenity Migration."
54. Molnar, "Climate Change and Societal Response."
55. Sorokin and Zimmerman, *Principles of Rural-Urban Sociology.*

56. Fischer, *Made in America.*
57. Albrecht, "The Industrial Transformation of Farm Communities."
58. Lobao and Meyer, "The Great Agricultural Transition."
59. Lyson, "Big Business and Community Welfare."
60. Vias, "Bigger Stores, More Stores, or No Stores."
61. Flaherty and Brown, "A Multilevel Systemic Model."
62. Smith and Krannich, "'Culture Clash' Revisited."
63. Brown, Cromartie, and Kulcsar, "Micropolitan Areas."
64. Cloke, "Conceptualizing Rurality."
65. Friedland, "The End of Rural Society."
66. Friedland, "Agriculture and Rurality."
67. W. K. Kellogg Foundation, *Perceptions of Rural America.*
68. Albrecht and Albrecht, "Metro/Nonmetro Residence."
69. Brown and Snyder, "Residential Differences."
70. Johnson et al., "Local Government Fiscal Burden."
71. Woods, "Rural Geography."
72. Clark et al., "Spatial Characteristics."
73. Brown et al., "Continuities in Size of Place Preferences."
74. Thomas and Howell, "Metropolitan Proximity."
75. Carrion-Flores and Irwin, "Determinants of Residential Land-Use Conversion."
76. White, Morzillo, and Alig, "Past and Projected Rural Land."
77. Belay, "Transmissible Spongiform Encephalopathies in Humans."
78. Bar-Massada et al., "Wildfire Risk in the Wildland-Urban Interface."
79. Goetz et al., "US Commuting Networks and Economic Growth."
80. Kurtz, "Scale Frames and Counter-Scale Frames."
81. Shriver and Webb, "Rethinking the Scope of Environmental Injustice."
82. Ruddell and Mays, *Rural Jails.*
83. Glasmeier and Farrigan, "The Economic Impacts of the Prison Development Boom."
84. Eason, "Mapping Prison Proliferation."
85. Besser and Hanson, "Development of Last Resort."
86. Hooks et al., "Revisiting the Impact of Prison Building."
87. Broadway, "Meatpacking and the Transformation of Rural Communities."
88. Tickamyer and Duncan, "Poverty and Opportunity Structure."
89. Beale, "Anatomy of Nonmetro High-Poverty Areas."
90. Farrigan, *Rural Income, Poverty, and Welfare.*
91. Jolliffe, *Rural Poverty at a Glance.*
92. National Center for Health Statistics, *Health, United States, 2011.*
93. Bluestone and Harrison, *The Deindustrialization of America.*
94. Leigh-Preston, *The Nation's Changing Earning Distribution.*
95. Tickamyer and Duncan, "Economic Activity and the Quality of Life."
96. Lichter, "Race and Underemployment."
97. Lichter, "Race, Employment Hardship, and Inequality."
98. Lyson, "Entry into Farming."
99. Molnar, *Agricultural Change,* 155–76.
100. Thompson, Yeboah, and Evans, "Determinants of Poverty among Farm Operators."
101. Colclough, "Uneven Development and Racial Composition."
102. Cho and Ogunwole, "Black Workers in Southern Rural Labor Markets."
103. Tickamyer and Bokemeier, "Sex Differences in Labor-Market Experiences."
104. Tickamyer and Tickamyer, "Gender and Poverty in Central Appalachia."
105. O'Hare and Johnson, "Child Poverty in Rural America."

106. Farrigan, "Rural Poverty and Well-Being."
107. O'Hare, *The Rise of Poverty in Rural America.*
108. Foulkes and Schafft, "The Impact of Migration on Poverty Concentrations."
109. Nord, "Poor People on the Move."
110. Slack et al., "Poverty in the Texas Borderland and Lower Mississippi Delta."
111. Massey and Denton, *American Apartheid.*
112. Quillian, "Why Is Black-White Residential Segregation So Persistent?"
113. Burton, Garrett-Peters, and Eason, "Mortality, Identity, and Mental Health."
114. Davidson, *Broken Heartland.*
115. Lobao, "Continuity and Change in Place Stratification."
116. National Center for Health Statistics, *Urban Rural Health Chart Book.*
117. Stamm, *Rural Behavioral Health Care.*
118. Berger, *The Devil Wagon in God's Country.*
119. Hollingshead, "The Life Cycle of Nebraska Rural Churches."
120. Johansen and Fuguitt, *The Changing Rural Village in America.*

STORIES OF
SMALL CITIES OF KANSAS

Small Cities of Kansas

Stories of Recent Changes

In Kansas, an area is either incorporated as a city or it is an unincorporated territory. Unincorporated areas are sometimes designated by a name, but they are not legally constituted entities and therefore have none of the legal powers to act as a properly established municipality. The state has no towns or villages. Constitutional home rule (Art. 12, § 5) [1] is the single most important source of a city's legal authority to act in the state. Home rule is a direct grant of the power of local self-government from the people of Kansas through the state constitution to each city. It gives the right to the people of every city to govern themselves by enacting and administering laws concerning local matters. Under home rule, cities have the power to initiate legislation without the need for authority granted by the state legislature. In addition, if a statute prohibits or restricts a particular activity but does not make that prohibition or restriction uniformly applicable to all cities, the city can use its home rule power to exempt itself by charter ordinance from the provisions of that statute.

Kansas state law provides for three classifications of cities in Kansas. When a city incorporates, it becomes a city of the *third class*. To be eligible for incorporation, either: (1) there must be 250 inhabitants or 250 or more platted lots, each of which is served by water and sewer lines owned by a nonprofit corporation, and 50 electors sign a petition for incorporation; or (2) the territory has been designated a national landmark by the Congress of the United States (K.S.A. 15–115, et seq.) [2]. To become a city of the *second class*, a city must have a population of more than 2,000 and fewer than 15,000. A city of more than 2,000 and fewer than 5,000 may remain a city of the third class until its population reaches 5,000 (K.S.A. 14–101) [2]. Finally, any city with a population of 15,000 or more may elect to become a city of the *first class*. When a city reaches a population of 25,000, it must certify that fact to the governor, who will then proclaim it to be a city of the first class (K.S.A. 13–101) [2].

In general, there are no special legal advantages or disadvantages for being in one class of city rather than another. This is particularly true since the adoption of constitutional home rule for all Kansas cities. Cities are incorporated as cities of the third class, and there are statutory procedures established for changing classification as the population of the city grows. Once a city has been proclaimed by the governor as a city of a certain class, there is no provision for changing the class in the event of a population loss, except in cities of the second class with a population of 1,000 or fewer (K.S.A. 14–901) [2]. Legally, there are 625 cities in Kansas. Out of these, 25 are cities of the first class; 97 are cities of the second class; and 503 are cities of the third class. Over 82.94% (2,416,195) of the state's population resides in an incorporated city. Of the total city population, approximately 68% reside in the first-class cities; 21% in the second-class cities; and 11% in the third-class cities. It should be noted here that the classification of cities based on Kansas state law is different from any other classification by the US Census Bureau, Office of Management and Budget (OMB), and the US Department of Agriculture (USDA) discussed in chapter 2. Therefore, cities defined as "small towns and cities" for the purpose of this book may include all three classes of cities defined by Kansas law.

The purpose of this chapter is to provide an account of recent economic, demographic, and environmental changes in small cities of Kansas using stories published in local and national news sources or in scholarly publications when available. Many other changes often follow or happen concurrently with economic, demographic, or environmental changes. For example, economic changes may transform, concurrently or not, employment patterns, class structure, rural-urban dependency, and the environment. Demographic changes may affect race relations, language, religion, and culture. Environmental changes and challenges may transform the livability and sustainability of a city. In a socio-ecological model of population health, none of these changes can be ignored (chapter 1). They interact in a complex manner. The complex web of these interactions determining population health cannot be easily sorted out. Therefore, this chapter does not provide a comprehensive account of all recent changes shaping small Kansas cities. Rather, it provides just enough information on recent changes to help the reader better understand the population health issues of these cities, which I describe in chapter 5.

Economic Challenges in Small Cities of Kansas

Economic challenges in small cities of Kansas are not unique. Like in many other US small towns and cities, traditional economic activities are declining in many small Kansas cities. In some of these cities, they are simply going away. In others, they are being replaced by something else as dictated by the needs of a globalized economy. Such replacements of economic activities often bring in new people and jobs, creating unavoidable tensions between the old and the new, much like in many other small cities.

Many of these recent economic trends in Kansas and elsewhere, however, are unlikely to change soon. One example is the meat industry. A few decades back, jobs in the meat industry were unionized and paid good wages, enough for a person to raise a family. Now, the meat industry is consolidated and is dominated by just a few enormous corporations that removed the unions, which clearly has long-term implications for rural labor market and economy.

Another example is the provision of commodity subsidy programs provided by the federal government. The provision has converted the previously diverse agricultural landscape of the United States to a series of large, highly industrialized farms that require far fewer workers than before. As a result, US agriculture has become less dependent on human labor. Without jobs on the farm, young people have been moving out, and poverty has set in in many places in Kansas. This, again, has long-term implications for the rural labor market and economy.

Yet another economic change came in the form of the North American Free Trade Agreement (NAFTA). The agreement devastated small farms across Mexico with American corn imports, so Mexican farmers left their country for the United States in search of farm jobs. Many instead found jobs in the meat industry of Kansas and other states. These low-paying jobs are bad, but they are better than having no jobs. More recently, NAFTA was replaced by the US-Mexico-Canada Agreement (USMCA). Only time will tell how this new agreement will affect rural economies in the United States.

Amid these persistent economic challenges, many small cities of Kansas remain resilient and continue to innovate and thrive. Some of these challenges and innovations, as reported in various news sources, are described in the following sections.

Changes in Agriculture

A common economic phenomenon impacting Kansas's small cities is changes in farming. Kansas farms are getting bigger and more technology dependent to meet the demands of a global market. The trend threatens many small cities in Kansas that were built in a different time, when larger numbers of small farmers depended on these cities for their everyday needs. These cities used to have banks, churches, grocery stores, and implement dealers. Today, they look weathered, worn, and neglected. In the 1950s, Atwood was a bustling town of about 2,000. It had well-kept shops lining Main Street, including grocery stores, car dealers, a pharmacy, and a thriving local newspaper. Since then, the town has lost nearly half its population. Most of the old businesses are gone, having taken the community's core of civic leaders with them. Several factors are responsible for the decline of the city, including consolidation in agriculture. In the 1950s and 1960s, a nearby farm would have employed many more people than it does now. Yet the same farm today is bigger and produces more grain than it did in the past by using more technology and less human labor. In the 1970s, one Kansas farmer could feed about 73 people annually. Today, one Kansas farmer feeds about twice that number of people annually [3].

In the United States, a vast consolidation of farms and changes in farming practices toward larger and less diverse farms have occurred over the past several decades. The number of farms has decreased from about 6 million to fewer than 2 million, and the average number of acres per farm has gone from 175 to close to 500. According to the USDA, as recently as 1987, midsize farms between 100 and 1,000 acres covered nearly 60% of the nation's cropland. By 2012, those midsize farms had lost about half their acreage to large farms—those with 2,000 acres or more [4]. Kansas followed a similar trend. It had 167,000 farms, with an average size of 272 acres, in 1920. In 2018, the number of farms in the state dropped to 58,900 while the average size increased to 778 acres [5].

In one example, a western Kansas farm, located just south of Dighton, covered 3,000 acres in 1973. It is now 14,000 acres, or nearly 22 square miles, and growing. According to its owner, getting bigger made him a more efficient farmer and a better steward of the land. He can afford the sophisticated equipment needed for the latest precision agriculture. He can map fields in great detail and analyze nutrient levels in different patches of soil and use satellite-guided planters and sprayers to deliver the smallest amount of seed and fertilizer to maximize crop production [3]. Critics among the farmers, however, argue that large-scale commodity farming, as described in this example, puts farmers at the mercy of markets that often fail to return break-even prices, burdens them with debt, and pollutes the environment at a faster rate.

Livestock production has also changed in Kansas, as it has elsewhere in the country. It has changed from being locally distributed on family farms to being a national operation in which feeding, processing, and packaging are done at a massive scale by large companies in different states. This takes money away from local communities while increasing their environmental problems. Since the decisions about how these facilities are operated are made by people who do not live in these communities, their decisions often lead to conflicts between the interests of the large companies and the local communities.

Decline in Economic Activities

Small-scale, family-owned commercial activities are among the ones hardest hit in small cities of Kansas. Most were dependent on small farms. Their economic base has shrunk significantly since the number of these farms has decreased. Some of them are hit even harder in small cities that are located close to big cities. To get a better deal, residents of these cities would rather drive to big cities for their commercial activities.

Independence, Kansas, has seen its economic activities waning in recent years [6]. At its peak in the early 20th century, with oil and gas money fueling prosperity, Independence was said to have many millionaires. The main business street in town, North Pennsylvania Avenue, is still lined with two-story brick buildings dating back to the early 20th century. Now, the street is a shadow of what it once was. "For rent" signs are taped to storefront after storefront. The city used to have a JCPenney department store, a furniture store, a RadioShack store, a Hallmark store, a sporting goods store, and more. They are all gone. But the biggest body blow came in 2015, when it lost the only hospital. Mercy Hospital had a shrinking patient base, but its closure became inevitable when Kansas decided not to expand Medicaid under the Affordable Care Act.

Mercy Hospital and the oil pipeline company Arco, which shut down its Independence headquarters in the 1990s, were major pillars supporting the Independence community. They sponsored events and gave money to schools and churches. The nicer houses that were built, the banks that loaned the money, and anything that worked for the good of Independence came from these two institutions. Gradually, Independence has lost its character and economic independence and has become a satellite town for other communities. Like in many other small Kansas cities, Independence's Main Street has become something like a highway ramp, where one finds hotels, fast food restaurants, agricultural implement and tool chain stores, a Walmart supercenter, a FedEx warehouse and distribution center, a metal factory, car dealerships, and convenience stores with gas.

Atchison, Kansas, is facing similar challenges. With a population of 11,000, it has some of the same challenges facing other small cities around the state and the country, but for different reasons. While most of Kansas is focused on agriculture, manufacturing has long been an economic driver in Atchison. For the last few decades, however, the city has had a hard time retaining jobs and attracting young people. Its manufacturing industry has declined significantly. Bradken Engineered Products began as the Atchison Foundry in 1872, making parts for train cars. In its heyday, the plant operated three shifts and ran 24/7. Today, there is one shift Monday through Friday. Another plant, Northwest Pipe Company, made steel pipes for oil and gas. It shut down for good in 2016 [7]. The Fargo Factory, a longtime parts supplier for Harley-Davidson, also shut down recently, putting up to 200 full-time and temporary employees out of work. The Lockwood Co. Inc. printing company and the Cash Saver grocery store were among others to close recently [8].

Factories and warehouses, if there were any, have been closing in many small cities of Kansas since the Great Recession of 2008. In Seneca, a small town north of Topeka with a population of just over 2,000 people, SKF USA shut down its factory that manufactured oil shaft seals for the industrial market, putting 170 people out of work [9]. In 2015, Amazon shuttered its 1 million-square-foot warehouse in Coffeyville, which had employed between 600 and 700 full-time workers [10]. Stories like these are common in small Kansas cities.

Negative Effects of Recent Economic Changes

When major economic activities in a small city are disrupted, closed, or added, the whole city is affected, most often negatively. For example, a factory or a warehouse may be all that a small city has as a stable source of employment. When that closes for an economic recession or a change in market demand, unemployment rises. Without employment, people feel worthless. They suffer from depression and anxiety. To get relief, some seek drugs. Consequently, a once-happy place soon becomes distressed. If a large employer manages to survive an economic recession or a change in market demand, it tends to hire temporary workers at lower wages with no benefits to cut expenses. As a result, the middle class declines and the number of people living in poverty increases in a small city.

Even when a large employer shuts down temporarily, the effects can be devastating for a small city. Recently, when a fire broke out and destroyed a part of the structure of the Tyson plant in Holcomb, ripples of uncertainty were felt not only in western Kansas but also in the cattle industry of the state and the nation. Before the fire, the Holcomb Tyson plant processed approximately 5,600 cattle per day, which represented 5% of the beef processed in the United States and nearly a quarter of beef processed in Kansas. The fire affected feedlots as well as livestock and meat supply chains. Without many trucks hauling livestock to feedlots and the plant itself, Garden City and Finney County did not have truckers fueling up their vehicles, eating in local restaurants, or staying in local hotels. The fire also affected the programs at the Garden City Community College, which held its Beef Empire Days contest at the Tyson plant. Since another plant was not found to sponsor the competition, it was canceled for only the second time in 30 years [11].

In Harper County, the city of Anthony, population 2,269, showed different kinds of negative effects due to short-lived changes in economic activities that existed for no more than five years. The community became divided over constant earthquakes from hydraulic fracturing during a short period of oil boom in the early 2010s. The oil companies employed many people in the town, so some went to great lengths to protect these companies at the displeasure of their friends, neighbors, or coworkers who were not happy with frequent earthquakes. The effects of drilling oil were not limited to earthquakes, however. Leasing land to oil companies impacted the entire community. Roads throughout the county were destroyed by oil trucks hauling heavy equipment. The people who lived on those roads were not necessarily the ones leasing land. Yet they were the ones who had to live with any negative effects [12].

Prior to the temporary oil boom, Harper County's population had been in a decade-long decline. During the oil boom, workers flocked to the area seeking high-paying jobs in nearby oil fields and wind farms. They stopped the decade-long population decline for a while but created a housing shortage in the small towns of the county, causing rent to skyrocket. Enterprising residents were renting out everything from double-wide trailers to rooms in an old bank for as much as $2,000 a month in a place where two-bedroom homes have rented for only $400 a month for years. The City of Anthony built new apartment complexes. The owners of a local motel built a new 45-room hotel to fit the overflow of guests. Local businesses that were destroyed by a 2009 fire bounced back. A new shopping center was built. Harper County even planned to transform the 101-year-old Carnegie library into an office for the workers of an oil company [13, 14].

Anthony was not the only city impacted by the short-lived oil boom of the early 2010s in Kansas. Many small cities in western Kansas counties, such as Barber, Ellis, Ness, Haskell, and Rooks, expected to turn their economies around using oil and gas revenues. In these counties, most property tax revenue had come from oil and gas for a few years at least until 2014. As oil and gas valuations dropped, jobs disappeared, workers were laid off, and many left. To put things in perspective, the Kansas oil industry was worth $5.8 billion in 2014, which supported 118,000 jobs along with $3 billion in family income. In 2015, the industry fell by nearly 50% to $2.8 billion [15]. A reduction in oil income affected everything—housing, streets, schools, hospitals, libraries, and all other city services. During the oil uptick, Barber County built a new Kiowa District Hospital, which opened in 2014. The county gave $4 million to this critical access hospital, and the community raised an additional $1.5 million through the local health foundation. The hospital also received a $3 million USDA loan. By 2016, however, officials of the county were projecting a $500,000 reduction in mill levy tax dollars. They were trying to put as much as they could in a reserve fund to prepare for the reduction [15].

Stories of Economic Successes

To survive in an increasingly harsh economic environment, many small Kansas cities have reinvented themselves, as did the city of Montezuma in Gray County. Back in 2001, Gray County was the first in Kansas to build a wind farm. For the first 10 years, Montezuma Unified School District 371 received $143,000 from the wind farm. The amount was renegotiated after 10 years, and it dropped to $103,000. In 2014, when the last three towers were added to the wind farm, the amount was renegotiated and increased to $115,000, which the school district will continue to receive if the turbines remain in operation. The fund is generally used for gifts and grants and for improvements and maintenance of the physical facilities of the school district. While the school district has been the biggest recipient, the recreation commission of Montezuma has also received some of the wind farm income [16].

Atchison, described earlier, despite having a persistent economic decline, also presents several stories of economic successes. As some industries are shutting down, others are getting better and bigger. The second-largest industry in Atchison is education. Benedictine College was started by the Benedictine order in the mid-19th century. The school struggled during the 1970s and 1980s, but aggressive marketing and a campus-wide facelift have given a new life to the college. Enrollment has tripled during the last several decades, adding revenue to the local economy [7]. Among other bright spots on the Atchison economy is MGP Ingredients. MGP was once the largest provider of industrial alcohol for fuel during World War II. The company is now well known for booze, both gin and vodka made from corn. The company also has a signature premium drink made strictly and totally from Kansas hard red winter wheat called Till American Wheat Vodka. Despite the overall sluggish economy of the city, MGP quadrupled its operating income during the last few years. Today, it employs 220 people [7].

It should also be noted that many small Kansas cities have used tax breaks and other economic incentives as tools to grow their populations. Marquette, a small city located southwest of Salina, gave away land for people to relocate and build homes in the early 2000s. The lot sizes ranged from 11,000 to 25,000 square feet. Originally, the town set aside 10 acres, divided into 70 lots, to give away for new homes. More than a decade later, the city still gets calls from people looking for free land. City leaders who designed the program believe that it saved their town. A small city of 650 people, Marquette still has grocery stores, family-owned shops, a bank, and other features characteristic a small city [17].

Demographic Challenges in Small Cities of Kansas

Population decline has been a trend in rural areas of Kansas and the Great Plains for generations. The loss of younger people constitutes a crisis in many areas. Between 2010 and 2017, rural areas of the state lost over 5% of their working-age population. It is noteworthy that many midwestern rural communities, including many in Kansas, hard hit by decades of population decline, have more young men than young women. Many young women leave rural communities for education, and for personal, social, and economic reasons they do not return home [18]. The trend negatively affects the natural growth of an already declining population.

Willowdale in Kingman County, Dubuque in Barton County, Lebanon in Smith County, Quinter in Gove County, and Windthorst (also known as Windhorst) in Ford County are among many small Kansas cities that have lost their population for similar reasons. Families had fewer children. Farms got bigger but did not need as many farmhands as when they were smaller and less mechanized. Youth moved to bigger cities in search of employment because of a lack of farm jobs in rural areas.

Built around religion and farming, Willowdale once was a thriving small community. It had a store, a church, a house for priests, a convent, a school, a blacksmith, a pool hall, an icehouse, a saloon, and a livery stable. Now, the dilapidated town has no more than a few families. It has lost everything except the church [19].

Located at the geographic center of the country, Lebanon, Kansas, attracts journalists and tourists from across the country and the world, who come to see the marker for the center of the United States. But visitors have been unable to save the falling population and economy of the city. Now, the city is trying to attract younger families with state tax incentives, student debt payment programs, and a summer celebration, known as the Lebanon Bash [20]. Similar programs exist in many other Kansas counties in an effort to stop population decline.

Quinter, Kansas, is among the small cities that have taken a comprehensive approach to combatting population decline [21]. When the 2010 US Census showed Quinter with a 4.5% population decline, the city put in place a plan for new businesses through a revolving loan fund, which was created by the sale of a factory building given to the city when the factory closed. The city also used a combination of federal, state, and regional grants to develop new civic infrastructure that promises an attractive lifestyle for new residents and workers.

With only a few exceptions, most cities in Kansas have been unable to revert depopulation trends. Those that have successfully reverted the trends did so for immigrants. In these cities, immigrants, mostly Hispanic, arrived in numbers large enough to offset or even exceed the decline in the white population. For example, in Crawford County, the Hispanic population grew by 94%, from 910 in 2000 to 1,762 in 2010. In Seward County, it grew by 37%, from 9,486 in 2000 to 12,990 in 2010. In Stevens, it grew by 57%, from 1,187 in 2000 to 1,866 in 2010. Cowley, Gray, Ford, Finney, Hamilton, Pratt, and Saline Counties observed similar growth.

In several small cities in the growing counties of Kansas, immigrants reopened closed storefronts with ethnic groceries, filled the empty schools with children, and added younger people to older communities. Examples include Dodge City in Ford County, Garden City in Finney County, and Liberal in Seward County, where meat processing and packing plants attract immigrants from Mexico, Central America, Asia, and Africa. Today, immigrants account for more than two-thirds of the total population in each of these cities. A city official in one of these small Kansas cities noted, "I think our community would be a dying community without the immigrants that have come in to fill in the gaps, and to grow business." [22]

Population increase due to immigration raises interesting issues in many small cities of Kansas, as it does in other small cities and towns around the country [23]. For example, the political and economic interests of an aging white and longtime resident population may not always align with those of immigrants, who may not have long-term attachment to place. Previous research in metropolitan communities, for example, has shown that older white residents are less likely to vote for a school bond referendum to raise property taxes if the school-aged population is disproportionately composed of minorities rather than white children [24].

The hostile political environments of the late 2010s also had significant effects on immigrants in small Kansas cities, as they did elsewhere. In interviews, Guatemalan immigrants in Kansas spoke about their fears and uncertainty surrounding their ability to stay in the United States, which could lead to indefinite separation from their families and children. One spoke of being afraid to even take out the trash and essentially remaining locked inside the house. A key effect of fear is that fewer immigrants will engage with others or social institutions, which could have intergenerational effects on their children's well-being or ability to earn an education [25].

New immigrants are often blamed for an eroding sense of community and shared values (that come from similar cultural experiences and backgrounds) in small communities [26]. It is argued that immigrants reflect the economic decisions of big multinational corporations that link these communities to the national and global economy. As a result, they replace the horizontal ties of a community with vertical ties that bind the community to the outside world [27]. Somewhat disassociated from the preexisting rural communities, therefore, new immigrants present a "symbolic threat" to cultural or national identity, as well as to traditional or nostalgic ways of life [28]. More recently, immigrants have become more than a "symbolic threat." This was exemplified by the plotting of a terrorist attack on a mosque and apartment complex in Garden City, Kansas, in 2016. It was reported, "The defendants had allegedly conducted surveillance of the housing complex, stockpiled firearms and bomb-making materials and had even written a manifesto that was to be published in conjunction with the attack" [29].

In small cities, new immigrants also raise concerns among others for crowded living conditions, occupational heterogeneity, ethnic and ancestral diversity, low educational attainment, poor health status, and fragmentation of values and behaviors [30]. In Finney County, where immigrants constitute most of the population, more than half (56%) of students qualify for free lunch in public schools, compared with 40% of students in public schools statewide. Educational attainment is significantly lower in this county than it is in the state and the nation, with racial/ethnic disparities mirroring those related to income. The county also does worse than Kansas as a whole on nearly all health indicators, especially access to health care, which coincides with the county's lower rate of health insurance coverage and shortage of primary care providers [31].

Economic threats, welfare dependence, and new taxes to build schools or hire more teachers are only a few among many concerns that breed hostile attitudes toward new immigrants [32]. Too often, politicians play on people's fears, especially during economic downturns. Even though immigrants in the country, legally or illegally, are less likely to be convicted of a crime than native-born residents and are not correlated with increased violent crime rates, many politicians, including some in Kansas, have made repeated false claims that undocumented immigrants are more prone to committing violent crimes to stoke fear in people.

As a result, during the past few years, many new local anti-immigrant city ordinances have been introduced to discourage unauthorized workers from settling in Kansas and elsewhere [33]. Anti-immigrant ordinances come in many forms. Some impose additional regulations on dayworker agencies, penalize employers who hire unauthorized immigrants, or require that all municipal business be conducted in English only. Other local ordinances restrict landlords from knowingly (or even unknowingly) renting to unauthorized immigrants, which can lead to racial profiling and housing discrimination based on race or ethnicity [34]. Of course, rhetoric on immigration is cheap, but laws can be very expensive. Localities that started testing these anti-immigration laws often find that they cost too much money to defend. By the time the courts hand down a decision, the laws themselves end up being toothless.

Environmental Pollution

Environmental pollution in small cities of Kansas tends to be less related to poor air quality due to ozone, sulfur dioxide, nitrogen oxide, and particulate matters—unless the area in question is close to a major metropolitan area. Instead, environmental pollution in these small cities is generally related to heavy use of fertilizers, herbicides, and pesticides in large-scale farming and industrialized livestock operations. In some cases, it is also related to environmentally insensitive mining and other extraction operations that have decreased significantly over the last several decades.

Chemical Pollution

With industrialized agriculture, the use of fertilizers, herbicides, and pesticides has increased significantly among farmers in the Midwest, a 12-state territory that includes Illinois, Indiana, Iowa, Kansas, Missouri, Nebraska, and North Dakota. Nationwide, the use of glyphosate, a weed killer, on crops has increased from 13.9 million pounds in 1992 to 287 million pounds in 2016, according to estimates by the US Geological Survey. About 65% of that was used on crops in the Midwest. Upward of 95% of corn and soybeans, which are among the major crops in the region, are treated with herbicides. In 2017, about 459 million acres of US agricultural land were also treated with some kind of pesticide [35].

Though the effects of fertilizers, pesticides, and herbicides on the population of small cities in Kansas are less known, environmental damages done by these chemicals are well known. Water pollution caused by high levels of nitrates from excess fertilizers is a problem in many rural areas. The High Plains aquifer, which provides drinking water and water for irrigating farm crops, shows many hot spots with high levels of nitrates. Nitrates can cause serious health problems among pregnant women, young children, and older adults. Many farmers are unable to grow specialty crops because of the damage caused by weed killer. In one of many similar lawsuits, a specialty producer sued and won against the agribusiness giants Monsanto and BASF for causing extensive damage to its orchard by weed killers [36].

With a billion pounds of chemicals applied to crops every year, stories about crop dusters accidentally spraying people are quite common in small midwestern cities. Also common is unlawful drifting of chemicals beyond their intended targets to human settlements [37]. Nine US states, including California, mandate buffer zones for certain pesticides near schools and waterways. In much of the Midwest, state-mandated buffer zones do not exist.

Every state has a designated lead pesticide agency responsible for enforcing federal and state regulations. Some of them keep track of misuse incidents, such as unlawful applications or products drifting beyond their intended targets. But these agencies do not necessarily distinguish between accidents involving human exposure and those that affect crops, trees, and other plants [35].

Pollution from Industrialized Livestock Operations

In Kansas alone, about 2.4 million cattle can be found in feedlots on any given day. At the Finney County Feedyard near Garden City, some 34,000 cattle fill pens lined with concrete feed bunks [38]. Industrialized livestock operations such as this are a significant source of pollutants, including hydrogen sulfide, methane, ammonia, and odoriferous vapors that result from animal husbandry activities and manure storage and handling. Ammonia, for example, can foul air quality and can contribute to potentially deadly respiratory diseases. It can also contribute to greenhouse effects. Ammonia-heavy water runoff from cattle operations can contribute to the nitrogen overload in lakes and rivers that triggers algae blooms. Those, in turn, can suck oxygen from waterways and create dead zones.

An emerging problem related to livestock operation is the contamination of water supplies with the growth-promoting agents used for raising livestock, which include nontherapeutic antibiotics—those used for purposes other than treating disease [4]. Antibiotics have been used in livestock feed since the 1940s, when studies showed that the drugs cause animals to grow faster and put on weight more efficiently. By killing off the bacteria in the animals' guts, the antibiotics make more of the energy in the food available for the animals themselves [39]. Because of this growth advantage, nontherapeutic antibiotics were routinely given to livestock, poultry, and fish on industrial farms [40]. While antibiotic misuse in medicine is subject to serious public scrutiny, antibiotic abuse in agriculture is both more widespread and subject to far less oversight. According to the Food and Drug Administration, more than 20 million pounds of antibiotics (or about 80% of all antibiotics) were sold for use on livestock farms in 2014 [41].

Disease-causing bacteria are more likely to develop in industrial livestock facilities than in small or backyard livestock farms because of cramped conditions, poor sanitation, and antibiotic overuse [42]. These bacteria can infect people through animals, food, the environment, and other people, both on and off the farm. Regulations for safer work conditions or worker exposure in concentrated animal feeding operations (CAFOs) are generally absent in the United States. CAFOs provide many opportunities for worker and community infection. Increased bacterial and viral pathogen exposure and infections have been reported among farmers, their families, and farmworkers at industrial poultry and swine operations as compared to control populations [42]. Workers at these facilities often (unknowingly) carry antibiotic-resistant bacteria into the general public. As one example, Methicillin-resistant Staphylococcus aureus (MRSA), a now-common staph bacteria resistant to many antibiotics, has been found to persist in the nasal passages of workers at industrial hog operations, even following extended periods away from these facilities [43].

Manure is another way both antibiotics and antibiotic-resistant bacteria enter the environment, contaminating drinking wells and endangering the health of people living close to large livestock facilities [42]. Industrial livestock operations produce a tremendous amount of animal waste: 369 million tons in 2012, almost 13 times more than that produced by the US human population. While human waste is treated at municipal treatment plants or by other means, there are very few regulations for animal waste and disposal, and no specific requirements for the treatment of animal waste [42, 44]. Most waste from CAFOs is stored in ponds (called lagoons) and ultimately applied untreated as fertilizer to farm fields. Bacteria can survive in untreated and land-disposed farm animal waste for two to twelve months. It is estimated that animals do not digest approximately three-quarters of the actual antibiotics, which then also necessarily pass from the animals into the environment, where they speed up the evolution of drug-resistant bacteria in soil and water [45]. Manure lagoons can also overflow or fail during natural disasters, like they did during Hurricane Florence in 2018, which adds an additional threat to health and safety when and where clean water and medical access are already limited [46].

Bacteria are also present in the air, where they travel with dust particles and water droplets. CAFOs are dusty places, and numerous studies have found high levels of antibiotics and antibiotic-resistant bacteria in air samples downwind of feedlots in dry regions. These airborne bacteria can be very persistent in the environment—E. coli in dust from industrial livestock barns can survive for more than 20 years [43, 47–49]. Flies and other insects that thrive around CAFOs can also carry disease off the farm and into communities [50, 51].

Pollution from Mining and Oilfields

Examples of small cities affected by mining operations that continued into the latter half of the 20th century include Baxter Springs, Galena, and Treece in Cherokee County, Kansas. Today, sites around these areas are covered with mine waste, water-filled subsidence craters, and open mineshafts. Founded around a mining operation, Treece served as a major supplier of lead, zinc, and iron ore for decades. The economy of this once-thriving city collapsed when the mining reserves dried up, but toxic waste left behind continued to make people sick. Most residents left Treece in 2012 as part of a government-funded relocation program after the Environmental Protection Agency (EPA) named it one of the most environmentally devastated places in the country. Where churches, a city hall, and small businesses once stood, torn-up roads and murky, orange waters remain.

Fracking, although it has subsided significantly in Kansas during the last four or five years, has been a more recent environmental concern for small cities in rural Kansas. Hydraulic fracturing is a method of enhancing oil and gas recovery from wells by injecting water, sand, and chemicals into rock formations under very high pressure to fracture the rock and release trapped hydrocarbons. As of May 2017, there were only 1,039 horizontal wells that were hydraulically fractured in Kansas, which is only a fraction of what the state used to have [52].

The impact of fracking on air quality is difficult to calculate. As with any type of energy production operation, however, the process of fracking can produce air pollutants at varying levels depending on the level of operations in a particular area. Air pollution sources during fracking can include road and pipeline construction, well drilling and completion, and natural gas processing, transportation, and storage. The main pollutants released during the fracking process include volatile organic compounds (VOCs), nitrogen oxides, sulfur dioxide, and particulate matter. VOCs react with nitrogen oxides to produce ground-level ozone, also known as smog. Though not conclusive, the EPA's 2016 study on hydraulic fracturing indicated that, in some circumstances, poorly constructed drilling wells and incorrect wastewater management also affected drinking water resources, particularly near drilling sites [53].

Another environmental problem related to fracking has been induced seismicity, which refers to seismic events that occur at higher-than-normal rates due to human activities. Earthquakes began occurring more frequently in southern Kansas and Oklahoma in 2013 after an increase of hydraulic fracturing. However, in 2016, the US Geological Survey found that oilfield wastewater disposal, rather than fracking, was the main cause of an increase in earthquakes throughout the central United States from 2009 to 2013. Nevertheless, the Kansas Corporation Commission (KCC) found that increased seismic activity due to fracking is an immediate danger to public health, safety, and welfare. In the two years since the KCC issued its first order limiting salt-water injections mostly in Harper and Sumner Counties, seismic activity has dropped from 1,967 earthquakes between March 2015 and August 2015 to 668 earthquakes between September 2016 and February 2017, a reduction of 66%. In 2021, it has further restricted the amount of oilfield wastewater that can be injected underground in Kingman, Sedgwick, and Barber Counties in southern Kansas to further reduce earthquakes in the region [54].

Conclusions

Small cities in Kansas are not all the same. Cities like Treece are almost deserted due to environmental pollution from mining industries that built the city. Cities like Willowdale were built on religious faith and agriculture but are dying due to changing agriculture, out migration, and shrinking family size. Against all odds, cities like Abilene, Anthony, Atwood, Cawker City, Independence, and Lebanon keep their hopes alive as new people and businesses continue to come for various perks and incentives. Small cities like Atchison, Baldwin, Montezuma, and Tribune are redefining themselves while holding on to their culture and tradition. Atchison has long been known for manufacturing and education; after a period of economic decline, it is reinventing its industrial and educational establishments. Montezuma is redefining itself as one of many small Kansas cities where wind farms are a new source of energy and economy. Some small cities like Dodge City, Garden City, and Liberal have completely reinvented themselves. Today, these cities thrive on large meatpacking plants powered by immigrant labor.

Despite differences, most small Kansas cities are facing economic, population, or environmental challenges. What happens to a small city in Kansas as it continues to lose population? Without doubt, the loss indicates an economic decline and a lack of employment opportunities. As unemployment rises, will there be more depression and anxiety and consequently higher drug addiction and suicide rates in the city? As younger residents move out, older population increases in the city. Will there be higher rates of mortality and morbidity, or will there be more socially isolated people in the city?

When the economy of a city declines, demographic shifts are only one of many challenges it faces. As a city becomes poorer, it is unable to provide essential services to its populations, which may include healthy food, health care services, and educational and recreational facilities. The city is also unable to maintain its streets and parks, to provide enough housing, and to ensure public safety. Will this result in decreased physical activity, increased obesity and chronic diseases, and higher rates of crime and social isolation in the city?

The good news is that population is not decreasing in every small city of Kansas. Several of these small cities are observing a rise in population due to immigration. What effects do immigrants have on the population health of a city? Does crime go up in cities with more immigrants, as some would like us to believe? Do immigrants cause anxiety and depression among residents? Do immigrants increase the burden of disease of a city? Do they overburden the health care system of a city?

Then, there are the population health effects of environmental pollution. Chemical pollution from fertilizers, herbicides, and pesticides; pollution from industrialized livestock operations; and pollution from mining operations are different. There is no doubt that these sources of environmental pollution negatively affect population health. Do we know enough about their effects on the population of small cities in Kansas?

There are no easy answers to these or many other questions because the relationships between economic, demographic, or environmental factors and health are not straightforward. To find the answers, we must first learn more about population health in small cities of Kansas. Chapter 5, therefore, will present the population health problems of small cities in Kansas. Chapters 8 through 11 will explore how these health problems may be associated with the spatial and geographical characteristics of these cities. These exploratory studies may not answer how the economic, demographic, and environmental problems discussed in this chapter affect the population health of small Kansas cities. Their findings should, however, provide some indications regarding how we can minimize population health problems in small cities through design and planning.

NOTES

1. State of Kansas. "Constitution of the State of Kansas."
2. Kansas Office of Revisor of Statutes. "Kansas Statutes."
3. McLean, "'Get Big Or Get Out.'"
4. Institute of Medicine, *Rebuilding the Unity of Health and the Environment.*
5. National Agricultural Statistics Service, "Kansas Farm Facts."
6. Block, "Despite Economic Troubles."
7. Ziegler, "Atchison, Kansas, Residents."
8. Clem, "Fargo Factory to Shut Down."
9. Chilson, "'A Huge Blow.'"
10. Greene, "Amid Rapid Expansion."

11. Boyer, "Tyson Plant Fire."
12. Dowd, "Fracking Divides Small Town."
13. Ellis, "Where Trailer Homes Rent for $2,000 a Month."
14. Ellis, "Oil Boom Strikes Kansas."
15. Bickel, "Downward Flow's Ripples."
16. Hanks, "Montezuma."
17. Sharp, "Land Giveaway Helps Keep Marquette Vibrant."
18. Reed, "Young Men Increasingly Outnumber Young Women."
19. Bickel, "Faith Still Strong in Ghost Town of Willowdale."
20. Newill, "For This Kansas Town."
21. Dreiling, "Small Town Works Together."
22. Morris, "A Thriving Rural Town's Winning Formula Faces New Threats."
23. Lichter, "Immigration and the New Racial Diversity."
24. Poterba, "Demographic Structure and the Political Economy of Public Education."
25. Diepenbrock, "Political Climate Spurs Kansas Immigarants to Fear Interactions."
26. Crowley and Lichter, "Social Disorganization in New Latino Destinations?"
27. Popke, "Latino Migration and Neoliberalism in the US South."
28. Fennelly, "Prejudice toward Immigrants in the Midwest."
29. Rott, "3 Men Charged with Plotting Attack."
30. Lichter and Brown, "Rural America in an Urban Society."
31. Robert Wood Johnson Foundation. "Finney County, Kansas."
32. Massey, *New Faces in New Places*.
33. Valverde, "Is Illegal Immigration a Problem in Kansas?"
34. Mexican American Legal Defense and Educational Fund. "Immigrants' Rights."
35. Mayer, "Across Midwest Farm Fields."
36. Ruff, "Monsanto, BASF Will Pay $250 Million."
37. Beck, "Wind-Blown Pesticides an Issue in Courtrooms, Communities."
38. Boyer, "Why the Cattle Industry Might Not Use a Drug That Cuts the Pollution."
39. Dibner and Richards, "Antibiotic Growth Promoters in Agriculture."
40. National Hog Farmer, "FDA Announces Implementation of GFI #213."
41. FoodPrint, "Antibiotics in Our Food System."
42. Graham et al., "The Animal-Human Interface and Infectious Disease."
43. Nadimpalli et al., "Persistence of Livestock-Associated Antibiotic-Resistant Staphylococcus aureus."
44. Link, "What's Wrong with Factory Farming?"
45. Chee-Sanford et al., "Fate and Transport of Antibiotic Residues and Antibiotic Resistance Genes."
46. Biesecker and Robertson, "Hurricane Florence Breaches Manure Lagoon."
47. McEachran et al., "Antibiotics, Bacteria, and Antibiotic Resistance Genes."
48. Ahmad et al., "Insects in Confined Swine Operations."
49. Schulz et al., "Antimicrobial-Resistant Escherichia coli Survived in Dust Samples."
50. Zurek and Ghosh, "Insects Represent a Link."
51. Graham et al., "Antibiotic Resistant Enterococci and Staphylococci Isolated."
52. Suchy and Newell, "Hydraulic Fracturing of Oil and Gas Wells in Kansas."
53. US Environmental Protection Agency, *Hydraulic Fracturing for Oil and Gas.*
54. Hoffman, *Commission Staff's Report.*

CHAPTER FIVE

Health in Small Cities of Kansas

Stories of Recent Concerns

The state of Kansas faces many health challenges, which have been amply reported in the literature, and some were briefly mentioned in the preface. According to America's Health Rankings [1], a joint effort by the United Health Foundation and the American Public Health Association, among all the US states, Kansas has seen the greatest decline in its health rankings over the past 30 years. According to the same source [2], in 2020 Kansas ranked:

- 40th for *public health funding* in the *community and family safety* category;
- 40th for *food insecurity* in the *economic resources* category;
- 35th for *physical environment*, which includes *air and water quality, climate change*, and *housing and transit*;
- 47th for *driving alone to work* in the *housing and transit* category, which is a significant risk factor for many chronic diseases;
- 28th for *clinical care*, which includes *access to care, preventative clinical services*, and *quality of care*;
- 36th for *dental care and mental care providers* in the *access to care* category;
- 26th for *behaviors*, which include *insufficient sleep, nutrition and physical activity, sexual health*, and *tobacco use*;
- 38th for *exercise* in the *nutrition and physical activity* category;
- 26th for *health outcomes*, which include *behavioral health, mortality*, and *physical health*; and
- 39th for *risk factors*, such as *high blood pressure, high cholesterol*, and *obesity* in the *physical health* category.

In fact, it is hard to find a population health category where Kansas does better than at least 50% of US states. The status of population health in small cities of Kansas is likely to be similar, but we cannot say that with certainty because nothing has been reported on this topic.

The purpose of this chapter, therefore, is to provide an account of population health in small cities of Kansas. It considers only a few factors and indicators of population health, which often show direct or indirect associations with the built environment in reported studies. Interestingly, these are also the factors and indicators for which Kansas ranks poorly. They include *obesity*, which is an important health risk factor, and *diabetes*, which is a common chronic disease. Both obesity and diabetes are common in rural areas, and they have been related to physical activity or lack thereof, which can be affected by where people live. These factors also include *depression, anxiety, substance abuse, social isolation*, and *suicide*, which can also be affected by the quality of a place. *Crimes* are included because they do not show similar patterns in urban and rural areas. Crimes that are prevalent in urban areas are not always prevalent in rural areas. *Diet and food environment* are included because unhealthy dietary habits and food deserts are prevalent in rural areas. *Physical activity* is included because it is affected by the built environment in different ways. *Challenges facing rural health care systems* are included because they show many problems in rural areas. *Health disparities* are included because population health seems to vary based on socioeconomic and demographic factors within and between places. Notably, *environmental pollution* is not included in the account of population health in small cities of Kansas. A serious threat in many small cities, environmental pollution rarely originates within a small city and often requires regional interventions.

Population Health Challenges

The population health of small cities in Kansas is rarely discussed in scholarly publications. Its coverage in local new sources is inconsistent at best. These sources cover some population health concerns, such as obesity and diabetes, more frequently than others. These local news sources also cover crime, drug use, and addiction as crimes more than as population and public health concerns. In the absence of reliable sources, this chapter uses a mixture of sources—local news, gray literature (e.g., reports, theses, dissertations, official documents, informal communication, research in progress, clinical trials, etc.), and some scholarly publications—for the description of population health in small Kansas cities.

Obesity

Obesity is an important health risk factor and morbidity indicator. It poses serious threats to the population health of rural America. Rural residents have higher rates of chronic diseases compared to their urban counterparts, and obesity may be a major contributor to this disparity. According to a 2012 national study of over 8,800 Americans that used body mass index based on measured height and weight [3], rural populations are more likely to be obese compared to those living in cities; and rural residence is associated with higher obesity prevalence above and beyond the effects of age, education, income, race/ethnicity, marital status, and diet and physical activity. According to the same study [3], the differences between rural and urban populations are most pronounced for younger adults between the ages of 20 and 39. Younger adults in rural areas may be more susceptible to weight gain due to many changes that have occurred over the last several decades. Rural residents traditionally have consumed high-fat, high-calorie diets that were offset to some extent by high-caloric expenditure during vigorous physical labor necessary for farming, logging, and other activities [4, 5]. Increased mechanization of rural occupations, however, has reduced their caloric expenditure. As a result, obesity has increased, impacting younger working adults the most.

Except for 2016, obesity has been rising in Kansas since 1995. In 1995, the adult obesity rate in Kansas was 13.3%. In 2018, that rate was 34.4%. According to the 2018 Kansas Behavioral Risk Factor Surveillance System (BRFSS) report [6], higher percentages of obesity in adults were seen among African Americans (41.5%), middle-aged adults (40.7% for adults between 45 and 54 years old), adults with income less than $15,000 (41.7%), adults with a high school diploma, a GED, or some college education (37.3%), adults with co-morbid conditions—asthma (43.5%), diabetes (57.5%) and arthritis (46.3%)— and adults living with a disability (44.7%).

Obesity specific to isolated small cities in Kansas has not been reported in the literature at an aggregate level. Therefore, it is hard to say how prevalent it is in these cities compared to in rural and urban areas of the state. These small cities often have many risk factors for obesity. Most are located far away from major urban centers. Residents often drive alone and for longer to their everyday destinations, which are risk factors for obesity. They generally lack access to healthy food, recreational facilities, and well-managed parks. In the absence of public transit, they depend on cars even for shorter trips. Residents of these cities are older, are socially isolated, and have comorbidity contributing to obesity.

Diabetes

Diabetes can be related to obesity, lack of access to healthy food, and physical inactivity. Diabetes has a significant impact on health, with high rates of associated morbidity and mortality [7, 8]. More specifically, it has been linked to many serious health complications, including cardiovascular disease, stroke, high blood pressure, blindness, kidney failure, neuropathy, and amputations [9]. Diabetes is the 7th leading cause of death in both the United States and Kansas according to death certificate data, which is likely to be an underrepresentation of the true incidence of diabetes-related deaths [10]. A comparison between states reveals that Kansas ranks 22nd in the total number of diagnosed cases of diabetes mellitus [9, 11].

In 2018, approximately 9.7% of Kansas adults reported having ever been diagnosed with prediabetes. That's more than 187,000 Kansans [10]. In Kansas, approximately 15.2% of adults with an average annual household income of less than $25,000 per year have diabetes, as compared to 8.9% in households earning more than $25,000 per year [10]. The incidence of diabetes is higher in people without a college degree at 12.3%, compared to those with a college degree at 9.4% [10]. Data of age-adjusted prevalence of diabetes indicate that the number of diagnosed cases are highest among Hispanics (16.7%), followed by non-Hispanic African Americans (15.3%), other/multi-race residents (10.1%), and non-Hispanic white Americans (8.6%) [10]. A comparison of diabetes prevalence by demographic location in Kansas reveals some minor differences between urban (10.1%) and rural populations (11.6%) [10].

In the United States, the total estimated cost of diagnosed diabetes in 2017 was $327 billion, including $237 billion in direct medical costs and $90 billion in reduced productivity [12]. After adjusting for inflation, economic costs of diabetes increased by 26% from 2012 to 2017 due to the increased prevalence of diabetes and the increased cost per person with diabetes. The growth in diabetes prevalence and medical costs occurred primarily among the population aged 65 years and older, contributing to a growing economic cost to the Medicare program [12]. The treatment of diabetes in Kansas costs an estimated $2.4 billion in both direct and indirect costs [10]. More than 5,000 hospital admissions were due to diabetes in Kansas in 2017 [10]. KanCare, Kansas's managed care program, spent $570 million on patients with diabetes in 2018 [10].

Diabetes cannot be treated in isolation. It requires a multifaceted approach that includes teams of physicians, nurse practitioners, physician assistants, nurses, diabetes educators, and registered dieticians along with fitness facilities, weight loss organizations, local agricultural resources, community leaders, local and state government representatives, and validated online tools and resources to help patients understand the disease and develop skills to promote overall health. Since small cities and rural areas lack most of these resources, the impact of diabetes on health is likely to be more severe than in urban areas. However, events to raise diabetes awareness remain commonplace in small Kansas cities [13–15].

Social Isolation

Social isolation is defined both subjectively, based on how people perceive their experience and whether they feel isolated, and objectively, based on quantifiable measurements, such as the size of one's social network or the frequency of engagement with it. Often, the objective components are referred to as "social isolation," while the subjective are called "loneliness" [16–18]. Therefore, they are related, but distinct, constructs. The relationship between social isolation (the experience of diminished social connectedness) and health status and all-cause mortality among older adults is well established [17, 19–21]. Similarly, there is strong evidence of the importance of social connectedness to overall quality of life [19, 22].

Having a married or partnered status, talking with family and friends about important things, visiting with family or friends, attending church service, and participating in a club are indicators of a lack of social isolation. Using these indicators, a 2017 study found that 21.9% of US adults 65 years and older are socially isolated [23]. The percentage is likely to be much higher in the isolated cities of rural areas with low population density, poor transportation, and fewer community services. A 2005 study in Alabama found that 22.1% of older adult Black women did not have reliable transportation, while only 3.2% of older adult white men reported not having reliable transportation [24]. Living in a rural, unsafe, or inaccessible location; living in a home that is inadequate for the person's needs (e.g., not accessible or with a high risk for a fall); and lack of access to affordable transportation could decrease both opportunities and capacity to engage in socially connecting activities [25–27].

Social isolation is more than just a common complaint of rural life. It can often be at the root of a host of social and health problems. One newspaper article published a story of three Catholic nuns, who converted a storefront in Concordia, Kansas, into a drop-in center for poor young mothers living in isolated areas to find support and resources. In this town of 5,000, about two dozen women, from a range of backgrounds, now come through the center each day. Since then, the idea has spread to other rural parts of Kansas. Recently, a new drop-in center opened in Abilene [28].

Day services for adults unable to be alone during the day are available in many small Kansas cities. Kansas Care Planning Council's website lists as many as 21 adult day services in 12 of the state's 105 counties [29]. Most of the state's rural counties, therefore, are not listed on the website. One wonders if these counties have adult day services at all. If not, how do these rural counties deal with social isolation among adults without day services?

Depression and Anxiety

Kansas recognizes mental health as one of the major public health concerns and as one of the 10 leading health indicators to monitor population health. Depression and anxiety are considered leading mental health disorders. They are associated with increased risk of morbidity, mortality, and poor quality of life. According to the 2018 Kansas BRFSS Report [6], about 1 in 3 (36.8%) adults aged 18 years and older with symptoms of depression over a period of two weeks or longer in the past 12 months received any treatment. About 1 in 7 females had ever been diagnosed with anxiety as compared to 1 in 12 males. The prevalence of ever receiving a diagnosis of anxiety was higher among adults who had lower annual household income (<$15,000) and were unable to work as compared to adults who had higher annual household income (≥$50,000) and were employed. The prevalence of ever receiving a diagnosis of anxiety was also high among adults who were divorced or separated and who were never married as compared to adults who were married.

Higher prevalence of ever being diagnosed with anxiety was also seen among current smokers, people with chronic disease such as asthma and coronary heart disease, and people who suffered stroke. About 1 in 4 adults who rated their health as fair or poor had ever been diagnosed with anxiety as compared to 1 in 11 who rated their health as excellent, very good, or good. One in 5 adults who needed to see a doctor in the past 12 months but did not because of the cost reported having anxiety. Diagnosis of anxiety was also higher among adults living with disability as compared to adults living without disability.

Mental health disparities exist in Kansas with respect to various socio-demographic subgroups and subgroups with chronic diseases and disability. A need for public and population health strategies to address mental health conditions among Kansas adults is strong. In this regard, the built environment of a city can be important. It can affect social isolation, which in turn can affect mental health. It can also affect how physically active people are, which in turn can affect physical and mental health and well-being. The availability of nature in and around a place for pleasure and recreational activities can reduce stress and anxiety among its inhabitants.

Substance Use and Abuse

Substance use and abuse are often related to illegal activities and can have physical, mental, and social health consequences, including increased crime and violence, vehicular crashes caused by driving while intoxicated, transmission of infectious diseases, fetal alcohol syndrome, risky sexual behavior, homelessness, and increased unemployment.

Drug poisoning remains a significant cause of injury deaths in Kansas. From 2012 to 2016, 1,583 drug poisoning deaths were reported in Kansas, and almost 85% of these deaths involved a specific pharmaceutical opioid [30]. Overdose deaths due to fentanyl and carfentanil, which are several hundred times more powerful than heroin, occur often in rural and small-city Kansas communities.

According to the Kansas Hospital Association, opioid-related emergency and inpatient visits are rising steadily in Kansas. From 2009 to 2018, the number of opioid-related emergency room (ER) visits increased by 0.1% of all ER visits; and the number of opioid-related discharges increased by 0.5% of all discharges [31]. Likewise, the percentage of hospital discharges related to drug poisoning has significantly increased for several Kansas counties, including Wyandotte (20%), Shawnee (46%), Dickinson (49%), Jackson (50%), Osage (64%), and Jefferson (82%), in 2010–2014 compared to 2005–2009 [32].

In many small Kansas cities, substance use is widespread, and overdose is commonplace. The effects of substance use are worsened by several unique challenges in these communities. Behavioral health and detoxification (detox) services may not be readily available in these communities, and their range of services may be limited. Patients who require treatment for substance use disorder may need to travel long distances to access services. First responders and hospital ER staff in small cities may have limited experience in providing care to a patient presenting with drug overdose. Law enforcement and prevention programs may be sparsely distributed or understaffed. Patients requiring substance use disorder treatment may be hesitant to pursue treatment because of privacy issues associated with smaller communities.

While unemployment, poverty, chronic diseases, disability, low educational attainment, social isolation, and a lack of mental health care are among the primary reasons for addiction, sometimes geographical location can help explain why addiction is more prevalent in some places than others in Kansas. Many of the state's meth lab incidents, which include lab, dump site, and other material seizures, are found in cities close to Oklahoma and Missouri in southeast Kansas. They include Caney, Coffeyville, and Dearing in Montgomery County; Independence in Doniphan County; Parsons in Labette County; and Cherokee and Pittsburg in Crawford County [33]. The locations of these cities allow people dealing with addiction to move from one state to another for ingredients or to escape the law easily.

Suicide

Suicide is a serious personal and public health problem that has far-reaching medical, economic, and psychosocial implications for Kansans [34]. According to the Kansas Violent Death Reporting System, there were 2,055 violent deaths among Kansas residents from 2015 to 2017. About three-quarters (73.9%) of these cases were suicide deaths (n=1,518) [35]. From 2015 to 2017, Kansas resident suicides cost an estimated $2.24 billion (2017 US dollars) in medical expenses and work loss and 46,837 years of potential life lost (YPLL) for people under age 75 [35]. The rate of suicide in Kansas increased from 12.02 per 100,000 persons in 1999 to 18.60 per 100,000 persons in 2018 [34]. The 2018 suicide rate was the highest in the last 20 years and is higher than the national rate (14.20 per 100,000 persons) [35]. In 2018, suicide was the ninth leading cause of death among all ages and the second leading cause of death following unintentional injuries for those age 15–34 years in Kansas [36].

In Kansas "frontier" counties—places with fewer than 6 people per square mile—about 26 out of every 100,000 people commit suicide per year. In 2020, Kansas had 556 suicides at a rate of 19.25 per 100,000 people, and the state ranked 13th in the country. The number of suicides in northwest Kansas has increased by more than 50% in recent years. Twenty counties in the region saw suicides climb by 57% from 2014 through 2018. That jump comes in a part of the state where people already commit suicide at a higher rate than in the rest of Kansas [37].

According to the Kansas Department of Health and Environment (KDHE), growing isolation, greater economic pressures, and increased untreated mental illnesses may be among the reasons why suicides are increasing in the state. Statistically, the use of alcohol or other substances can increase suicide risk, as can chronic physical illness or pain and mental illness. Easy access to firearms and opioids also adds to the chances of suicide. Suicide risk is highest when people feel like they are a burden on others, feel outcast or isolated from others, and have ready access to lethal means. Though the Centers for Disease Control and Prevention (CDC) retracted a report in 2018 suggesting suicide is higher among farmers than any other occupation, it still concludes that farmers suffer a higher suicide rate than most workers [38]. Given that the suicide rate is high in Kansas and in its counties, the rate is likely to be high in its small cities as well.

Crime

In the Federal Bureau of Investigation (FBI) Uniform Crime Reporting (UCR) Program [39], violent crimes are defined as those offenses that involve force or threat of force. They include four offenses: murder and nonnegligent manslaughter, rape, robbery, and aggravated assault. According to the same source, property crimes include the offenses of burglary, larceny-theft, motor vehicle theft, and arson. Arson is included in this category because it involves the destruction of property; however, arson victims may be subjected to force. Because of limited participation and varying collection procedures by local law enforcement agencies, only limited data are available for arson. Therefore, arson statistics are not included in any estimated volume data throughout the FBI's UCR website.

According to the UCR [39], in 2018, Kansas had an estimated 439 violent crimes per 100,000 inhabitants, whereas the United States as a whole had an estimated 368.9 violent crimes per 100,000 inhabitants. In 2018, Kansas had an estimated 2,634 property crimes per 100,000 inhabitants, whereas the United States had an estimated 2,200 property crimes per 100,000 inhabitants. According to the website SafeWise [40], although Kansans are less concerned about crime, the state sees the second-highest crime rates in the midwestern region behind only Missouri. In 2020, Kansas was ranked 40th among all states for violent crimes by United Health Foundation's America's Health Rankings [2].

The UCR [39] also reports that both violent and property crime rates seem to decrease as the rurality of a region increases in Kansas. The estimated violent crimes per 100,000 people in metropolitan statistical areas, cities outside metropolitan areas, and nonmetropolitan counties are 501, 343, and 224, respectively. Likewise, the estimated property crimes per 100,000 people in metropolitan statistical areas, cities outside metropolitan areas, and nonmetropolitan counties are 2,894, 2,580, and 1,098, respectively. According to SafeWise

[40], 18 out of the 20 safest cities in Kansas have fewer than 49,999 people. Conversely, many small cities are also among the most dangerous cities in Kansas, including Independence, Arkansas City, Coffeyville, Salina, Junction City, Iola, and Augusta [40].

Social science literature provides many clues as to how and why crimes or social pathologies may be different in small cities and rural areas than in urban areas. They include differences in pecuniary benefits [41]; chances of being reported, recognized, and arrested [41]; numbers of female-headed households [42]; population density [43]; population growth and migration leading to differences in racial and ethnic diversity [42, 44]; and differences in the proportion of younger people [42].

The literature reports many findings on how and why the built environment may affect crime in urban areas: In mixed-use urban locations, it is easier for offenders to remain anonymous [45]. Mixed-use communities exhibit weaker social cohesion and higher crime rates [46]. Single-use residential environments show lower rates of crime than areas with mixed uses [47, 48]. Proximity to a range of mixed land uses generates crime [49]. Increased densities are associated with higher rates of violent crime and social pathologies [50–52]. Larger numbers of onlookers ("eyes on the street") are linked with less intervention in a crime situation [53]. Most of these findings, however, are not related to small cities in the United States and elsewhere.

Challenges Related to Diet and Food Environment

There are many challenges related to diet and food environment in the rural areas and small cities of Kansas. In these areas, access to healthy food is decreasing due to changes in agriculture. As farms in Kansas become bigger, they focus more on national and international markets and less on local markets. Crops that can be produced easily in this and other midwestern states for national and international markets are wheat, corn, soybeans, milo, and hay. As a result, many rural and small-city residents in Kansas may not get enough locally grown fresh produce.

An added challenge is that traditional diet in rural areas of the state and the region contains significantly high fat [3]. This creates population health problems as large-scale agriculture takes over. On today's mechanized farms, people do not do as much manual labor as they did on their small farms before mechanization took over. As a result, rural populations are not burning the fat they consume, creating an obesity epidemic.

Along with a lack of fresh produce and unhealthy diet, food insecurity remains a significant problem in Kansas's rural areas and small cities. According to Feeding America's Map the Meal Gap, in 2019, approximately 1 in 8 Kansans, or 351,090 people (12.1% of total population), struggled to have enough food, and 41% of Kansans were living below the Supplemental Nutrition Assistance Program (SNAP) threshold of 130% poverty [54]. According to the 2015 Food Access Research Atlas of the United States Department of Agriculture (USDA) [55], 498,144 Kansans (17.46% of the total population) do not have access to healthy food sources, such as grocery stores, within a reasonable distance from their home. This distance is 1 mile for urban areas and 10 miles for rural areas.

The declining number of local grocery stores is notable because it affects both the food and community environments in rural and small-town Kansas. These small grocery stores are no match for big-box grocery stores and are closing at an alarming rate. In Iowa, for example, 43% of grocery stores in towns with populations under 1,000 have closed, while in Kansas, nearly one in five rural grocery stores has gone out of business since 2006. Local grocery stores' decline creates a crisis because they represent a critical piece of community infrastructure [56, 57].

Local grocery stores are a vital source for nutrition and health, providing a supply of fresh fruits, vegetables, dairy, and protein. With no grocery store, many rural and small-town residents might be living in what is known as a food desert. Residents in these food-deprived rural areas struggle simply to find healthy and nutritious food for their families and themselves. In "severe" food desert counties, residents must drive more than 10 miles to a grocery store. Approximately 40% of Kansas counties are severe food desert counties [55].

Local grocery stores are a part of the economic engine that sustains rural and small-town communities. They are a significant source of local taxes, powering the creation and maintenance of civic services and amenities. They provide essential, stable jobs—butchers, cashiers, managers, and stockers. Dollars spent at a local, independently owned grocery store cycle through the local economy more than dollars spent at an out-of-town big-box market.

Local grocery stores are also important vehicles for community development. They serve as gathering places, where residents see one another and talk about the latest issues affecting their towns. Just like local schools, cafes, and post offices, rural grocery stores are important community assets, providing tangible evidence of local strength and stability.

Declining rural and small-town population, increasing competition from

larger chain stores, changing shopping patterns, and changing food distribution models are among many trends that hurt rural and small-town grocery
stores' chances to remain profitable in states like Kansas. To understand the
significant challenges local grocery stores face, Kansas State University and
the Kansas Sampler Foundation—a Kansas nonprofit dedicated to preserving
rural Kansas—conducted a study involving local grocery stores in rural areas
that used a mail-in survey, a summit, and in-depth interviews [56]. The study
identified many challenges facing the local grocery store owners, including
competition with big-box grocery stores; high maintenance, insurance, and
shipping costs relative to revenue; a lack of reliable workers and resources to
follow federal and state regulations governing alcohol sales, food handling,
SNAP and SNAP for Women, Infants, and Children (WIC) participation,
proper labeling, and workers' compensation; a lack of local demand and community support; and a low purchase volume that does not justify the service
of wholesale distributors.

Despite the many challenges facing local grocery stores, the significance of
these stores does not go unnoticed by small-town residents. For example, a
proposed Walmart Express in Baldwin City faced strong opposition from
local residents. Although much smaller than traditional Walmart stores, the
proposed project would have offered general merchandise, a pharmacy, fuel
pumps, and a grocery with dairy, meat, and produce sections. About 1,000 of
the city's 5,000 residents signed a petition against the project. They believed
that the new store would threaten the survival of the city's existing grocery
store, pharmacies, convenience stores, and hardware store. In the end, Walmart withdrew the proposal [58, 59].

Challenges Related to Physical Activity

Many Kansas residents do not get the recommended amount of physical activity. According to the 2018 Kansas BRFSS report [6], approximately 22.5%
of Kansas adults ages 18 years and older did not participate in leisure-time
physical activity in the past 30 days. Even higher percentages were seen among
females (24.7%), non-Hispanic African Americans (25.8%), older adults (26.7%
for adults between 55 and 65 years old), Hispanics (27.2%), uninsured adults
(30.5%), adults with lower annual household income (37.4% for adults with
less than $15,000 income), and adults with less education (38.7% for adults
with less than high school education). Many adults with comorbid conditions
also do not get the recommended amount of physical activities, including
those with asthma (27.3%), obesity (29.1%), arthritis (32.5%), adults living with

disabilities (39.7%), and diabetes (39.9%). According to KDHE, only 16.5% of Kansas adults met both aerobic and strengthening exercise guidelines in 2011. In 2020, only 20.8% met the guidelines [1].

Physical activity is important because physically active people tend to live longer and have a lower risk of chronic health conditions, including but not limited to obesity, diabetes, heart disease, depression, and some cancers. In contrast, inactive adults are more likely to be obese and have a higher risk of living unhealthy lives. Due to economic constraints, many small cities do not have sidewalks, walking and biking paths, or well-kept parks to encourage recreational physical activities among residents. Small-city residents do not always have access to health care support and resources to help them maintain a healthy and active lifestyle. Their physical isolation also poses a barrier to healthy living [3]. Physical isolation makes it difficult for them to get to a gym in another location if there is no gym in their own city.

Physical activity for health improvement is being considered by many small cities in Kansas. Many, including Abilene, Iola, and Greensburg [60], provide bike share programs to promote active lifestyles. Park City, Kansas, used a grant from the Wichita Area Metropolitan Planning Organization for the Planning Walkable Places Program [61]. To improve physical activity among its residents, Coffeyville, a small southeast Kansas community, used funding from a federal program designed to revitalize disadvantaged neighborhoods [62]. Volunteers built a foot trail at Douglas County State Lake (also known as Douglas State Fishing Lake, or simply Douglas Lake) providing recreational opportunities for the Baldwin City community [63]. In partnership with the CDC, the Association of American Indian Physicians, and the Sunflower Foundation, the Kickapoo tribe built a walking trail on its reservation near Horton [64]. In a survey regarding future development in the city, Bel Aire residents prioritized street development projects. In contrast, they were generally against any sort of commercial development in downtown [65]. Though these and other spatial design and planning strategies to promote active living are commonly found in small Kansas cities, their effectiveness remains unknown due to a lack of studies.

Challenges Facing Rural Health Care Systems

According to a report by the American Hospital Association, rural health care systems face a mixture of *long-term problems*, such as staff shortages and aging infrastructure; *more recent problems*, such as rising drug costs and federal regulation changes; and *emerging problems*, such as the opioid crisis and cyber threats [66]. Beginning in 2020, the COVID-19 pandemic created additional problems, including costs of pandemic-related preparations and uninsured patients seeking hospital care and loss of income for postponed non-emergency procedures. Taken together, these problems have created a perfect storm that threatens the survival of many critical community health care facilities.

Small rural hospitals always have higher risks of going out of business because they have fewer patients, have fewer revenue streams, and serve populations that are older, sicker, and either underinsured or uninsured. Medicare introduced critical access hospitals in 1997 to help preserve access to health care in rural areas [67]. By federal law, critical access hospitals cannot have more than 25 beds, must offer around-the-clock emergency room services, and must not keep patients more than four days. These hospitals used to receive 101% of their Medicare-allowable costs from Medicare. Now, they receive 99% of their allowable costs, which still is generous compared to what hospitals can collect from patients—largely the working poor—who have no insurance at all.

Since 2005, as many as 180 rural US hospitals have closed, according to the North Carolina Rural Health Research Program [68]. Out of these, 136 closures occurred since 2010; 97 were completely closed; and 83 were converted closures—facilities that no longer provide inpatient care but continue to provide some health care services, including primary care, emergency care, and skilled nursing care. The US Government Accountability Office (GAO) report found that states that had expanded Medicaid had fewer hospital closures [cited in 68].

Kansas is one of the 14 states that have not expanded Medicaid under the Affordable Care Act. So, in Kansas, critical access hospitals do not receive the cost-based Medicare reimbursements they need. Eight of the 180 closures were in Kansas, which took away 243 hospital beds. After closures, there are still at least 84 critical access hospitals in Kansas. Critical access hospitals are not just providers of medicine and health care but also are often major employers and a massive part of a town's tax base. Without them, many Kansans would have to travel long distances for care. It would help if Kansas would expand Medicaid eligibility, as envisioned in the Affordable Care Act. Despite an aggressive lobbying campaign by hospitals, Kansas has not taken that step. Nearly 1 in 6 rural hospitals in Kansas has some of the same financial characteristics as those that have already closed and would be considered at-risk. That means as many as 15 Kansas hospitals could be struggling to keep their doors open.

Small-town residents know the importance of their hospitals and are often willing to pay higher taxes to support them. But as rural populations decline and tax bases shrink, resident support might not be enough to save many financially stressed hospitals and health care facilities across the state [69]. When asked, 65% of the farmers and ranchers of Sedgwick County, Kansas, responded that the cost of health care was the single greatest threat to their operations and was most likely to force them out of business. In this county, the cost of purchasing individual coverage has led many farm families to take town jobs just to secure health insurance and has prevented young adults from coming back to their families' operations. In the face of increasing health insurance costs, many of the county's farmers and ranchers have chosen to remain uninsured, putting their health and businesses at incredible risk [70].

Health Disparities

Vast health disparities exist among cities and counties of Kansas. The disparities are most apparent in two neighboring Kansas counties: Johnson and Wyandotte. These are not rural counties but are useful examples to illustrate that even the more urbanized counties in the state have serious health disparities. According to county health rankings by the University of Wisconsin Population Health Institute [71], the two counties' relative health rankings have remained essentially unchanged over the last several years, with Johnson County at or near the top and Wyandotte County—along with the state's southeastern counties—at or near the bottom among all of the state's counties. In 2021, Wyandotte County ranked 104th and Johnson County 1st for *health outcomes, health factors, quality of life, health behaviors*, and *social and economic factors* among Kansas's 105 counties (table 5.1). Wyandotte County performed worse than Johnson County for all but two important measures: *percent of adult residents who drive alone to work* and *percent of adult residents with long commutes who drive alone* (table 5.2).

Wealth and poverty may help explain health disparities between the two counties. An immense body of research shows that social determinants—including economic factors—have a much greater impact on health than medical interventions. Generally, people with more wealth are better educated and thus better informed about health. Wealthier people also have better access to health care. In contrast, it is hard for people with less wealth to be healthy

TABLE 5.1.
Health rankings for Johnson and Wyandotte Counties, Kansas

	Johnson	Wyandotte
Health outcomes	1	104
Health factors	1	104
Length of life	1	90
Quality of life	1	104
Health behaviors	1	104
Clinical care	1	91
Social and economic factors	1	104
Physical environment	56	94

Source: 2021 County Health Rankings, University of Wisconsin Population Health Institute

without education, access to health care, and amenities that promote health. As a result, wealthier people have higher life expectancies and lower morbidity than poorer people.

Johnson County is the most affluent county in the state, with a median household income of $73,733, according to the 2010 Census. (In fact, out of 3,143 counties in the entire country, Johnson County is the 81st richest.) Wyandotte County, on the other hand, is the 8th poorest of Kansas's 105 counties. Its median household income of $38,503 is about half that of Johnson County. When compared with Johnson County, Wyandotte County has more unemployment, more children in poverty, fewer residents with high school and college diplomas, and more severe housing problems (table 5.2). It is true that there are pockets of poverty in Johnson County, but Wyandotte County has generational poverty, where generations of families have been living in poverty. Of course, the county averages and aggregates do not account for the differences among different population subgroups within each county. For example, the figures for African Americans and some Hispanics in Johnson County are quite like what one would see in the counties with the lowest average incomes in Kansas [71].

Initiatives to Identify Health Priorities

A survey conducted by the Healthy Kansans 2020 initiative of about 1,700 health professionals, KDHE partners, legislators, and other interested parties found 12 areas of health improvement in Kansas: lifestyle behaviors such as smoking, nutrition, and physical activity; chronic diseases; access to health services; social determinants of health; environmental health; mental health;

TABLE 5.2.
Measures for different health outcomes and factors
for Johnson and Wyandotte Counties, Kansas

	Johnson	Wyandotte	Kansas
Years of potential life lost rate[1]	4,424	**9,684**	7,079
Fair or poor health	11%	**26%**	16%
Average number of physically unhealthy days	2.7	**5.1**	3.6
Average number of mentally unhealthy days	3.5	**5.1**	4.1
Smokers	13%	**23%**	18%
Adults with obesity	26%	**40%**	33%
Food environment index[2]	8.8	**6.5**	6.7
Physically inactive	17%	**33%**	24%
With access to exercise opportunities	95%	**90%**	80%
Uninsured below age 65	7%	**16%**	10%
Primary care physicians rate[1]	124	**46**	78
Primary care physicians ratio	810:1	**2,175:1**	1,278:1
Dentists rate[1]	87	**41**	60
Dentists ratio	1,154:1	**2,469:1**	1,661:1
Mental health providers[1]	242	**161**	205
Mental health providers ratio	414:1	**622:1**	489:1
Preventable hospitalization rate[3]	3,790	**5,862**	3,959
Completed high school	96%	**79%**	91%
Some college	84%	**51%**	70%
Unemployed	2.8%	**4.3%**	3.2%
Children in poverty	6%	**31%**	14%
Income ratio[4]	3.9	**4.4**	4.3
Children in single-parent households	16%	**32%**	21%
Social association rate[1]	8.6	**10.0**	13.6
Violent crime rate[1]	157	**704**	365
Injury death rate[1]	51	**81**	76
Average daily PM2.5[5]	6.9	**8.5**	6.7
Severe housing problems	11%	**19%**	13%
Drive alone to work	**85%**	82%	82%
Long commute—drive alone	**24%**	23%	21%

Source: 2021 County Health Rankings, University of Wisconsin Population Health Institute
Note: Bold numbers indicate which of the two counties has the worst result for each of the health outcomes and factors.
1. Per 100,000 population
2. 0 is worst; 10 is best
3. Per 100,000 Medicare enrollees
4. Ratio of household income at the 80th percentile to income at the 20th percentile
5. Fine particulate matter of 2.5 microns or less in diameter; higher levels are more harmful for health

maternal, infant, and child health; violence prevention; oral health; disabilities; injuries; and immunizations and infectious diseases [72]. Though not included in the areas needing improvement, many rural areas and small cities are hit hard by the increase of older and sicker patients, the lack of Medicaid expansion, and the decline of Medicare reimbursements. A recent report from Trust for America's Health and the Robert Wood Johnson Foundation finds Kansas in the bottom half in federal and state allocations in disease prevention and public health [73].

Like the state, many Kansas counties and cities face similar health challenges. In their study involving more than 1,500 residents, the Lawrence-Douglas County Health Department identified 13 areas of health improvement [74]:

1. *Inadequate access to affordable nutritious foods.* Residents listed transportation as being a barrier. Eighty-one percent of residents reported consuming fewer than five servings of fruits and vegetables daily. Other problems related to healthy food include that some cities did not have a farmers' market; that some neighborhoods lacked grocery stores and/or restaurants that offer healthy foods; and that food pantries in many places lacked healthy offerings.

2. *Inadequate access to dental services.* In this county, one in five residents did not see a dentist in the past 12 months. In 2011, there were more than 470 cases of preventable emergency room visits to local hospitals for dental problems. Some cities also did not provide dental services based on a sliding-income scale, creating additional burden for low-income population.

3. *Inadequate access to general health care services.* In this county, 35% of adults did not have a general checkup in the past year, and 20% did not identify a primary care physician.

4. *Poverty and few job opportunities.* Between 20 and 30% of the county's population lived in poverty. The rate exceeded the state average.

5. *Limited access to safe and affordable housing.* The study estimated that 13% of homes in the county had an increased risk of lead exposure.

6. *Abuse of alcohol.* In the county, 14% of youth and 10% of adults had engaged in binge drinking in the past 30 days. More than 250 cases of preventable ER visits in 2011 were due to excessive alcohol use.

7. *Lack of access to health insurance coverage.* Nearly 15% of the county's residents did not have health coverage.

8. *Disparities in health care outcomes and quality of life.* There were schools

where 10% of students qualified for free and reduced lunch and others
where 75% of children qualified. One resident commented, "Health depends on who you are and where you live."

9. *Inadequate access to mental health services.* About one-third of residents
   reported having one or more days in the past 30 days in which their
   mental health was not good.
10. *Limited knowledge of available health and other services.* Residents of
    several cities in the county noted a lack of venues for events, activities,
    and services.
11. *Lack of physical activity.* More than 50% of residents did not meet rec-
    ommendations for weekly exercise. Many residents noted a lack of side-
    walks and recreational facilities.
12. *Inadequate transportation linking people to services, jobs, and recre-
    ation.* Inadequate transportation was a prominent theme among many
    residents. They noted that the implications are widespread, including
    limiting employment opportunities and ability to access services and
    recreation facilities.
13. *Prevalence of abuse and intimate partner violence.* Intimate partner vio-
    lence and bullying were top concerns for many residents. In 2010, there
    were 7.2 cases of domestic violence per 1,000 people reported in the
    county.

Notably, the study found that most emergency room visits for dental, asthma,
diabetes, and alcohol treatment came from areas associated with poor housing and poverty.

Conclusions

Small cities in Kansas have many population health challenges, including
poor diet and lifestyle behaviors, diabetes, obesity, depression and anxiety,
drug abuse, crime, and suicide. They exist due to food deserts or areas with
limited availability of healthy food and food outlets, limited opportunities for
physical activities, extreme social isolation, limited access to health care, and
limited resources to ensure a safe and healthy environment to live, work, and
recreate.

Due to a shift in agriculture from small farms to large farms, employment
opportunities on local farms have diminished in several small Kansas cities.
Since local businesses were organized around communities of small farmers
and farm workers, they are also going out of business. As local job markets

shrink, residents of these cities are forced to find jobs elsewhere. They drive alone and for longer to their jobs. It is necessary to know if these trips contribute to obesity, diabetes, and other chronic diseases in small Kansas cities.

Access to healthy foods has diminished in many rural areas of Kansas in the recent years due to increasing monocrop agriculture. Many small cities have turned into food deserts. Fresh food, when available, is more expensive in local stores than it is in chain stores many miles away. Limited access to healthy food promotes cooking at home, but rural cooking generally contains more fat and is less healthy. Due to a lack of local grocery stores and food outlets, transit time of food and "food miles" has increased. Therefore, it is also necessary to know if a lack of grocery stores contributes to obesity, diabetes, and other chronic diseases in these cities.

Depression and anxiety are common among those without jobs. Chronic depression and anxiety often lead to addiction and suicide among socially isolated residents of economically depressed small cities. One wonders if similar mechanisms could help explain addiction and suicide in small cities of Kansas.

Limited availability and access to community gyms or exercise facilities, sidewalks, walking and biking paths, and well-kept parks may be among other reasons why population health is poor, but we do not know that yet. Health care providers can help individuals lead healthy lives and can engage community members to help establish programs and provisions for walking, biking, or exercise, but there is a chronic shortage of health care providers in many small Kansas cities. Many local hospitals are closing because of changes in medical treatments, the increased number of uninsured patients, and a lack of Medicare and Medicaid benefits in the state. Such closures are often harmful not only to the local economy but also to the population health of a small city.

Clearly, there are many population health problems in small Kansas cities. There are also many place-based differences in population health problems. Based on the evidence from two neighboring counties—Johnson and Wyandotte—presented in this chapter, similar place-based differences among small cities in Kansas should not be surprising.

This book's studies exploring the relationship between the built environment and population health are needed to understand how best to use spatial design and planning as a tool to promote population health in small cities of Kansas based on their challenges and differences. These studies provide much-needed evidence on effective spatial design and planning strategies concerning some of the population health priorities already identified through local initiatives. Even though spatial design and planning strategies may not solve the more persistent economic, demographic, and environmental challenges of these small cities described in chapter 4, they may at least help us rethink and redesign the built environment of a city, which is yet another source of persistent challenges affecting the population health of a city. Before presenting the studies exploring the relationships between the built environment and population health in small cities of Kansas, chapter 6 presents the approaches and methods of these studies, and chapter 7 presents the sample of cities selected for these studies using spatial, lifestyle, and health data collected from various publicly available sources.

NOTES

1. United Health Foundation, *America's Health Rankings: Annual Report 2020.*
2. United Health Foundation. "America's Health Rankings Analysis of America's Health Rankings Composite Measure."
3. Befort, Nazir, and Perri, "Prevalence of Obesity."
4. Flora, Flora, and Gasteyer, *Rural Communities.*
5. Pearson and Lewis, "Rural Epidemiology."
6. Kansas Behavioral Risk Factor Surveillance System, *Health Risk Behaviors of Kansans 2018.*
7. Schwasinger-Schmidt et al., "The State of Diabetes in Kansas."
8. Fowler, "Microvascular and Macrovascular Complications of Diabetes."
9. Centers for Disease Control and Prevention, *National Diabetes Statistics Report.*
10. Bureau of Health Promotion, "Diabetes Control and Prevention."
11. Ablah et al., "Prevalence of Diabetes and Pre-Diabetes in Kansas."
12. American Diabetes Association, "Economic Costs of Diabetes in the U.S. in 2017."
13. News Staff, "Community Health Fair Set."
14. Heilman, "Medical Center Marks Diabetes Month."
15. News Staff, "'Biggest Loser' Father and Son."
16. Steiner et al., *Disrupting Disparities in Kansas.*
17. Steptoe et al., "Social Isolation, Loneliness, and All-Cause Mortality."
18. Courtin and Knapp, "Social Isolation, Loneliness and Health in Old Age."
19. Holt-Lunstad, Smith, and Layton, "Social Relationships and Mortality Risk."
20. Holt-Lunstad et al., "Loneliness and Social Isolation as Risk Factors for Mortality."
21. Taylor, "Social Isolation's Influence on Loneliness."
22. Ashida and Heaney, "Differential Associations of Social Support and Social Connectedness."
23. Pohl et al., "Measuring Social Isolation."
24. Locher et al., "Social Isolation, Support, and Capital and Nutritional Risk."
25. Elder and Retrum, *Framework for Isolation in Adults over 50.*
26. Smith, "Portraits of Loneliness."
27. Cornwell, "Social Resources and Disordered Living Conditions."
28. Thompson, "Rural Drop-In Centers."

29. Kansas Care Planning Council, "Kansas Adult Day Services."
30. Kansas Injury and Violence Prevention Program, *Kansas Trends in Drug Poisoning Deaths.*
31. Kansas Hospital Association, "Opioid Crisis."
32. Kansas Hospital Association, "All Drugs-Related Poisoning Hospital Discharges by County."
33. Hittle, "Losing the Meth War."
34 Kansas Prevention Collaborative, *Kansas Suicide Prevention Plan.*
35. Kansas Violent Death Reporting System, *2015–2017 Death Circumstances Data.*
36. Kansas Information for Communities, "2013–2017 Vital Statistics Data."
37. Kansas Violent Death Reporting System, *Suicide Statistics in Kansas (2015–2017).*
38. Centers for Disease Control and Prevention, "Suicide Increasing among American Workers."
39. Federal Bureau of Investigation, "Crime in the U.S."
40. McEntire, "Kansas's 20 Safest Cities of 2021."
41. Glaeser and Sacerdote, "Why Is There More Crime in Cities?"
42. Ladbrook, "Why Are Crime Rates Higher in Urban than in Rural Areas?"
43. Danzinger, "Explaining Urban Crime Rates."
44. Miethe, Hughes, and McDowall, "Social Change and Crime Rates."
45. Stark, "Deviant Places."
46. Goldsmith et al., *Analyzing Crime Patterns.*
47. Greenberg, Rohe, and Williams, "Safety in Urban Neighborhoods."
48. Greenberg and Rohe, "Neighborhood Design and Crime."
49. Buck, Hakim, and Spiegel, "Endogenous Crime Victimization."
50. Cozens, "Crime and Community Safety."
51. Calhoun, "Population Density and Social Pathology."
52. Dye, "Population Density and Social Pathology."
53. Banyard, "Measurement and Correlates of Prosocial Bystander Behavior."
54. Feeding America, "Food Insecurity in Kansas."
55. Economic Research Service, "Food Access Research Atlas."
56. Kansas State University, "Rural Grocery Initiative."
57. Procter, "The Rural Grocery Crisis."
58. Jones, "Top-Five Stories of Baldwin City for 2014."
59. Jones, "Walmart Withdraws Plans for Store."
60. Thrive Allen County, "Thrive's Innovative Approach to Rural Bike Share."
61. Messick, "Park City Hoping to Improve Sidewalks."
62. Thompson, "Coffeyville Trail Project Gets Boost."
63. Jones, "Volunteers See Community Benefits."
64. Kansas Health Institute, "Kickapoo in a Race to Stem the Tide of Diabetes."
65. Messick, "Bel Aire Residents Want Good Roadways."
66. American Hospital Association, *Rural Report 2020.*
67. Medicare Learning Network, *Critical Access Hospital.*
68. Cecil G. Sheps Center for Health Services Research, "Rural Hospital Closures."
69. Thompson, "Kansas Rural Hospitals Struggle to Stay Afloat."
70. Seiler, "Farmers Struggle with Health Care."
71. University of Wisconsin Population Health Institute, *2021 County Health Rankings Key Findings Report.*
72. Cauthon, "Health Improvement Initiative Launched."
73. Trust for America's Health, "A Funding Crisis for Public Health and Safety."
74. Britt, "New Health Assessment Identifies 13 Challenges."

PART THREE

APPROACHES, METHODS, AND STUDY SAMPLE

Approaches and Methods

How to Study Spatial Associations of Population Health in Small-Town America

As a field of study, public health has its foundation in infectious disease epidemiology and control. Therefore, it is not surprising that urban health has been at the forefront of research in public health. After all, urban areas were and, in many cases, still are the places where infectious diseases spread more easily due to high population density and poor environmental and sanitary conditions. Over the last several decades, however, public health concerns have grown beyond infectious diseases to include mortality, morbidity, chronic diseases, obesity, lifestyle, mental health, and social health. Population health as an area of study recognizes these growing concerns, but the focus has not changed significantly from urban areas to include less urbanized and rural areas.

Given the history of the field of study, it is not surprising that the population health of rural and small-town America has not been studied as much as the population health of urban America [1]. Although limited in volume and scope, the recent population health literature does agree that rural and small-town America have unique qualities that ultimately result in persistent health disparities between rural and urban groups and between rural subgroups. Much of this literature, however, assumes that findings in urban areas are usable in rural areas and in small towns and cities. This is simply not the case.

As small but somewhat urbanized units of sociological significance, small towns and cities are different from urban, suburban, and rural areas, and they are different from one another [2]. They vary in distance from large metropolitan areas. They vary significantly in terms of their built, social, and natural environments. Unlike large metropolitan areas, small towns and cities often have singular functional concentrations, such as recreational, educational, health care, manufacturing and food processing, or military functions. These differences can combine to affect population health differently in small towns and cities. Attention needs to be given to scale- and place-specific differences to prevent unintended consequences of "one-size-fits-all" approaches to population health in small-town America.

Highlighting the significance of scale- and place-specific features in population health, studies have consistently found significant differences in the associations between spatial design and planning factors and population health outcomes for urban and rural areas. For example, studies have found that the association between perceived residential density with recreational walking is positive at lower values of perceived density, which may be found in small towns; but the same association is negative at higher values of perceived density, which may be found in urban areas [3]. Studies have also found that the associations between built environment features and population health in urban areas are different from the relatively compact small towns in rural areas [4–6]. Additionally, studies have found that processes for spatial planning and design related to population health may differ in urban areas, suburban areas, small towns, and rural areas [7]. (More examples of these studies can be found in chapters 8–11.)

Therefore, using the socio-ecological perspective described in chapter 1, this chapter describes the methodology of research used in the analytic studies of the book (chapters 8–11). In describing the methodology, first, an individual-level study is distinguished from an area-level study in population health, emphasizing that the scale- and place-specific features of population health are more readily considered in the latter than the former. Second, using the pathways for spatial factors to influence health presented in chapter 1, the pathways of influence explored in the book's studies are identified. Third, different spatial, lifestyle, and health data used in the analytic studies of the book are identified. Finally, the methods of analysis used in the book's analytic studies are briefly described.

Individual- and Area-Level Studies in Population Health

According to the socio-ecological approach presented in chapter 1 and in the literature [e.g., 8, 9], the built environment is only one of several environments affecting population health. Still, it can have remarkably broad effects on population health. At the individual level, it can affect health through living and working conditions and through lifestyle. At the neighborhood level, it can affect health through the availability of local amenities and healthy food, through safe and equitable environments, and through social integration and support. At the community and regional levels, it can affect health through city size and density, through road network and accessibility, and through the quality of air, water, and soil [10]. Also, according to the socio-ecological approach, health care services are only one of many categories of intervening factors that can affect the associations between spatial factors and population health. Examples of other important categories of intervening factors include people's attitudes and preferences, social and cultural norms, rurality or urbanicity of a place, demography, and socioeconomic status.

For the socio-ecological approach, it is important to note that many studies on the relationships between built environments and population health raise concerns because they commonly use individual-level data to show how differences in individual features (e.g., supermarkets, sidewalks, parks, etc.) influence individual health and health-related decisions. In many cases, therefore, it is not known whether any individual-level influences scale up to the neighborhood or community level or whether a city or a city area as an environmental type or as a settlement unit influences population health differently from those reported at the individual level. This is important because, due to many unknown and unrecognized interactions, the aggregate effect of the built environment on population health can be different from the effects of individual features on individual health.

For the socio-ecological approach, it is also important to note that any individual-level health and environmental data are rarely complete due to the sheer number of individuals to be considered in a study. For example, it is difficult to collect the lifestyle and health data of every individual within a population, and it is even more difficult to associate every piece of individual health data with individual environmental features. With big data analytics, this may become possible in the future, but the validity of these tools will still depend on smaller samples that humans can inspect and verify. Until validated tools for big data analytics are available, it is important to find an unbiased way to select some parts of a population and some features of the built environment for population health studies. Yet when a study is focused on some environmental features instead of others or on some parts of a population instead of others, the complementary as well as the contradictory effects of different parts in relation to one another remain unexplored.

For the socio-ecological approach, an area-level study involving aggregate data of many areas may be appropriate. Such a study may help describe population health differences based on differences among areas rather than based on differences among individuals within an area. Findings of such area-level studies, for example, may support the idea that the abundance of food outlets that generally provide healthy diet not only influences obesity at the individual level but also at the scale of broad urban areas. Such a relationship may exist due to greater provision and availability of food with varying nutritional quality within an area that people can access on a regular basis [11], or it may exist due to varying demand for types of food among adults living in different areas within a city [12]. Whichever the case may be, an area-level study may provide us a perspective of population health that we may not get from an individual-level study.

A focus on the area-level study may also facilitate a systematic comparison of the effects of the built environment on population health by directing our attention to the overall features of an area as an environment type (e.g., a residential neighborhood, a campus, or a business district) or a settlement unit (e.g., a rural, an urban, or a suburban area). Systematic comparison, in turn, may facilitate hypothesis testing and strengthen scientific studies on the role of different areas representing different environment types or settlement units in defining population health. For example, it may help us identify a functional threshold for some features, such that areas above the threshold are significantly more likely to experience beneficial population health outcomes than those below the threshold. Put simply, it may help us define, build, and support "good" cities and city areas to enhance population health.

In presenting area-level studies on the relationships between built environment and population health, this book is guided by two generic principles. First, the studies remain focused on the effects of small towns and cities as an area representing a very specific place, context, or settlement type with distinct physical, social, and cultural realities. Though not exhaustive in its scope and approach, the book includes factors as varied as the size and type of these areas, their distance from large urban areas, their street networks and land use patterns, their key facilities, and their population health described using lifestyle, morbidity and mortality, and physical, mental, and social health. Second, through emphasis on the area as the unit of analysis, I hope to reinforce that important factors of health-related behaviors and health are defined by relationships that tie individuals not only to other individuals but also to organizations, neighborhoods, and communities within a given place or locality [13].

A Review of Area-Level Studies in Population Health

Area-level population health studies are not new. In the United Kingdom, the Black Report of 1980 was a significant landmark concerning area-level population health studies. By integrating socioeconomic status, health inequalities, and premature deaths with census-level data, the report helped scholars understand the significance of the neighborhood-level determinants of health [14–16]. Since then, the importance of area-level studies has continued to grow, with an increasing consensus among epidemiologists that risk factors can operate at area levels and that there is a need to assess cumulative area-level factors [17–20].

Today, there are numerous area-level population health studies covering many topics [21–30]. Briggs and Leonard [21] observed a significant association between mortality differentials and place-based socioeconomic disadvantages. Fox and Goldblatt [22] reported significant variations in mortality across 36 types of places defined based on regional and local geographies. Wing et al. [29] reported a lower population-weighted and age-adjusted rate of ischemic heart disease mortality for communities with higher fractions of white-collar employment for both men and women. Britton et al. [24] reported significant differences in mortality among 30 socio-residential clusters based on housing tenure and social class. Eames et al. [25] reported higher mortality from all causes, coronary heart diseases, and smoking-related diseases with increasing area-level deprivation. Raleigh and Kiri [27] reported lower longevity and higher gender differentiation with increasing area-level deprivation. Morris et al. [26] reported area-level educational attainment and deprivation as significant predictors of all-cause, coronary, and infant mortality in 107 local educational authorities of England. Shouls et al. [28] reported limiting long-term illness and premature mortality to be significantly associated with area-level socioeconomic conditions and the urban-rural divide.

In these and other studies, epidemiologists generally theorize that, in addition to individual factors, area-level factors, such as specific socioeconomic, cultural, physical, and built environment attributes of a place, can influence health-related behaviors and exposure to risk factors and thereby can affect health outcomes and mortality [31]. Their theorization has sociological underpinnings in that social processes generally are manifested over areas within which social groups function, and these area effects configure an individual's exposure and vulnerability to risks. Area-level factors also reflect how the cumulative health-defining characteristics of individuals, such as education, employment, income, deprivation, socioeconomic status, social capital, and so on, are distributed in a specific place and over a specific population. It has been highlighted that these contextual macro-level factors have independent effects on an individual's health outcomes [32].

In addition to having sociological underpinnings, for epidemiologists, the area-level study design is an important tool for investigating population health that cannot be addressed with individual-level study design [30]. Through the aggregation effects of selection, distribution, interaction, adaptation, and so on, an area-level study design can capture contextual effects that an individual-level study design cannot capture, thereby allowing the researcher to test the usefulness of an ecological model in identifying population health patterns and studying the impact of contexts and policies on population health.

Despite their theoretical underpinning and methodological advantages, well-intentioned area-level epidemiological studies are often deemed less meaningful by their critics [33, 34], who argue that the relationships observed at the aggregate level cannot provide an accurate manifestation of individual-level relationships. Already in the 1950s, Selvin [35] coined the term "ecological fallacy" to illustrate the bias associated with attempts to make inferences at an individual level using area-level analysis. Acknowledging such limitations, epidemiologists interested in an area-level study design have used many recent developments in statistical techniques that can handle hierarchical data structures [36, 37]. These multilevel or contextual analysis techniques allow the researcher to use macro-level group or area (contextual) variables simultaneously with the micro-level individual (compositional) variables [38, 39].

In recent years, an increasing number of epidemiological studies have used a multilevel contextual analysis. Some of these multilevel studies have attempted to evaluate the magnitude of area effects by partitioning the variances into *between-individuals (within-area)* and *between-area* effects in addition to adjustments for individual- and area-level variables [40–42]. Stressing the significance of within-area correlations in the population context, it has been argued that a higher correlation is synonymous with a greater homogeneity in the health outcomes of individuals within a neighborhood, which in turn reflects the potential effects of neighborhood context on the determinants of individual health [43].

In one of these multilevel contextual studies, Haan et al. [44] observed significantly higher rates of mortality among the residents of poverty areas as compared to non-poverty areas in Alameda County, California. The differences persisted even after subsequent statistical adjustments for individual-level sociodemographic, lifestyle, and health factors. In another study, Humphreys and Carr-Hill [45] found significant area-level variability in health outcomes after controlling for individual socioeconomic characteristics and health-related behaviors. In yet another study, Diehr et al. [46] reported significant areal variations in smoking, consumption of alcohol, consumption of dietary fat, and use of seatbelts, independent of individual characteristics. Diez-Roux et al. [39] found that neighborhood contexts shaped the population distribution of coronary heart disease such that living in deprived neighborhoods was associated with increased odds of coronary heart disease and exposures to risk factors. The associations persisted after adjustments for individual-level variables. Smith et al. [47] observed that both individual social class and area-level deprivation were independently and inversely associated with all-cause and cardiovascular disease mortality. Sundquist et al. [48] identified higher hazards of coronary heart diseases among individuals living in neighborhoods associated with lower area-level income and education independent of individual-level variables.

Some studies, however, have reported negligible contextual effects. Sloggett and Joshi [49] found that all-cause mortality was significantly associated with area-level deprivation for both men and women. Adjustments for areas and a wide range of individual socioeconomic factors, however, progressively minimized and explained away the effect of area-level deprivation in men, while it was strongly attenuated in the case of women. The study thus could find no evidence supporting that living within deprived areas was independently associated with higher rates of mortality. In a subsequent study, Sloggett and Joshi [50] similarly found no evidence of area-level deprivation on adverse fertility events in women. Smith et al. [51] found that areal variations in mortality originated in the distribution of deprivation among individuals in areas rather than in the differences between areas per se.

Like any research design, a multilevel contextual design for population health studies has several conceptual and methodological challenges. One challenge is the lack of theory explaining how neighborhood-level factors affect health risks and thereby health outcomes [52, 53]. Another is the lack of optimized definitions of areal units or neighborhoods with respect to size and degree of heterogeneity so that these units can accurately capture the population-level socioeconomic, political, cultural, environmental, and institutional processes within them [37, 52]. Nevertheless, exploring the independent associations of both objective and subjective area-level built environment factors with health outcomes after adjustments for individual-level covariates has become an important field of research in public and population health in recent years. In following this tradition, the studies in this book use a multilevel contextual study design exploring a few among many pathways through which spatial factors may influence population health (see chapter 1 for details).

Pathways of Influence Considered

Figure 6.1 shows the pathways of influence considered in the studies of this book. The items in lighter font will not be considered. From the spatial design and planning factors of the built environment in column 1 of the figure, the studies will only consider macro-level spatial planning and design factors, which include city size and density, availability of key destinations and facilities, land use type and mix, and route accessibility defined using properties of street systems. From intervening factors in column 2, the studies will only consider the rural-urban status of a small city defined based on population size, population density, population change due to daytime travel, distance from the nearest large city of ≥50,000 people, and commute time. From lifestyle behaviors in column 3, the studies will consider work-related travel behaviors, food shopping and eating behaviors, and different types of physical and sedentary activities. From health risk factors and outcomes in columns 4 and 5, the studies will consider several indicators of mortality and morbidity, as well as several indicators of physical, mental, and social health. The definitions of the factors, indicators, or variables in each of the categories are provided in the next section of this chapter.

Concerning the pathways of influence, the book's analytic studies ask two sets of simple questions. The first set of questions explored in chapters 8 and 9 relates to lifestyle:

1. How are spatial design and planning factors (column 1) associated with lifestyle (column 3) in small towns and cities?
2. How does rurality (column 2) affect spatial associations of lifestyle in small towns and cities?

The second set of questions explored in chapters 10 and 11 relates to health:

1. How are spatial design and planning factors (column 1) associated with health (columns 4 and 5) in small towns and cities?

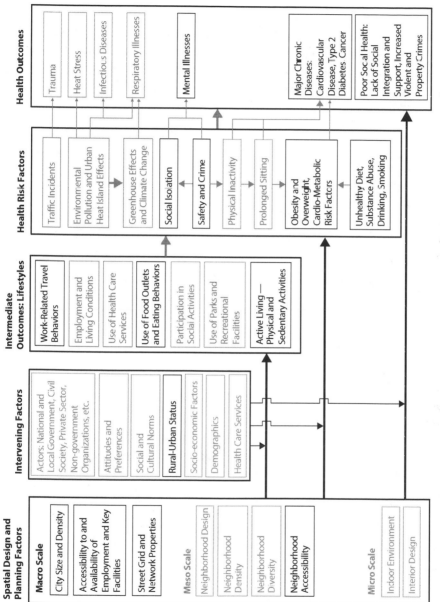

Figure 6.1. Potential pathways through which spatial design and planning factors may influence health and health-related behaviors. The pathways being considered in this book's studies are shown in darker font.

2. How does rurality (column 2) affect spatial associations of health in small towns and cities?

Variables

Dictated by an ecological approach to population health described in chapter 1 and as presented in figure 6.1, the studies of this book use several spatial design and planning factors, indicators of lifestyle and health, and factors of rurality that may affect spatial associations of lifestyle and health, which are described below.

Spatial Design and Planning Factors

This category includes different variables in the following subcategories: city size, density, availability of key services and destinations, land use type and mix, and street properties.

CITY SIZE

City size is important because a bigger city is generally less rural. However, this may not always be correct. Some large cities with low population density may be more rural than some small cities with high population density. The studies of the book consider one variable in this subcategory:

1. *The total land area of a city.*

DENSITY

Density is one of the most widely used measures in studies on population health and spatial planning and design. It refers to the quantity of people, dwelling units, jobs, or specific destinations distributed per unit of land area such as acre, square kilometer, or square mile. It is generally suggested that as density increases, things are brought into greater proximity to one another, improving accessibility. For example, high-density, compact places tend to shorten trip lengths while increasing the number of trips. If density is high enough, then the number of motorized trips may decrease, resulting in higher demand for walking and cycling. There is consistent evidence that high-density developments are associated with more walking—particularly walking for transport—across all age groups [54].

Handy [55] observes that it is not density per se that increases physical activities such as walking and cycling. Rather, density works in combination with other built environment features. Walking for transport or recreation is largely dependent on having somewhere to walk to—that is, a mix of shops, services, and transport connections. However, without sufficient residential density, we cannot ensure that destinations are proximate to housing and that local businesses are viable.

As reported in chapters 8 and 10, high density is not always good for population health. In many cases, a high density of activities may increase crime and diminish safety with negative effects on lifestyle and health. The studies of this book use two variables of density:

1. *Census block density*: the number of census blocks per square mile.
2. *Housing density*: the number of housing units per square mile.

These variables are important not only because they may affect lifestyle and health but also because they may indicate the level of rurality of a city.

AVAILABILITY OF KEY SERVICES AND DESTINATIONS

Availability of key services and destinations is an important determinant of population health (for details, see chapters 8 and 10). It measures how easy it is to reach employment and other key destinations required for daily living. Among the destinations frequently included in the literature are transit stops, retail functions, green space, physical activity facilities, and food environments. These are not homogeneous categories. For example, physical activity resources include, among other things, sport and recreation centers, gyms and fitness facilities, golf courses, tennis courts, swimming pools, parks, and other forms of public open space, biking and walking paths and trails, beaches, and riverfronts. They provide opportunities for different kinds of physical activities.

Availability of key destinations and services are computed *per 10,000 people* and *per square mile*. A value per 10,000 people describes the availability of a facility in terms of people—that is, how many people can potentially use a facility, even though all of them may never use it. Without any reference to area, the value per 10,000 people does not describe how spread out these people are. In some cases, they may live in a 10-square-mile area, whereas in other cases they may live over a 1-square-mile area. In contrast, a value per 1 square mile describes how frequently some facilities are distributed in a city; however, it does not describe how many people can potentially use a facility. In some areas a facility may be available for 10,000 people, whereas in other areas it may be available for 1,000 people. Together these variables should provide a better description of the availability of a facility in a city. The studies of the book use several variables in this subcategory:

1. *The number of health care facilities per 10,000 people.*
2. *The number of health care facilities per square mile.*

These variables measure the availability of health care facilities, which can be used as proxy measures for health care access in a city. High values of either of these variables in a city may indicate better health care access.

3. *The number of parks per 10,000 people.*
4. *The number of parks per square mile.*

These variables measure the availability of parks in a city. The availability of more parks and recreation facilities has been linked to more physical activity among residents. Regular physical activity has a wide array of health benefits, including weight control, muscle and bone strengthening, improved mental health and mood, and improved life expectancy. Regular physical activity also reduces the risk of cardiovascular disease, type 2 diabetes and metabolic syndrome, and some cancers. High values of either of these variables in a city may indicate more opportunities for active living and health equality.

5. *The number of supermarkets/grocery stores per 10,000 people.*
6. *The number of supermarkets/grocery stores per square mile.*

These variables measure the availability of supermarkets or grocery stores in a city. A lack of access to healthy foods is often a significant barrier to healthy eating habits. Low-income and underserved areas often have limited numbers of grocery stores that sell healthy foods. People living farther away from grocery stores are less likely to have access healthy foods on a regular basis and thus are more likely to consume less-healthy foods, which are readily available at convenience stores and fast food outlets. High values of either of these variables in a city may indicate that residents have better access to healthy foods.

7. *The number of convenience stores per 10,000 people.*
8. *The number of convenience stores per square mile.*

These variables measure the availability of convenience stores in a city. High values of either of these variables in a city may indicate that residents of the city have better access to less-healthy or unhealthy foods.

9. *The number of convenience stores with gas per 10,000 people.*
10. *The number of convenience stores with gas per square mile.*

These variables measure the availability of convenience stores with gas. High values of either of these variables in a city may indicate that residents have easy access to gasoline and have easy access to less-healthy or unhealthy foods.

11. *The number of full-service restaurants per 10,000 people.*
12. *The number of full-service restaurants per square mile.*

These variables measure the availability of full-service restaurants in a city. High values of either of these variables in a city may indicate that residents have easy access to healthy foods and healthy eating behaviors. The effects may depend on income, however, because people with lower income do not often get the benefits of eating at full-service restaurants.

13. *The number of businesses per 10,000 people.*
14. *The number of businesses per square mile.*

These variables measure the availability of businesses in a city. In this case, a business is a single physical location at which business is conducted or where services or industrial operations are performed. It is not necessarily identical with a company or enterprise, which may consist of one establishment or more. High values of either of these variables in a city may indicate that the city provides more employment opportunities, which may be related to improved health and well-being.

Finally, it should be noted that the *availability of transit stops* is not included in these studies because public transit systems are commonly absent in small cities and towns of America.

LAND USE TYPE AND MIX

Land use type and mix are important factors of population health. Land use types refer to the proportion of the area occupied by different categories of land uses, whereas land use mix refers to the composition of land uses in a city or city area. Studies show that different types of land use affect lifestyles and health differently. Studies also show that mixed-use urban form with fine-grained neighborhood blocks provides enhanced permeability, connectivity, and accessibility. As a result, it may reduce the need for longer vehicular trips, increase nonmotorized (e.g., walking, bicycling) trips, create a more even distribution of trips throughout the day and week, and provide new opportunities for shared parking arrangements [56]. (See chapters 8 and 10 for additional information.) The studies of the book use several variables in this subcategory.

1. *Open area as a percentage of total city area.* High values may indicate more active living and better health equality in the city.
2. *Industrial area as a percentage of total city area.* High values may indicate poor environmental qualities but better employment opportunities in the city.
3. *Residential area as a percentage of total city area.* High values may indicate more residential areas in the city.
4. *Commercial area as a percentage of total city area.* High values may indicate better economic opportunities in the city.
5. *Institutional and other city amenities as a percentage of total city area.* High values may indicate better social health, active living, and health equality in the city.
6. *Land use mix* (LUM) is a measure widely used in studies on the associations between built environment and health.

LUM is quantified as follows:

$$LUM = \frac{\sum_{i=1}^{n} P_i \cdot \ln P_i}{\ln N}$$

Where P_i is the proportion of estimated square footage of land use i, and N is the number of land use types. The land use mix values normally range from 0 to 1, with 0 representing a homogeneous, single land use environment, and 1 representing a perfectly heterogeneous neighborhood comprising all possible permutations and combinations of a set of land use categories. [57, 58]

STREET PROPERTIES

As a major determinant of morphological patterns, land use patterns, and movement patterns (trip route choices and modes of transportation), street properties can shape travel and physical activity behaviors, thereby significantly affecting population health. Typically, dense urban grids of highly interconnected straight streets crisscrossing at right angles can give rise to fine-grained urban blocks and can increase permeability, connectivity, and accessibility. In contrast, with numerous loops, three-way intersections, and dead ends formed by narrow curving residential streets, sparse suburban grids can reduce permeability, connectivity, and accessibility. (For more on the importance of street properties for lifestyle and health, see chapters 8 and 10.)

One important property of street systems is route accessibility, which indicates the ease with which various routes and route segments are reached and used. In studies assessing the effects of route accessibility on physical activity and health, researchers frequently use objectively defined network measures, as well as intersection density, percentage of different intersections, and number of intersections. When computing these measures, some use buffers around a destination or an origin [59–63], while others use no buffer [64–67]. In this book, two metric variables and several network variables are used for describing street properties, including route accessibility.

Metric Variables Describing Street Properties. Two metric variables describing street properties in the studies of the book are:

1. *Total street length* (in miles) of a city is a variable that can be related to the level of urbanicity of the city, as well as the level of movement opportunities within the city. Higher values can indicate higher levels of urbanicity as well as movement opportunities.
2. *Street density* (i.e., street length per square mile) is a variable that more accurately describes the level of urbanicity of a city, as well as the level of movement opportunities within a city. Higher values should indicate higher levels of urbanicity as well as movement opportunities.

Network Variables of Space Syntax Describing Street Properties. These studies use several network variables defined using "space syntax," which is a body of theories, methods, techniques, and measures for describing the configurations of street networks. The theoretical foundations of space syntax were first provided by Hillier and Hanson in *The Social Logic of Space* [68] and were later elaborated by Hillier in *Space Is the Machine* [69] as well as in several other articles that followed [70–72]. Among the many techniques of space syntax, the techniques of linear map analysis have been used most frequently in studies on how centrality or accessibility (physical, visual, or both) of streets, districts, and neighborhoods affects empirical phenomena as diverse as pedestrian and vehicular flows, wayfinding, crime, urban liveliness, walkability, and pollution. For a review of some of these studies, see the article by Peponis and Wineman on spatial structure of environment and behavior, my article on space syntax, and my book on the geometry of urban layouts [73–75].

The techniques of linear map analysis include the axial map and segment map analysis. Both techniques involve representing the street systems of a city as a linear map, which includes the fewest number of lines needed to cover every street and complete every circulation ring of the system. So defined, a linear map is more commonly known as the axial map in space syntax. When needed, a segment map can be generated by breaking the lines of an axial map into segments at their intersections. In the next stage of analysis, software programs use different centrality measures to describe patterns of connections, differentiation, and centrality in axial and segment maps. Finally, correlations between any empirical phenomena along the axial lines or segments and the syntactic or network measures of the lines or segments are studied to explore the effects of spatial patterns on these phenomena.

A key syntactic measure of space syntax is integration. The integration value (or the closeness value) of a line indicates how well the line is connected to all other lines in a linear map, or how close the line is to all other lines in the map. A higher integration value of a line indicates stronger connections of the line to the network. In space syntax, the integration value is relativized to allow direct comparison between networks of different sizes [68]. The integration value of the system is given by the mean of the integration values of the lines in the system. In theory, linear maps with higher mean integration values should provide better accessibility.

Another key syntactic measure of space syntax is choice. While integration is about closeness, choice is about betweenness. Unlike integration, choice gives the degree to which a line lies on the simplest paths from one line to another line in the network. In simple words, integration measures how easy it is to go from a line to all the other lines of a network, thus indicating the line's *to-movement* potential (or, simply, accessibility). In contrast, choice indicates the likelihood of a line being chosen on all the paths from one line to every other line in a network, thus indicating the line's *through-movement* potential (or, simply, movement opportunities) [76]. The choice value of the system is given by the mean of the choice values of the lines in the system. In theory, linear maps with higher mean choice values should provide better movement opportunities.

Yet another syntactic measure of space syntax is *node count*, which describes the number of nodes of an axial or segment map. Different from street intersections, nodes in the axial or segment map include street intersections as well as all the intersections of lines where significant directional changes occur. In this sense, node counts in an axial or segment map are experientially more robust than intersection counts in relation to directional choices available in a street system.

Using space syntax techniques, it is possible to compute integration, choice, and nodes at different radii. For example, the integration value at radius 3 (R3) of a line uses only those lines that are three steps away for the given line; the integration value at radius 5 (R5) uses only those lines that are five steps away for the given line; and so on. The integration value at radius n (Rn) of a line considers n steps needed to cover all the lines in the system. The integration, choice, or nodes computed at a lower radius describe more local syntactic property than that computed at a higher radius. The most local of any syntactic property of a line, however, is its connectivity value, which is the number of lines directly connected to the line. Readers interested in the mathematics of space syntax measures should consult "Space Syntax: A Network-Based Configurational Approach for Urban Morphological Studies" and *The Geometry of Urban Layouts: A Global Comparative Study* [75, 77].

The book's studies consider several syntactic or network measures of the street system of a city generated using axial and segment map techniques of space syntax, which are described below.

VARIABLES MEASURED ON AXIAL MAPS

1. *Mean axial choice (Rn)* describes the global through-movement potential of the street system of a city. Higher values indicate higher levels of movement potentials of the streets within the city.

2. *Mean axial choice (R3)* describes the through-movement potential of a local street system of the city that includes lines up to 3 steps away from any line. Higher values indicate higher levels of movement potentials of the streets within the local areas of the city.

3. *Mean axial choice (R5)* describes the through-movement potential of a local street system of the city that includes lines up to 5 steps away from any line. Higher values indicate higher levels of movement potentials of the streets within the local areas of the city.

4. *Mean axial connectivity* provides the mean number of direct connections streets have with other streets. Higher values may indicate higher levels of movement opportunities at the street level.

5. *Mean axial integration (Rn)* describes the global accessibility of the street system of a city. Higher values may indicate higher levels of accessibility within the city.

6. *Mean axial integration (R3)* describes the accessibility of a local street

system of the city that includes lines up to 3 steps away from any line. Higher values may indicate higher levels of accessibility within the local areas of the city.

7. *Mean axial integration (R5)* describes the accessibility of a local street system of the city that includes lines up to 5 steps away from any line. Higher values may indicate higher levels of accessibility within the local areas of the city.

8. *Axial node count (RN)* is a global descriptor of directional changes within a city. Higher values may indicate more changes in directions within the city.

9. *Axial node count (R3)* is a descriptor of directional changes within a local area of the city that includes lines up to 3 steps away from any line. Higher values may indicate more changes in directions within the local areas of the city.

10. *Axial node count (R5)* is a local descriptor of directional changes within a local area of the city that includes lines up to 3 steps away from any line. Higher values may indicate more changes in directions within the local areas of the city.

VARIABLES MEASURED ON SEGMENT MAPS

1. *Mean segment choice (Rn)* describes the global through-movement potential of the street system of a city. Higher values may indicate higher levels of movement potentials of the streets within the city.

2. *Mean segment choice (R3)* describes the through-movement potential of a local street system of the city that includes lines up to 3 steps away from any line. Higher values may indicate higher levels of movement potentials of the streets within the local areas of the city.

3. *Mean segment choice (R5)* describes the through-movement potential of a local street system of the city that includes lines up to 5 steps away from any line. Higher values may indicate higher levels of movement potentials of the streets within the local areas of the city.

4. *Mean segment integration (Rn)* describes the global accessibility of the street system of a city. Higher values may indicate higher levels of accessibility within the city.

5. *Mean segment integration (R3)* describes the accessibility of a local street system of the city that includes lines up to 3 steps away from any line. Higher values may indicate higher levels of accessibility within the local areas of the city.

6. *Mean segment integration (R5)* describes the accessibility of a local street system of the city that includes lines up to 5 steps away from any line. Higher values may indicate higher levels of accessibility within the local areas of the city.

7. *Segment node count (Rn)* is a global descriptor of directional changes within a city. Higher values may indicate more changes in directions within the city.

8. *Segment node count (R3)* is a descriptor of directional changes within a local area of the city that includes lines up to 3 steps away from any line. Higher values may indicate more changes in directions within the local areas of the city.

9. *Segment node count (R5)* is a descriptor of directional changes within a local area of the city that includes lines up to 5 steps away from any line. Higher values may indicate more changes in directions within the local areas of the city.

Lifestyle

Population health studies consider different lifestyle behaviors, including physical and sedentary activities, work-related travel behaviors, recreational behaviors, food shopping behaviors, and eating behaviors, such as having or not having breakfast and consuming sugar-sweetened beverages, fruits, vegetables, dairy products, meat and beans, and food with fiber. These behaviors are important because they can affect health. For example, physical activity can affect weight, mental health, and risk of diseases such as stroke, heart disease, type 2 diabetes, depression, and some cancers. It can also affect social well-being by enhancing social cohesion and economic well-being by reducing health care costs [78] and transportation costs. Yet only one in five adults meets the Centers for Disease Control and Prevention's physical activity guidelines [79], while almost 30% of adults remain physically inactive [80].

Three subcategories of lifestyle behaviors are considered in this book: work-related travel behaviors, food shopping and eating behaviors, and physical and sedentary activities.

WORK-RELATED TRAVEL BEHAVIORS

Work-related travel behaviors have population health significance. For example, walking to work is a good way to incorporate exercise into a daily routine. In addition to various health benefits, walking helps people get in touch with their communities, reduces commute costs, and helps protect the environment by reducing air pollution from car trips. Studies have shown that walking to work improves employees' overall attitude and morale, and it reduces stress in the workplace. In contrast, driving alone to work consumes more fuel and resources than other modes of transportation, such as carpooling, public transportation, biking, and walking. Driving alone also increases traffic congestion, especially in areas of greater population density. The sedentary habit of driving to work has been associated with decreased levels of physical activity and cardiorespiratory health and with increased body mass index (BMI) and hypertension. Stress-inducing traffic congestion may further exacerbate these negative health effects. Alternatives to driving alone—carpooling, taking public transportation, and biking—may help reduce the number of commuters who drive alone to work each day.

Workers commuting by public transportation is not included as a work-related travel behavior in this book's studies because most small cities in rural America are not large enough in terms of population and economy to run public transportation at scale without significant government subsidies. This is even though public transportation generally offers mobility to residents, particularly people without cars. It can help bridge the spatial divide between people and jobs, services, and training opportunities. Public transportation is also beneficial because it reduces fuel consumption, minimizes air pollution, and relieves traffic congestion.

This book uses the following variables of work-related travel behaviors:

1. *Workers who live and work in this city* (as percentage of total population).
2. *Workers who work at home* (as percentage of working population).
3. *Workers who drive alone to work* (as percentage of working population).
4. *Workers who carpool to work* (as percentage of working population).
5. *Workers who bicycle to work* (as percentage of working population).
6. *Workers who walk to work* (as percentage of working population).

FOOD SHOPPING AND EATING BEHAVIORS

Diet and food environment are among the root causes of rural obesity. Rural people generally consume significantly higher fat because of the culture of their eating patterns (e.g., "country cooking") [81–83], as well as less access to healthy foods [84]. Even though many would like to believe that rural areas have better access to fresh food and vegetables, this is not necessarily true.

Nowadays, monocrop agriculture has reduced access to a wide variety of vegetables in rural areas. The declining number of grocery stores also affects food environments in rural areas.

Along with unhealthy diet, food insecurity remains a significant problem in rural areas. The US Department of Agriculture defines food insecurity as "limited or uncertain availability of nutritionally adequate and safe foods, or limited or uncertain ability to acquire acceptable foods in socially acceptable ways" [85]. Poverty and unemployment are frequently predictors of food insecurity in the United States. Rural households face considerably deeper food insecurity than those in metropolitan areas. Millions of working families, veterans, people with disabilities, seniors, and children in rural communities cannot always afford and access enough food for active, healthy lives [86]. Food insecurity is often associated with chronic health problems in adults, including diabetes, heart disease, high blood pressure, hyperlipidemia (high cholesterol), obesity, and mental health issues, including major depression [87–89].

The studies of this book use the following food shopping and eating behaviors as health risk factors:

1. *Income spent on food at supermarket/grocery store* (as percentage of total income).
2. *Income spent on food at other stores* (as percentage of total income).
3. *Income spent on eating out* (as percentage of total income).
4. *Income spent on carryout/delivered foods* (as percentage of total income).
5. *Healthy diet rate* (people taking healthy diet as percentage of total population).

PHYSICAL AND SEDENTARY ACTIVITIES

Physical activity itself is a broad term used to describe "any force exerted by skeletal muscle that results in energy expenditure above resting level" [90]. It generally includes any form of human movement, including walking, cycling, play, active hobbies, or manual occupations, as well as structured exercise or sport. In this sense, sport and exercise are subsets of physical activity.

As noted previously, physically active adults reduce their risk of many serious health conditions, including obesity, heart disease, diabetes, colon cancer, and high blood pressure. In addition to reducing the risk of multiple chronic diseases, physical activity helps maintain healthy bones, muscles, and joints and helps to control weight, develop lean muscle, and reduce body fat

[91]. Adults must engage in at least 2 hours and 30 minutes of moderate-intensity exercise or 1 hour and 15 minutes of vigorous-intensity aerobic exercise (or any combination thereof) per week and work out all major muscle groups two or more days per week to fully meet the Centers for Disease Control and Prevention physical activity recommendations. Despite the growing body of evidence of the health benefits of physical activity, most US adults and children do not get enough physical activity [79, 92].

In contrast, sedentary lifestyles—that is, too much sitting, as distinct from too little physical activity—increase all causes of mortality, double the risk of cardiovascular diseases, diabetes, and obesity, and increase the risks of colon cancer, high blood pressure, osteoporosis, lipid disorders, depression, and anxiety [93–96]. Prolonged periods of sitting include time spent in cars, which can be associated with increased cardiovascular disease risk [97, 98] and poorer mental health [99]. In high-income countries, time in cars, television viewing, and other screen use account for up to 85% of adults' nonoccupational sitting time [100]. Working adults, who sit for 10 hours or more per day, can face increased health risks, even if they meet physical activity guidelines [101, 102].

Worldwide, sedentary behaviors are rapidly rising as low- and middle-income countries shift from agricultural to manufacturing and service economies with increased use of labor-saving devices and more motorized forms of transport [103]. Globally, some 5 million people die annually because they are physically inactive [91]. It is estimated that around 60% of the world population get insufficient physical activity to benefit their health. Apart from the direct impact on chronic disease, this is important because around 20 million children (aged five and under) and 1.3 billion adults are now either overweight or obese [104]. Thus, even a modest increase in the number of physically active people could produce significant societal benefits, with substantial savings to global health systems [105].

The studies of this book include the following physical and sedentary activities as health risk factors:

1. *People doing vigorous-intensity work activities* (as percentage of total population). These activities cause large increases in breathing or heart rate, like carrying or lifting heavy loads, digging, or construction work for at least 10 minutes continuously.
2. *People doing moderate-intensity work activities* (as percentage of total population). These activities cause small increases in breathing or heart

rate, such as brisk walking or carrying light loads for at least 10 minutes continuously.

3. *People walking or bicycling* (as percentage of total population). Riding a bike and walking have demonstrated a wide range of health benefits, such as lowering the risk of death, heart disease, and colon cancer and reducing the chances of being affected by diabetes as well as by depression, anxiety, and other mental health issues.

4. *People doing vigorous-intensity recreational activities* (as percentage of total population). These activities cause large increases in breathing or heart rate, like running or playing basketball for at least 10 minutes continuously.

5. *People doing moderate-intensity recreational activities* (as percentage of total population). These activities cause a small increase in breathing or heart rate, such as brisk walking, bicycling, swimming, or golfing for at least 10 minutes continuously.

6. *Average hours a day doing sedentary activities.* These activities include sitting at work, at home, getting to and from places, or with friends, including time spent sitting at a desk, traveling in a car or bus, reading, playing cards, watching television, or using a computer.

7. *Average hours a day watching TV or videos.* Prolonged TV viewing can increase the risk of type 2 diabetes, cardiovascular disease, and premature death. It can also increase memory loss and decrease fine motor skills.

8. *Average hours a day using a computer.* Prolonged computer use can lead to obesity, sleep problems, chronic neck and back problems, depression, anxiety, and lower test scores in children.

Health

The studies of this book consider the following subcategories of health factors: mortality and morbidity, physical health, mental health, and social health.

INDICATORS OF MORBIDITY AND MORTALITY

Four indicators are included in this subcategory:

1. *People reporting general health conditions* (as percentage of total population). This indicator shows the percentage of adults 18 years and older who self-report fair/poor health. People's subjective assessment of their health status is important. When people assess themselves to be healthy,

they are more likely to feel happy and to participate in social and economic activities. Healthy residents are essential for creating a vibrant and successful community. Areas with unhealthy populations lose productivity due to lost work time.

2. *People under 65 with disability* (as percentage of total population). People with a disability have difficulties performing activities due to a physical, mental, or emotional problem. The extent to which a person is limited by a disability is heavily dependent on the social and physical environment in which he or she lives. Without sufficient accommodations, people with disabilities may have difficulties living independently or fulfilling work responsibilities. Several federal agencies use information on the size, distribution, and needs of the disabled population to develop policies, distribute funds, and develop programs for individuals with disabilities.

3. *Death rate per 100,000 people.* This indicator shows the total age-adjusted death rate per 100,000 people due to all causes. Mortality or death rates are often used as measures of health status for a population. Many factors affect the risk of death, including age, race, gender, occupation, education, and income. One of the strongest factors affecting the risk of death is age. Age-adjusted rates are valuable when comparing the mortality experience between different geographic areas, causes, races, ethnic groups, or time periods.

4. *Age-adjusted suicide mortality rate per 100,000 people.* This indicator shows the total age-adjusted death rate per 100,000 people due to suicide. Suicide results in the tragic loss of human life as well as agonizing grief, fear, and confusion in families and communities. Its impact is not limited to an individual person or family but extends across generations and throughout communities. The breadth of the problem and the complexity of its risk factors make suicide prevention well suited to a population health–based approach that engages multiple systems and reaches all citizens.

INDICATORS OF PHYSICAL HEALTH

Four indicators are included in this subcategory:

1. *Adult diabetes rate* (as percentage of total adult population). This indicator shows the percentage of adults who have ever been diagnosed with diabetes. Women who were diagnosed with diabetes only while preg-

nant are not included in this count. Diabetes is the seventh leading cause of death in the United States. In 2010, an estimated 25.8 million people, or 8.3% of the population, had diabetes. Diabetes disproportionately affects minority populations and the elderly, and its incidence is likely to increase as minority populations grow and the US population becomes older. Diabetes can have a harmful effect on most of the organ systems in the human body; it is a frequent cause of end-stage renal disease and nontraumatic lower-extremity amputation and a leading cause of blindness among working-age adults. Persons with diabetes are also at increased risk for ischemic heart disease, neuropathy, and stroke. According to the American Diabetes Association, the total costs of diagnosed diabetes rose to $327 billion in 2017 from $245 billion in 2012, when the cost was last examined. The 2017 cost includes $237 billion in direct medical costs and $90 billion in reduced productivity. Diabetes costs tend to vary in specific populations. For example, total per capita health care expenditures are higher among men than women ($10,060 vs. $9,110), lower among Hispanic Americans ($8,050), and higher among non-Hispanic Black Americans ($10,470) and non-Hispanic white Americans ($9,800).

2. *Average BMI.* Body mass index is a measure of body fat based on height and weight that applies to adult men and women. Different weight categories—underweight, healthy weight, overweight, obesity—are easily and inexpensively screened by BMI. Studies show that BMI is moderately correlated with direct measures of body fat, even though BMI does not measure body fat directly [106–108]. Studies also show that BMI is strongly correlated with various metabolic and disease outcomes [109–115].

3. *Adult overweight rate* (as percentage of total adult population). Being overweight can affect quality of life and put individuals at risk for developing many adverse health conditions, including heart disease, stroke, diabetes, and cancer. Losing weight can help to prevent and control these diseases. Being overweight can also carry significant economic costs due to increased health care spending and lost earnings.

4. *Adult obesity rate* (as percentage of total adult population). This indicator shows the percentage of adults 18 years and older who are obese (body mass index ≥30 kg/m²). The term "obese" generally means a much higher amount of body fat than "overweight." Obesity increases the risk

of many diseases and health conditions, including heart disease, type 2 diabetes, cancer, hypertension, stroke, liver and gallbladder disease, respiratory problems, and osteoarthritis. Losing weight and maintaining a healthy weight can help to prevent and control these diseases. Obesity can lead to significant economic costs due to increased health care spending and lost earnings.

It should be noted here that BMI, overweight, and obesity are related measures, but they apply to increasingly smaller samples of population: BMI includes a sample of the whole population, overweight includes a subsample of the whole sample, and obesity includes a subsample of those who are overweight. Therefore, all three indicators are included in the exploratory studies in this book.

INDICATORS OF MENTAL HEALTH

Five indicators are included in this subcategory:

1. *People feeling badly about themselves* (as percentage of total population).
2. *People who have little interest in doing things* (as percentage of total population).
3. *People feeling down, depressed, or hopeless* (as percentage of total population).
4. *People having thoughts they would be better off dead* (as percentage of total population).
5. *People who have ever used marijuana or hashish* (as percentage of total population).

These are common symptoms of depression, which is a chronic disease that negatively affects a person's feelings, behaviors, and thought processes and is associated with increased risk of morbidity, mortality, and poor quality of life. Many people with depression never seek treatment; however, even those with the most severe depression can improve with treatments, including medications, psychotherapies, and other methods.

According to the National Comorbidity Survey of mental health disorders [116], people over the age of 60 have lower rates of depression than the general population: 10.7% of people over the age of 60 compared to 16.9% overall. The Centers for Medicare and Medicaid Services estimates that depression in older adults occurs in 25% of those with other illnesses, including arthritis, cancer, cardiovascular disease, chronic lung disease, and stroke.

People who have ever used marijuana or hashish is used as an indicator of addiction. The National Institute on Drug Abuse classifies drug addiction as a mental illness [117]. Addiction can change the brain in fundamental ways, disturbing a person's normal hierarchy of needs and desires and substituting new priorities connected with procuring and using drugs. Drug abusers are often diagnosed with mental disorders and vice versa. The high prevalence of this comorbidity has been documented in multiple national population surveys since the 1980s. Data show that persons diagnosed with mood or anxiety disorders are about twice as likely to also suffer from a substance use disorder (abuse or dependence) compared with respondents in general. The same is true for those diagnosed with antisocial personality or conduct disorder. Similarly, persons diagnosed with substance use disorders are roughly twice as likely to also suffer from mood and anxiety disorders [117].

INDICATORS OF SOCIAL HEALTH

Two types of indicators are included in this subcategory:

1. *Crime.*
2. *Social isolation.*

Crime. Two types of crime are considered for these studies—violent crime and property crime. *Violent crimes* are defined as those offenses that involve force or threat of force. They include four offenses: murder and nonnegligent manslaughter, rape, robbery, and aggravated assault. *Property crimes* include the offenses of burglary, larceny-theft, motor vehicle theft, and arson. Because of limited participation and varying collection procedures by local law enforcement agencies, only limited data are available for arson. Therefore, arson statistics are not included in any estimated volume data throughout the Federal Bureau of Investigation's Crime in the U.S. records [118].

Measurement of crime for a given area (state, county, or city) allows law enforcement agencies to determine where, when, and what types of crimes have taken place within their jurisdiction. With this knowledge, agencies can determine the trend of crime over time, develop operations to address a particular type of crime, determine necessary manpower numbers, and develop defensive environmental design approaches. Population health experts view violent crimes as a health issue to any community. These measurements can assist these experts in quantifying health impacts that crimes have on an area and help establish crime prevention efforts to improve population health.

The variables included in the studies are:

1. *Murders per 100,000 people.*
2. *Rapes per 100,000 people.*
3. *Robberies per 100,000 people.*
4. *Assaults per 100,000 people.*
5. *Violent crimes per 100,000 people.*
6. *Burglaries per 100,000 people.*
7. *Thefts per 100,000 people.*
8. *Auto thefts per 100,000 people.*
9. *Property crimes per 100,000 people.*

Social Isolation. Only one indicator is included in this subcategory: *people 65+ living alone* (as percentage of total population).

People over age 65 who live alone may be at risk for social isolation, limited access to support, or inadequate assistance in emergency situations. Older adults who do not live alone are most likely to live with a spouse, but they may also live with a child or other relative, a nonrelative, or in group quarters. The Commonwealth Fund Commission on the Elderly Living Alone indicated that one-third of older Americans live alone and that one-quarter of those living alone are poor and report poor health [119]. Rates of living alone are typically higher in urban areas and among women. Older people living alone may lack social support and are at high risk for institutionalization or losing their independent lifestyle. Living alone should not be equated with being lonely or isolated, but many older people who live alone are vulnerable due to social isolation, poverty, disability, lack of access to care, or inadequate housing [120–122].

Factors of Rurality

The studies of this book include several factors of rurality. The significance of these factors is discussed in chapter 2. Factors include:

1. *The total population of a city* is important because most federal, state, and other administrative organizations make a simple assumption that more population may indicate less rurality or more urbanicity for a place. The population size of a region or a city is also important in planning for the future of a community, particularly for schools, community centers, health care, and childcare. Total population figures allow professionals to model fluctuations of a population over time and de-

termine stability, variation, and capacity to adapt to environmental changes; to find out the effects of social determinants on health; and to find out the effects of many other factors on the well-being of a given population.

2. *Population density* describes a city using the number of people per square mile. This is important because high population density may indicate low rurality. Population density is also one important indicator for how the land of an area is used. High population density may increase land use density.

3. *Daytime population change due to commuting* (as percentage of total population) is important because more population change may indicate fewer employment opportunities and more rurality for a place.

4. *Distance to the nearest city with 50,000 or more people* is important because longer distance may indicate more rurality for a place. Longer distance requiring longer commute is a health factor. It can cut into workers' free time and can contribute to health problems such as headaches, anxiety, and increased blood pressure. Longer distance also requires workers to consume more fuel, which is both expensive for workers and damaging to the environment.

5. *Mean travel time to work* (or commute time in minutes) is the average daily travel time to work for workers 16 years of age and older. In many cases, longer commutes may be a better indicator of rurality than distance. Some places near urban areas can remain rural if they lack accessibility to these urban areas due to difficult terrain or poor road conditions. Regardless of distance, longer commutes are a health factor. They can cut into workers' free time and can contribute to health problems such as headaches, anxiety, and increased blood pressure. Longer commutes also require workers to consume more fuel, which is both expensive for workers and damaging to the environment.

Analysis

The book's studies use a convenience sample of small cities from the state of Kansas. In chapter 7, the spatial design and planning, lifestyle behaviors, and health of the sample cities are described using the variables listed in this chapter. Since the studies include many variables, only the mean, maximum, and minimum values of each variable are considered in the description. For the description of the spatial design and planning factors, the distribution pattern of each variable is also considered.

Presented in chapters 8 through 11, the studies of the book explore the spatial associations of lifestyle and health in the sample of small cities using correlational analyses. The analyses are performed for the whole sample first and then for the two subsamples, defined based on high and low values of each factor of rurality described above. Reporting of the findings remains focused on significant correlations and their effect size. The total numbers of significant correlations between spatial factors and lifestyle behaviors and between spatial factors and health indicators and outcomes for the two sub-samples of small cities defined based on a rurality factor are used to see if there are any differences between the subsamples.

Conclusions

A gradual shift has occurred from traditional public health concerns to population health concerns among researchers working in urban areas, but a similar shift has not occurred among those working in rural areas and small towns and cities. Therefore, we observe a lack of studies on population health in rural areas and small towns and cities. Due to differences in scale and place, it is unlikely that models, methods, and findings of urban population health studies will be useful for population health studies in rural areas and small towns and cities.

Emphasizing the scale- and place-specific qualities of small-town America, this book uses an area-level study design in its population health studies. Unlike an individual-level study that considers individuals within an area as units of analysis, an area-level study uses aggregate data to understand population health differences between areas representing environmental or settlement units. Despite some theoretical and methodological challenges, public and population health studies in urban areas have frequently used such a study design since the 1980s.

The studies here consider small cities as units of analysis to avoid the common problem of areal definition in area-level studies. Limiting their scope, the studies consider only some pathways for spatial planning and design factors to influence population health among the many pathways indicated by a socio-ecological model of population health described in chapter 1. These pathways consider how rurality factors may affect spatial associations of lifestyle and health in small towns and cities.

Described in this chapter, the studies include four sets of variables—spatial factors, lifestyle, health outcomes and indicators, and the factors of rurality—in a two-level statistical analysis. At one level of analysis, these studies consider all the small cities in the study as one sample. At another level of analysis, the sample is divided into two subsamples based on high and low values of each factor of rurality to study the effects of rurality on spatial associations of lifestyle and health in these small cities. The two-level studies should not only provide simple methodological innovations, but they should also provide new ways to explore spatial associations of population health in small towns and cities. Before the findings of these analytic studies are presented in chapters 8 through 11, the sample of small Kansas cities included in the studies of the book are presented in chapter 7.

NOTES

1. Warren and Smalley, "What Is Rural?"
2. Wuthnow, *Small-Town America*.
3. Sugiyama et al., "Perceived Neighbourhood Environmental Attributes."
4. Ameli et al., "Do Better Urban Design Qualities Lead to More Walking?"
5. Hirsch et al., "Discrete Land Uses and Transportation Walking."
6. Stewart et al., "Comparing Associations between the Built Environment and Walking."
7 King-Shier, Mather, and LeBlanc, "Understanding the Influence of Urban- or Rural-Living."
8. Corburn, *Toward the Healthy City*.
9. Dannenberg, Frumkin, and Jackson, *Making Healthy Places*.
10. Barton and Tsourou, *Healthy Urban Planning*.
11. Swinburn et al., "Diet, Nutrition and the Prevention of Excess Weight Gain."
12. Pitts et al., "Formative Evaluation for a Healthy Corner Store Initiative."
13. Eng, Salmon, and Mullan, "Community Empowerment."
14. Macintyre, "The Black Report and Beyond."
15. Macintyre, Maciver, and Sooman, "Area, Class and Health."
16. Macintyre, Ellaway, and Cummins, "Place Effects on Health."
17. Rose, "Sick Individuals and Sick Populations," 1985.
18. Rose, "Sick Individuals and Sick Populations," 2001.
19. Susser, "The Logic in Ecological: I."
20. Susser, "The Logic in Ecological: II."
21. Briggs and Leonard, "Mortality and Ecological Structure."
22. Fox and Goldblatt, *Longitudinal Study*.
23. Fox, Jones, and Goldblatt, "Approaches to Studying the Effect of Socio-Economic Circumstances."
24. Britton et al., *The Influence of Socio-Economic and Environmental Factors*.
25. Eames, Ben-Shlomo, and Marmot, "Social Deprivation and Premature Mortality."
26. Morris, Blane, and White, "Levels of Mortality, Education, and Social Conditions."
27. Raleigh and Kiri, "Life Expectancy in England."
28. Shouls, Congdon, and Curtis, "Modelling Inequality in Reported Long Term Illness."
29. Wing et al., "Changing Association."
30. Wing et al., "Geographic and Socioeconomic Variation."
31. Whitehead et al., *The Health Divide*.
32. Blalock and Wilken, *Intergroup Processes*.

33. Thorndike, "On the Fallacy of Imputing the Correlations Found."
34. Robinson, "Ecological Correlations and the Behavior of Individuals."
35. Selvin, "Durkheim's Suicide and Problems of Empirical Research."
36. Duncan, Jones, and Moon, "Context, Composition and Heterogeneity."
37. Diez-Roux, "Investigating Neighborhood and Area Effects."
38. Von Korff et al., "Multi-Level Analysis in Epidemiologic Research."
39. Diez-Roux et al., "Neighborhood Environments and Coronary Heart Disease."
40. Duncan, Jones, and Moon, "Do Places Matter?"
41. Duncan, Jones, and Moon, "Psychiatric Morbidity."
42. Jones and Duncan, "Individuals and Their Ecologies."
43. Merlo, "Multilevel Analytical Approaches in Social Epidemiology."
44. Haan, Kaplan, and Camacho, "Poverty and Health."
45. Humphreys and Carr-Hill, "Area Variations in Health Outcomes."
46. Diehr et al., "Do Communities Differ in Health Behaviors?"
47. Smith et al., "Individual Social Class."
48. Sundquist et al., "Neighborhood Socioeconomic Environment."
49. Sloggett and Joshi, "Higher Mortality in Deprived Areas."
50. Sloggett and Joshi, "Deprivation Indicators as Predictors."
51. Smith et al., "Explaining Male Mortality Differentials."
52. O'Campo, "Invited Commentary."
53. Oakes, "The (Mis) Estimation of Neighborhood Effects."
54. Giles-Corti, Ryan, and Foster, *Increasing Density in Australia.*
55. Handy, *Critical Assessment of the Literature.*
56. Cervero, "Land-Use Mixing and Suburban Mobility."
57. Frank, Andresen, and Schmid, "Obesity Relationships."
58. Frank et al., "Many Pathways from Land Use to Health."
59. Norman et al., "Community Design and Access."
60. Nelson et al., "Built and Social Environments."
61. Gomez et al., "Built Environment Attributes and Walking Patterns."
62. Wells and Yang, "Neighborhood Design and Walking."
63. Troped et al., "The Built Environment and Location-Based Physical Activity."
64. Forsyth et al., "Design and Destinations."
65. Li et al., "Neighborhood Influences on Physical Activity."
66. Boer et al., "Neighborhood Design and Walking Trips."
67. Li et al., "Built Environment, Adiposity, and Physical Activity."
68. Hillier and Hanson, *The Social Logic of Space.*
69. Hillier, *Space Is the Machine.*
70. Hillier, "Studying Cities to Learn about Minds."
71. Hillier, "A Theory of the City as Object."
72. Hillier and Iida, "Network and Psychological Effects in Urban Movement."
73. Peponis and Wineman, "Spatial Structure of Environment and Behavior."
74. Rashid, "Studies on the Geometry of Urban Layouts."
75. Rashid, "Space Syntax."
76. Hillier, "The Art of Place and the Science of Space."
77. Rashid, *The Geometry of Urban Layouts.*
78. Carlson et al., "Inadequate Physical Activity and Health Care Expenditures."
79. Centers for Disease Control and Prevention, "Physical Activity."
80. Blackwell, Lucas, and Clarke, "Summary Health Statistics for US Adults."
81. Befort, Nazir, and Perri, "Prevalence of Obesity."
82. Nothwehr and Peterson, "Healthy Eating and Exercise."

83. Ely et al., "A Qualitative Assessment of Weight Control."
84. Larson, Story, and Nelson, "Neighborhood Environments."
85. US Department of Agriculture, "Key Statistics and Graphics."
86. Coleman-Jensen et al., *Household Food Security.*
87. Cummins and Macintyre, "Food Environments and Obesity."
88. Morland and Evenson, "Obesity Prevalence and the Local Food Environment."
89. Seligman, Laraia, and Kushel, "Food Insecurity Is Associated with Chronic Disease."
90. Casperson, Powell, and Christenson, "Physical Activity, Exercise and Physical Fitness."
91. Lee et al., "Effect of Physical Inactivity."
92. Centers for Disease Control and Prevention, *Strategies to Prevent Obesity and Other Chronic Diseases.*
93. Owen, "Sedentary Behavior: Understanding and Influencing."
94. Owen et al., "Sedentary Behaviour and Health."
95. Dunstan et al., "Television Viewing Time and Mortality."
96. Thorp et al., "Sedentary Behaviors and Subsequent Health Outcomes."
97. Sugiyama, Ding, and Owen, "Commuting by Car."
98. Sugiyama, Neuhaus, and Owen, "Active Transport, the Built Environment, and Human Health."
99. Vallance et al., "Associations of Objectively-Assessed Physical Activity."
100. Kazi et al., "A Survey of Sitting Time."
101. Healy et al., "Television Time and Continuous Metabolic Risk."
102. Owen et al. "Sedentary Behavior: Emerging Evidence."
103. Ng and Popkin, "Time Use and Physical Activity."
104. World Health Organization, *Obesity and Overweight.*
105. Stephenson and Bauman, *The Cost of Illness Attributable to Physical Inactivity.*
106. Garrow and Webster, "Quetelet's Index (W/H2) as a Measure of Fatness."
107. Freedman, Horlick, and Berenson, "A Comparison of the Slaughter Skinfold-Thickness Equations and BMI."
108. Wohlfahrt-Veje et al., "Body Fat throughout Childhood."
109. Steinberger et al., "Comparison of Body Fatness Measurements."
110. Sun et al., "Comparison of Dual-Energy X-Ray."
111. Lawlor et al., "Association between General and Central Adiposity."
112. Flegal and Graubard, "Estimates of Excess Deaths."
113. Freedman et al., "Relation of Body Mass Index and Skinfold Thicknesses."
114. Willett et al., "Comparison of Bioelectrical Impedance and BMI."
115. Centers for Disease Control and Prevention. "Healthy Weight, Nutrition, and Physical Activity."
116. Harvard Medical School, "National Comorbidity Survey."
117. National Institutes of Health, "National Institute on Drug Abuse."
118. Federal Bureau of Investigation, "Crime in the U.S."
119. Commonwealth Fund Commission on Elderly People Living Alone, *Old, Alone, and Poor.*
120. Wilson, Mottram, and Sixsmith, "Depressive Symptoms in the Very Old Living Alone."
121. Hughes, Bennett, and Hetherington, "Old and Alone."
122. Evans et al., "Living Alone and Cognitive Function in Later Life."

CHAPTER SEVEN

The Study Sample

A Description of Its Spatial, Lifestyle, and Health Data

According to the definition of small towns and cities given in chapter 2, a small town or city is *an incorporated town or a civil township that falls in the category of urban clusters (UCs) with US Census Bureau population between 2,500 and 49,999 and that is formed under the general laws of a US state or under a charter adopted by the local voters.* In Kansas, 95 cities fall in this category. The largest of these small cities is Salina, with a population of 47,230, and the smallest is Sterling, with a population of 2,515 [1].

Since it is almost impossible to find reliable spatial, lifestyle, and health data for some of the very small Kansas cities, the studies of this book will be limited to cities with 5,000 people or more. According to the US Census Bureau, 52 cities in Kansas have a population between 5,000 and 49,999. Again, not all 52 small cities are included in this book's studies. Only those that remain geographically isolated from other cities are considered here. Small cities that are generally considered suburbs of larger metropolitan areas are excluded. Cities are also excluded if the necessary data are not available for them. A list of the 36 cities selected for these studies is provided in table 7.1. Their locations are shown on a map of Kansas in figure 7.1. Nearly 560,000 people live in these cities, which is about 20% of the state's population.

This chapter describes the sample of 36 small Kansas cities selected for the studies using spatial, lifestyle, and health data collected from different sources. These sources are described first, then the built environment of these cities is described using spatial data on city size and density, key facilities and destinations, land use type and mix, and street systems. Finally, the lifestyles of the people of these cities are described using data on work-related travel behaviors,

TABLE 7.1.
Population and land area of the sample of cities

City	County	Population	Land area (square miles)
Abilene	Dickinson	6,590	4.13
Andover	Butler	12,509	6.85
Arkansas City	Cowley	12,205	7.51
Atchison	Atchison	10,771	6.83
Augusta	Butler	9,242	4.03
Chanute	Neosho	9,295	6.14
Coffeyville	Montgomery	9,876	7.60
Colby	Thomas	5,388	3.34
Concordia	Cloud	5,311	3.38
Derby	Sedgwick	23,234	7.45
Dodge City	Ford	28,117	12.60
El Dorado	Butler	12,879	6.37
Emporia	Lyon	24,560	9.90
Fort Scott	Bourbon	7,874	5.43
Garden City	Finney	27,004	8.53
Great Bend	Barton	15,840	10.60
Hays	Ellis	21,044	7.59
Hutchinson	Reno	41,642	21.10
Independence	Montgomery	9,162	4.97
Iola	Allen	5,553	4.21
Junction City	Geary	9,295	7.55
Leavenworth	Leavenworth	36,000	23.50
Liberal	Seward	21,012	11.10
McPherson	McPherson	13,189	6.14
Mulvane	Sedgwick	6,289	2.28
Newton	Harvey	19,120	9.58
Ottawa	Franklin	12,403	6.69
Paola	Miami	5,593	4.07
Parsons	Labette	10,174	10.40
Pittsburg	Crawford	20,394	12.40
Pratt	Pratt	6,963	7.42
Salina	Saline	47,867	22.70
Ulysses	Grant	6,160	2.89
Valley Center	Sedgwick	7,057	3.33
Wellington	Sumner	7,942	5.65
Winfield	Cowley	12,258	11.10

Source: City-Data.com

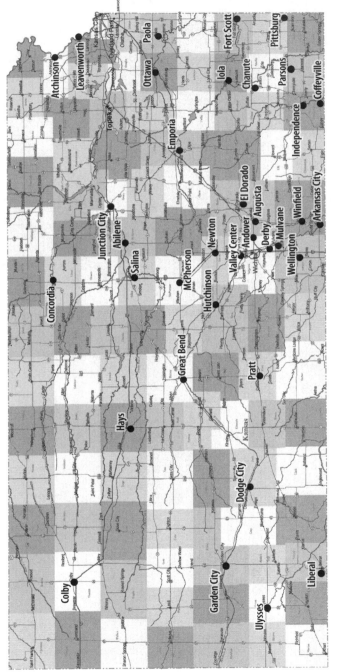

Figure 7.1. Locations of the small Kansas cities in the study sample shown as dots on a map from the Kansas Department of Transportation.

food shopping and eating behaviors, and physical and sedentary activities; and the residents' health is described using data on mortality and morbidity and physical, mental, and social health. The goal of this chapter is to provide a general understanding of the spatial characteristics of the sample of small cities, as well as the lifestyle and health in these cities in relation to the state.

Data Sources

Relevant data on the built environment and population health of small towns and cities are not easily available. When available from different sources, they have different formats, which makes them hard to use. Therefore, most studies on population health that use data collected by individual researchers generally have a very small sample size and have been limited to individual-level data [e.g., 2–10]. In contrast, most population health studies involving national or regional samples often use US Census or Centers for Disease Control and Prevention (CDC) data [e.g., 11–17]. Notably, population health studies rarely use spatial data that require researchers to do further work over and above what is already available through geographic information system (GIS) databases of individual cities, which are often inconsistent and are not updated regularly. In the absence of a common database, therefore, the data for these studies were collected from several primary and secondary (or gray) sources. In addition, I generated most spatial data for these studies through spatial network analysis performed using space syntax software programs (chapter 6). A brief description of these data sources is provided below.

Sources for Social, Economic, Housing, and Demographic Data

Some data for these studies were collected from the US Census Bureau's American Community Survey (ACS) [18]. The ACS is an ongoing survey by the US Census Bureau that collects various social, economic, housing, and demographic data on the US population. The data from the survey are available on the Census Bureau's website.

The ACS is designed to meet the needs of US federal agencies. For example, questions about how people get to work, when they leave, and the length of their commutes are used for planning improvements to roads, highways, rail lines, and bus routes and for planning emergency response routes. Because participation in the ACS is mandatory, the Office of Management and Budget (OMB) will approve only necessary questions for inclusion in the ACS. The ACS helps determine how government funds are distributed each year to communities around the country to support their projects and programs related to art and education, economic opportunities, criminal and justice systems, emergency services, health care, transportation, and many other services.

The annual ACS sample is smaller than the Census long-form sample. As a result, the ACS needs to combine population or housing data from multiple years to produce reliable numbers for geographic areas of different size. Data from the ACS are tabulated for a variety of different geographic areas that range in size from broad regions (Northeast, Midwest, South, and West) to states, cities, towns, census tracts, and block groups.

The ACS currently provides one-year estimates for geographic areas with at least 65,000 people and five-year estimates for smaller geographic areas down to the census tract and block group level. Census tracts are small geographic areas—with an average of about 4,000 people each—that are commonly used to present information for small towns, rural areas, and neighborhoods. For example, in Vermont, there are 184 census tracts with data available through the ACS five-year data products.

Sources for Crime Data

Crime statistics for these studies were abstracted from the Kansas Bureau of Investigation (KBI) report for 2018, which was the most current year for which the data was available at the time of writing. The full report may be found on the Statistics page at the KBI website [19]. Kansas crime statistics have been aggregated into two broad categories: violent crime and property crime. As described in chapter 6, *violent crimes* include murder and nonnegligent manslaughter, rape, robbery, and aggravated assault. *Property crimes* include burglary, larceny-theft, motor vehicle theft, and arson. For reasons described in chapter 6, arson data are not considered in this study. Crime rates are calculated using population estimates for each law enforcement jurisdiction provided by the Federal Bureau of Investigation. When summed to the county level, these estimates are close but not identical to the population estimates obtained by Kansas Department of Health and Environment (KDHE) from the US Census Bureau. Readers may want to refer to the original KBI report for breakdowns of the data by individual law enforcement jurisdiction and individual crime type.

Sources for Health Data

Most data on health for these studies were gathered from Kansas Health Matters [20]. Created by the Kansas Partnership for Improving Community

Health, this website brings many community health–related statistical data to one accessible, user-friendly location. The partners of Kansas Health Matters include Community Care Network of Kansas, Kansas Association of Local Health Departments, KDHE, Kansas Health Foundation, Kansas Health Institute, Kansas Hospital Association, and Kansas Foundation for Medical Care.

Kansas Health Matters presents public health data that affect the quality of Kansas residents' lives. Hospitals, health departments, community members, and policymakers can use the data to improve the health of the community. Community groups, schools, health associations, chambers of commerce, tourism bureaus, and many other organizations can use the data to show the benefits of living in Kansas. Master planners and government representatives can use the data to establish community goals on a variety of platforms.

Kansas Health Matters collects data from CDC Places [21], CDC Behavioral Risk Factor Surveillance System [22], US Census Bureau [23], ACS [24], KDHE, and KBI [19].

Sources for Spatial Data

I generated the spatial data describing street systems and networks, land use patterns, and the availability of different key facilities and destinations based on the documents prepared by local planning or GIS agencies and based on the information collected from online sources such as Google Maps and OpenStreetMap (OSM) [25]. Built by a community of mappers around the world, OSM provides and maintains very detailed spatial data on small cities to vary large metropolitan areas around the world in uniform map formats. The OSM mappers generally use aerial imagery, GPS devices, and low-tech field maps to verify if OSM is accurate and up to date. OSM is *open data*. People are free to use it for any purpose as long as they credit OSM.

Street network data for this book were generated using Depthmap [26], which includes open-source software programs for spatial analysis. Depthmap was developed based on a body of theories, methods, techniques, and measures of space syntax, some of which were described in chapter 6.

Additional Notes on Data Sources

In addition to the sources described above, some data were also collected from Data USA [27] and CensusViewer [28]. When using data from these websites, several precautions were taken. First, random tests were completed to check if these interactive websites were able to correctly identify the boundaries of small cities and towns. Second, the data from these websites were used only when they came from publicly available data sources so that the data can be independently verified. Third, data from these websites were not used in these studies if they were generated for commercial purposes using undisclosed, copyrighted formulas.

Finally, it should be noted that some temporal discordance exists in the data used for the book since they were collected by different federal, state, and nonprofit organizations in different but closely spaced years. Some spatial discordance exists in the data since different organizations often use samples of different sizes. For example, the US Census, the CDC, and the ACS use samples of different sizes.

Spatial Factors in Small Cities of Kansas

Table 7.2 provides some descriptive statistics for city size and density, availability of key destinations and facilities, land use type and mix, and properties of street systems of the sample of cities included in this study. The significance of these findings in relation to population health is difficult to assess and evaluate because the literature does not provide benchmarks. It is hoped that the findings reported here will serve as benchmarks for any future studies on the topic.

Though not shown here, histograms were used to study the patterns of distribution of the values of each spatial factor of the cities in the study sample. These patterns should help define different spatial design and planning strategies for promoting population health in these cities. For example, small cities with high housing densities may require different strategies for reducing crime than those with low densities.

The histograms showed that except for a few outliers with uncommonly large values, the values of *city size* for most small cities were clustered around the mean. The values of *census block density* did not show any extremes. The values of *housing density* showed a strong peak around the mean and a few extreme values on the higher side of the distribution.

According to the histograms showing the distributions of the values of the availability of different key facilities and destinations per 10,000 people and per square mile, except for a few cities, most of the sample cities had values clustered around the mean for these indicators.

The histograms of the distributions of the values of open areas, industrial areas, and commercial areas for the sample cities showed a few outliers on the higher side of the distribution. The distribution of residential areas was

TABLE 7.2.
Descriptive statistics for different measures of the spatial factors in the sample cities

	Minimum	Maximum	Mean	Standard deviation
Land area in square miles	2.28	23.50	8.20	5.14
Census block density (census block per square mile)	38.69	178.89	102.14	38.64
Housing density (houses and condos per square mile)	447.00	1,316.00	785.78	202.99
Health care facilities per 10,000 people	1.63	16.95	6.06	3.54
Health care facilities per square mile	0.38	3.07	1.06	0.62
Parks per 10,000 people	1.09	28.62	8.44	4.87
Parks per square mile	0.20	7.89	1.59	1.26
Grocery stores per 10,000 people	0.95	89.27	7.12	14.75
Grocery stores per square mile	0.18	18.92	1.46	3.29
Convenience stores per 10,000 people	0.00	22.67	1.84	4.34
Convenience stores per square mile	0.00	4.80	0.36	0.89
Convenience stores with gas per 10,000 people	3.70	160.12	16.14	26.06
Convenience stores with gas per square mile	0.81	33.93	3.20	5.81
Businesses per 10,000 people	9.92	70.53	30.93	10.66
Businesses per square mile	0.21	206.57	32.85	37.32
Full-service restaurants per 10,000 people	6.48	433.61	31.84	71.89
Full-service restaurants per square mile	1.08	91.89	6.58	16.01
Open area as % of total city area	0.48%	30.94%	10.19%	6.87%
Industrial area as % of total city area	0.00%	36.50%	11.67%	8.24%
Residential area as % of total city area	22.56%	79.46%	52.96%	13.47%
Commercial area as % of total city area	1.88%	29.88%	11.74%	7.39%
Institutional and other city services as % of total city area	0.00%	30.24%	10.06%	7.19%
Land use mix	0.42	0.89	0.74	0.12
Total street length (in miles)	183.43	1,566.43	487.43	239.32

(continued)

TABLE 7.2. *Continued*

	Minimum	Maximum	Mean	Standard deviation
Street length per square mile	26.67	112.44	66.80	20.03
Mean axial choice (RN)	2,203.29	43,028.00	10,289.16	9,076.99
Mean axial choice (R3)	28.04	96.66	55.78	17.81
Mean axial choice (R5)	195.78	890.09	440.03	175.52
Mean axial connectivity	2.35	5.59	3.05	0.53
Mean axial integration (RN)	0.53	1.24	0.90	0.19
Mean axial integration (R3)	1.23	1.74	1.51	0.14
Mean axial integration (R5)	1.08	1.52	1.30	0.13
Axial node count (RN)	366.00	2,775.01	1,013.41	601.63
Axial node count (R3)	20.26	59.41	36.54	10.27
Axial node count (R5)	68.55	279.32	143.36	52.92
Mean segment choice (RN)	16,221.90	292,300.92	78,967.95	63,366.82
Mean segment choice (R3)	25.11	20,715.10	6,232.19	7,136.84
Mean segment choice (R5)	120.99	83,746.60	21,275.46	24,617.39
Mean segment integration (RN)	243.20	1,627.97	643.79	284.64
Mean segment integration (R3)	17.71	458.27	168.96	155.08
Mean segment integration (R5)	29.02	795.82	289.21	266.81
Segment node count (RN)	990.00	6,928.00	2,639.95	1,440.57
Segment node count (R3)	20.57	987.18	349.21	339.47
Segment node count (R5)	47.43	2,738.37	887.09	883.59

Note: N=36

almost normal. The distribution of institutional areas had a light tail, indicating a lack of outliers.

Finally, the distribution of the values of street length showed a few outliers. With the exception of *mean axial choice at radius-n* and *axial connectivity*, most syntactic values measured on axial maps were somewhat normally distributed. In contrast, most syntactic values measured on segment maps were positively skewed with some very high values.

Lifestyle in Small Cities of Kansas

The descriptive statistics of the three categories of lifestyle in small cities of Kansas are provided in table 7.3. These categories are work-related travel behaviors, food shopping and eating behaviors, and physical and sedentary

TABLE 7.3.
Descriptive statistics for different measures of lifestyle in the sample cities

	N	Minimum	Maximum	Mean	Standard deviation	Kansas Mean	US Mean
Work-related travel behaviors							
Workers live and work in this city[1]	34	16.80	86.90	64.06	17.09	N/A	N/A
Work at home[2]	35	0.00	4.00	2.55	0.88	5.10	5.30
Drive alone to work[2]	36	72.00	89.30	81.80	4.63	82.20	76.30
Carpool to work[2]	36	7.00	22.00	11.53	3.99	9.10	9.00
Bicycle to work[2]	35	0.00	3.00	0.50	0.68	0.40	N/A
Walk to work[2]	36	0.00	6.00	2.70	1.64	2.30	2.60
Food shopping and eating behaviors							
Income spent on food at supermarket / grocery store[3]	36	19.30	27.70	23.61	1.89	24.50	N/A
Income spent on food at other stores[3]	36	3.40	70.00	6.13	10.95	4.20	N/A
Income spent on eating out[3]	36	5.70	9.30	7.24	0.85	7.00	N/A
Income spent on carryout / delivered foods[3]	36	1.00	23.00	1.88	3.62	1.30	N/A
Healthy diet rate[1]	36	45.40	53.20	48.96	1.93	48.50	N/A
Physical and sedentary activities							
People doing vigorous-intensity work activities[1]	36	19.80	24.50	22.26	1.15	22.10	N/A
People doing moderate-intensity work activities[1]	36	34.70	42.90	38.64	2.30	37.80	N/A
People walking or bicycling[1]	36	24.20	34.00	29.58	2.42	30.30	N/A
People doing vigorous-intensity recreational activities[1]	36	9.80	25.40	18.54	3.65	18.60	N/A
People doing moderate-intensity recreational activities[1]	36	32.20	49.90	41.56	3.95	41.60	N/A
Average hours a day doing sedentary activities	36	5.70	6.50	6.02	0.20	6.00	N/A
Average hours a day watching TV or videos	36	2.50	3.10	2.80	0.16	2.80	N/A
Average hours a day using a computer	36	1.00	1.40	1.22	0.09	1.20	N/A

Notes: The shaded behaviors are not considered in the studies in this book. N/A: Not available.
1. Percentage of total population
2. Percentage of working population
3. Percentage of total income

activities. When available, Kansas means and US means for these lifestyle behaviors are included.

The findings on *work-related travel behaviors* show that the mean of *workers drove alone to work* for the sample is slightly lower than the Kansas mean, but higher than the US mean; the mean of *workers carpooled to work* for the sample is higher than the Kansas and US means; the mean of *workers bicycled to work* is higher than the Kansas mean; and the mean of *workers walked to work* is higher than the Kansas and US means. In general, work-related travel behaviors for the sample of cities are somewhat similar to the state. Some of these behaviors, however, show notable variability as indicated by wide ranges. Since the percentages of *workers worked at home, workers bicycled to work,* and *workers walked to work* are small, they are not considered for further exploratory studies here.

The findings on *food shopping and eating behaviors* show that the mean of *percentage of income spent on food at supermarket/grocery store* for the sample is slightly lower than the Kansas mean; the means of *percentage of income spent on food at other stores, percentage of income spent on eating out,* and *percentage of income spent on carryout/delivered foods* are slightly higher than the Kansas means. The mean of *healthy diet rate* for the sample is also slightly higher than the Kansas mean. In simple words, the food shopping behaviors are slightly worse, but the eating behavior is slightly better in these small cities than in the state as a whole. Again, some of these behaviors have notable variability among small cities as indicated by their wide ranges. Since the percentage of *income spent on carryout/delivered foods* is small, it is not considered for further exploratory studies here.

According to the findings on *physical and sedentary activities,* in most cases the mean values of different physical and sedentary activities for the sample of small cities are close to the means of Kansas, indicating that the state as a whole may not be different from its small cities in terms of these activities. Once again, some of these behaviors have notable variability as indicated by their wide ranges. Since the values for *average hours a day watching TV or videos* and *average hours a day using computer* are small, they are not included in these exploratory studies.

Health in Small Cities of Kansas

The descriptive statistics of morbidity and mortality, physical health, mental health, and social health in the sample cities are provided in table 7.4. Again, when available, Kansas and US means for these indicators are included.

According to the findings on *morbidity and mortality*, general health conditions for the sample are similar to those of the state; the percentage of people under 65 with disability for the sample is lower than for the state; all-cause death rate per 100,000 is much higher for the sample than the state; and suicide rate for the sample is a little lower than the state rate but much higher than the national rate. It should be noted here that a wide range of variability of each indicator for the sample indicates variability in mortality and morbidity.

As the findings on *physical health* show, the means of the adult diabetes rate, obesity rate, and average body mass index (BMI) are slightly higher for the sample than for the state. In contrast, the percentage of overweight people for the sample is lower than for the state. Among these indicators, adult diabetes has a narrow range, indicating a lack of variability; but adult obesity, average BMI, and overweight have wide ranges, indicating variability.

According to the findings on *mental health*, the means of the mental health indicators for the sample are similar to those of Kansas. These indicators lack variability, as shown by their narrow ranges.

Based on the findings on *crime*, the means of the rates of murder, robbery, assault, and auto theft are lower than the state's, and those of rape, burglary, theft, and arson for the sample are higher than the state's. As shown by a very wide range, each of these indicators shows notable variability in small cities. According to the data, both violent crime rates and property crime rates are lower in small cities than in the state as a whole; but the state values are much higher than the national values. As noted, *arson* is not included in the calculation of property crime and is excluded from further studies here.

Finally, according to the findings, *people over 65 living alone* has higher values for the sample than the state, indicating more social isolation in small cities than in the state as a whole.

Conclusions

A sample of 36 of 52 small Kansas cities with a population between 5,000 and 49,999 is featured in these studies, representing 20% of the population of Kansas. Altogether, I collected data for 44 spatial factors, 19 lifestyle factors, and 24 health indicators and outcomes from several sources and used Depthmap to generate street network data.

According to the findings of the descriptive analyses of the spatial data on city size and density, key destinations and facilities, land use type and mix, and street properties, a few spatial factors have extremely high values in one

TABLE 7.4.
Descriptive statistics for different measures of health in the sample cities

	N	Minimum	Maximum	Mean	Standard deviation	Kansas Mean	US Mean
Mortality and morbidity							
People reporting general health conditions[1]	36	50.20	59.10	55.30	2.12	55.20	N/A
Percentage of people with disability under 65 years (2013–2017)[1]	35	3.30	18.70	10.16	3.48	12.70	N/A
Death rate (2016)[2]	36	10.00	2,380.00	1,290.00	560.00	934.70	N/A
Suicide rate (2018)[2]	36	0.00	57.14	18.16	15.60	18.60	14.20
Physical health							
Adult diabetes rate[3]	36	7.10	10.50	8.69	0.77	8.50	N/A
Average BMI	36	21.20	49.00	28.81	3.83	28.60	N/A
Overweight people[1]	36	6.80	36.40	32.89	4.81	33.60	N/A
Adult obesity rate[3]	36	27.80	91.30	31.02	10.37	32.30	N/A
Mental health							
Feel badly about themselves[1]	36	19.00	24.40	21.54	1.31	21.60	N/A
Have little interest in doing things[1]	36	24.10	29.40	26.26	1.43	26.50	N/A
Feel down, depressed, or hopeless[1]	36	24.00	30.90	27.50	1.66	27.50	N/A
Have thoughts that they would be better off dead[1]	36	3.50	5.30	4.44	0.46	4.40	N/A
Ever used marijuana or hashish[1]	36	61.30	68.20	65.22	1.37	65.50	N/A
Social health							
Crime[4]							
Murders	36	0.00	24.50	3.73	6.30	4.98	N/A
Rapes	36	0.00	114.70	57.52	29.39	45.95	N/A
Robberies	36	0.00	111.40	25.09	26.87	54.59	N/A
Assaults	36	42.50	911.60	284.93	189.11	316.67	N/A
Violent crimes	36	85.00	1,114.20	371.28	225.08	439.00	389.90
Burglaries	33	127.60	2,046.00	683.56	413.25	425.33	N/A
Thefts	36	793.80	5,175.70	2,535.28	900.49	2,010.26	N/A
Auto thefts	36	24.50	342.60	161.28	72.88	285.09	N/A
Property crimes	33	1,476.40	7,525.60	3,419.32	1,331.72	2,634.00	2,200.00
Arsons	36	0.00	108.90	25.52	23.10	21.30	N/A
Social isolation							
Age 65+ living alone (%) (2013–2017)	36	19.90	50.90	32.81	6.10	28.60	N/A

Note: The shaded behaviors are not considered in the studies in this book. N/A: Not available.
1. Percentage of total population
2. Per 100,000 population
3. Percentage of total adult population
4. Per 100,000 in 2014

or more cities. Therefore, when suggesting spatial strategies promoting population health, the small cities with extreme values should be considered differently from the cities without extreme values. A few spatial factors show strong peaks with values dropping sharply from a high mean, and others show weak peaks with values dropping slowly from the mean. Spatial factors with strong peak distributions should also be considered differently than spatial factors with weak peak distributions in spatial strategies aimed at affecting the built environment of these cities for health promotion.

The descriptive analysis of lifestyle shows similar work-related travel behaviors in small Kansas cities and statewide. The analysis also shows worse food shopping behaviors but better eating behavior in these small cities than in the state as a whole. Additionally, the analysis shows similar patterns of physical and sedentary activities in small cities and statewide. Based on these findings, it may be suggested that spatial strategies should focus on food shopping behaviors more than the other lifestyle behaviors in these small cities if the goal is to improve them to the state level. However, since lifestyle behaviors are generally worse in Kansas than the United States [20], spatial strategies should be considered for improving all lifestyle behaviors in small Kansas cities. These spatial strategies should also be considered on a case-by-case basis because several lifestyle behaviors show notable variability among these cities.

Findings of the descriptive analysis show that people reporting general health conditions and the percentage of people under 65 with disability may need less attention in small Kansas cities if the goal is to keep their values close to those of the state. Findings also show wide variability of these morbidity indicators in these cities, showing a need to reduce variability using spatial strategies. In contrast, all-cause death rate is much higher in small Kansas cities than in the state as a whole, and suicide rates in these small cities remain close to the state rate but higher than the national rate, showing a need to reduce these rates using spatial strategies.

The descriptive analysis shows that the means of the values of physical health indicators are close to Kansas means. This indicates that physical health in small cities may be similar to that in the state, but when compared nationally, physical health in these cities is generally worse than in the United States overall [20]. Whenever possible, spatial strategies should be considered for improving physical health in small Kansas cities. Spatial strategies should also be considered for reducing high variability in physical health indicators observed in the study.

The descriptive analysis shows that the means of the values of mental health indicators are also close to Kansas means, indicating that mental health in these small cities may be similar to mental health in the state. When compared nationally, however, mental health in these cities remains generally worse than that in the United States [20]. Whenever possible, spatial strategies should be considered for improving mental health status in small Kansas cities. Since these indicators show less variability, similar spatial strategies can be used for mental health promotion in these small cities.

The descriptive analysis shows notable differences in the values of crimes between small cities and the state. The means of some crimes are lower, whereas the means of the others are higher than the means of the state. The analysis also shows wide variability for all the crimes in these cities, which indicates that spatial strategies must be developed and used carefully to reduce crime in response to variability in these cities. Interestingly, violent crimes are lower and property crimes are higher in these cities than in the state or the nation. Therefore, more attention is needed to reduce property crimes in these cities.

Finally, social isolation, described using people 65 and older who are living alone, is higher in these cities than in the state. Again, more attention is needed to reduce social isolation in small Kansas cities.

The next few chapters explore the spatial associations of lifestyle and health using correlational analyses. Chapter 8 presents the correlational analyses between spatial factors and lifestyle for the whole sample, and chapter 9 presents the analyses for the subsamples defined based on the factors of rurality. Following this, chapter 10 provides the correlational analysis between spatial factors and health outcomes and indicators for the whole sample, and chapter 11 provides analysis for the subsamples defined based on the factors of rurality.

NOTES

1. Cubit Planning, "Kansas Cities by Population."
2. Boehmer et al., "What Constitutes an Obesogenic Environment?"
3. Brownson et al., "A Multilevel Ecological Approach to Promoting Walking."
4. Collins et al., "The Impact of the Built Environment on Young People's Physical Activity Patterns."
5. Doescher et al., "The Built Environment and Utilitarian Walking."
6. Evenson et al., "Assessing Urban and Rural Neighborhood Characteristics."
7. Huang et al., "Neighborhood Environment and Physical Activity."
8. Joens-Matre et al., "Rural-Urban Differences."

9. Li, Chi, and Jackson, "Perceptions and Barriers to Walking."

10. Stewart et al., "Comparing Associations between the Built Environment and Walking."

11. Befort, Nazir, and Perri, "Prevalence of Obesity among Adults."

12. Bennett, Olatosi, and Probst, *Health Disparities*.

13. Bethea et al., "The Relationship between Rural Status, Individual Characteristics, and Self-Rated Health."

14. Cohen et al., "A Closer Look at Rural-Urban Health Disparities."

15. Davis et al., "Obesity and Related Health Behaviors."

16. Fan, Wen, and Kowaleski-Jones, "Rural-Urban Differences in Objective and Subjective Measures of Physical Activity."

17. Fan, Wen, and Wan, "Built Environment and Active Commuting."

18. US Census Bureau, "About the American Community Survey."

19. Kansas Bureau of Investigation, "Statistics."

20. Kansas Health Matters, "Kansas Health Matters."

21. Centers for Disease Control and Prevention, "Places."

22. Centers for Disease Control and Prevention, "Behavioral Risk Factor Surveillance System."

23. US Census Bureau, "United States Census Bureau."

24. US Census Bureau, "American Community Survey (ACS)."

25. OpenStreetMap, "OpenStreetMap."

26. Varoudis, "DepthmapX."

27. Data USA, "Data USA."

28. Moonshadow Mobile, "CensusViewer."

PART FOUR

RURALITY, SPATIAL FACTORS, AND LIFESTYLE IN SMALL CITIES OF KANSAS

Spatial Associations of Lifestyle in Small Cities of Kansas

Correlational Analyses

In this chapter, the associations of spatial (design and planning) factors with lifestyle in small Kansas cities are studied using correlational analyses. As noted in chapters 6 and 7, work-related travel behaviors, food shopping and eating behaviors, and physical and sedentary activities are considered in lifestyle. Based on the findings reported in chapter 7, from work-related travel behaviors, *workers worked at home, workers bicycled to work*, and *workers walked to work*; from food shopping and eating behaviors, *income spent on carryout/delivered foods*; and from physical and sedentary activities, *average hours a day watching TV or videos* and *average hours a day using computer* are not considered in these studies.

As noted in chapters 6 and 7, the categories of spatial factors include city size and density defined in spatial terms, availability of key destinations and facilities, land use types and mix, and various street properties. In the literature, these spatial factors generally show frequent associations with lifestyle in urban areas. Similar studies in rural counties and small towns, however, are almost absent. A brief review of some of these studies is provided here. Following this, the findings of correlational analyses involving spatial factors and lifestyle for small cities of Kansas are reported using correlation coefficient (Spearman's rho) and their significance level (p-value).

The correlational analyses include 44 spatial factors and 13 lifestyle behaviors, producing 572 correlations to report. Given this large number, the correlations are not reviewed separately in reporting the spatial associations of lifestyle. Instead, the correlations of each spatial variable are aggregated by the lifestyle categories for review (work-related travel behaviors, food shopping and eating behaviors, and physical and sedentary activities). The total numbers of significant correlations for each category are considered as way to determine how sensitive a lifestyle category is to spatial factors. In general, a lifestyle category with more correlations is considered to be more sensitive to spatial factors than a category with fewer correlations. The findings of the correlational analyses are presented in tables 8.1 and 8.2 (available online at https://hdl.handle.net/1808/34227) and are explained shortly.

City Size and Lifestyle

Cities grow by taking advantage of agglomeration economies, where firms and people locate near one another to save cost and gain efficiency. From this viewpoint, small cities are inefficient because they do not have agglomerations large enough to drive their economies upward. As population and firms in a city increase, however, so do economic opportunities, which attracts more people. The process continues until a time when the economies of agglomeration return no significant benefit because of inefficiencies related to size—a phenomenon that has received significant attention in the literature [1–9].

More notably, the growth of cities has been greatly accelerated by mass car ownership during the last century or so. The greater freedom available to car owners has meant that people are able to travel farther, combining where they live, work, play, and learn in ways that would be difficult or impossible by other modes of transportation. As result, we observe significant geographic dispersion not only of residential areas but also of commercial functions and public facilities and amenities. Most often, developers of these facilities, amenities, and services use mobility to exploit economies of scale. They invest at fewer, better-equipped locations separated by significant spatial distance.

Very big cities inevitably become inefficient. They have many desirable locations separated by undesirable spatial distance. Often moderated by planning policies, cultural norms, density, land use and economic diversity, and spatial structure, they generally force people to drive more and longer. On many occasions, these cities produce too much traffic, which causes congestion. Uneven distribution of resources in big cities gives rise to environmental and social justice issues. Predicated on car dependence, large cities create problems of land-take (loss of countryside); wasteful energy use, pollution, and CO_2 emissions; deterring active travel (walking and biking); and severely restricting opportunities among groups within the population who do not and cannot have or use cars [10–19]. These problems lead to poor lifestyle behaviors for many residents.

In contrast, small cities remain inefficient for different reasons. Without the benefits of agglomeration economies, they cannot develop physical and social institutions and infrastructures that promote good living conditions. Since there is never enough for anyone in these cities, people with some mobility seek opportunities elsewhere. To access these opportunities, people travel to other—usually larger—cities or take frequent "between-town" journeys. These journeys are generally long, often impracticable for walking and biking and for public transport service because of relatively low levels of demand.

We therefore observe higher volumes of car use in smaller towns and rural settlements as a product of longer average journeys and as a greater proportion of journeys by car. Some car use is also a product of socioeconomic differences between settlements, but a clear overall gradient remains even when these differences are accounted for [20, 21]. In practice, a small city is likely to be "self-contained" if it is a service center within an extensive rural area. In contrast, relatively close alternative economic and other opportunities prompt a higher proportion of external journeys for small-city residents within an urbanized region. As the proportion of external journeys grows, a small city observes a greater decrease in daytime population, which translates into less economic activity—a process that creates additional negative impacts on a city that rarely has enough resources to provide better lifestyles and to deal with its population health problems.

Overall, the literature indicates numerous potential and empirical associations between city size and lifestyle, focusing primarily on commuting behaviors using cars only. The associations of city size with many other work-related travel behaviors, food shopping and eating behaviors, and physical and sedentary activities remain unknown, however, for both large and small cities. In this regard, findings reported in this chapter may be relevant.

Things We Observe in Small Cities of Kansas

According to the findings of this study, city size measured using land area shows no statistically significant association with different work-related travel behaviors. Even though we do not know why no correlation exists, it is quite possible that these cities are simply not large enough to provide economic benefits needed for an impact on work-related travel behaviors. If that is indeed the case, then the larger ones among these cities, if considered separately, may show some associations with work-related travel behaviors—something that will be explored in the next chapter.

City size, however, shows statistically significant associations of moderately large effect size with two out of four different food shopping and eating behaviors. The association is positive for *income spent at supermarkets or grocery stores*, and it is negative for *healthy diet rate*. A separate analysis shows a positive correlation between city size and poverty, indicating that the larger of these small cities are poorer; therefore, it is possible that people in these cities spend a larger part of their income at supermarkets and grocery stores. For the same reason, *healthy diet rate* may show a negative association with city size. As cities get bigger, they get poorer; as a result, *healthy diet rate* decreases. This will be explored further in the next chapter.

Finally, city size shows statistically significant associations with two out of six different physical and sedentary activities with moderate to large effect size. The association is negative for *people doing moderate-intensity work activities*, and it is positive for *people walking and bicycling*. The former association can be explained in terms of safety—as cities get bigger, they may have more safety issues, which may negatively affect *people doing moderate-intensity work activities*, assuming that these are mostly outdoor activities in small cities. The latter association may be explained using poverty. Since people in bigger small cities tend to have less wealth, they may simply drive less and walk and bike more. More studies are necessary on these issues.

We do not know exactly why correlations are found between city size and lifestyle in small cities. Given the frequency of these correlations, however, city size should not be overlooked in matters related to lifestyle in small cities of Kansas. More studies are needed to find out why work-related behaviors are not consistently associated with city size.

Density and Lifestyle

Numerous studies report associations between density and lifestyle [22–34]. Several of these studies report consistent positive relations between density and walking for transportation and recreation [35]. Several others report significant associations between density and travel mode choices, even when controlling for nonurban form factors for both work and shopping trips. Still others report significant relationships between population and employment density and mode choice for single-occupancy vehicle (SOV), transit, and walking for both work and shopping trips. Others report an increase in transit usage and walking and a decrease in SOV usage with an increase in density and land use mix [26].

More specifically, in low-density developments, longer journey distances and an accompanying sparseness of public transport result in personal dependence on car use, reducing physical activity (PA). In low-density developments, distance can also deter active travel, such as walking and biking, partly due to out-of-town commercial, recreational, and work activities. As a result, longer journeys can have malign effects on PA. Unsurprisingly, the prevalence of obesity and chronic diseases is higher in low-density developments [36, 37]. In contrast, in high-density developments, short average journey distances reduce the overall volume of travel. In these developments, different activities are placed within convenient walking or biking distance. High-density developments create greater intensity of travel demand, supporting the conditions for more frequent and commercially viable transit services. In combination, therefore, car use per head is much lower in high-density developments. The creation of higher-density compact cities, however, needs to be paired with an understanding of the impacts of increasing density on crime and residents' feelings of safety. Indeed, one key ingredient that facilitates local PA is how safe residents feel.

The results on the links between density and lifestyle are rarely straightforward. For example, higher residential densities and land use mix are often interdependent. It is not density per se that increases physical activities such as walking and biking; rather, density works in combination with other built environment features [38]. Walking for transport and, sometimes, for recreation is largely dependent on having somewhere to walk to—that is, a mix of shops, services, and transport connections. At the same time, neighborhoods require sufficient residential density to ensure that destinations are proximate to housing and that local businesses are viable. How much density is required to optimize physical activity outcomes? If residential density were viewed through a "health" lens, then the priority performance criterion for density would be the level that promotes health and well-being. Using a case study approach of compact developments that optimize walking outcomes, Campoli [39] concluded that the lower end of the optimum range of densities *begins* at eight units of housing per acre, or 20 dwellings per hectare. This threshold is consistent with empirical Australian evidence where densities of at least 20 dwellings per hectare were observed to be critical for health promotion through PA [40].

In summary, a certain level of density in a neighborhood is essential. It determines the presence, proximity, and viability of local amenities, such as public transport, shops, and services, which promote health and well-being. Conducted in urban areas, most studies on the relationships between density and lifestyle may not be relevant to small cities because the density of an urban area within a metropolitan region and the density of a small city in a rural area may not be comparable. Therefore, a need to study these associations in small cities exists. This book may help fulfill that need.

Things We Observe in Small Cities of Kansas

According to the findings of this study, except one behavior, census block density and housing density do not show any correlations with lifestyle, which includes work-related travel behaviors, food shopping and eating behaviors, and physical and sedentary activities. *Income spent on food at other stores* is the only behavior that shows a positive correlation of a moderate effect size with census block density in small Kansas cities. It is possible that people have less access to conventional grocery stores in dense small cities. As a result, they end up spending more on food in other stores.

That the density of small cities of Kansas may not be associated with lifestyle indicates a need for future studies on the topic. It is possible that density, as defined in this study, is different from that used in studies involving urban areas. It is also possible that density in these cities is too low to have any impact on lifestyle. Like urban areas, there may be a threshold value for density to have an impact on lifestyle in small cities. If that is the case, then small cities with higher density may show better associations with lifestyle behaviors than small cities with lower densities—something that will be explored in the next chapter.

Availability of Key Destinations and Functions and Lifestyle

Retail functions such as shops and commercial facilities are choice destinations, so it is expected that they would affect lifestyle. Likewise, the literature generally shows close proximity to potential amenities, such as shops and service, destinations as an important predictor of walking [41], but some studies report no significant association [30, 42]. The literature also shows a beneficial association between the total walk time, indicating PA, and the number of commercial and select establishments within buffers at different walking distances [43, 44], and between the amount of retail floor area and PA among adolescent boys [45]. Additionally, the literature shows that an increase in commercial floor area increases active travel in the form of transit and ride-sharing commutes [46]. In summary, the evidence presented in the literature indicates that accessibility and availability of (expressed as proximity to, number of, or density of) retail and commercial functions may encourage walking and other forms of PA among adults and adolescents.

According to a large body of literature, proximity to parks and green spaces is associated with increased PA [47–51], though the strength of association may vary for people of different socioeconomic status and age [52]. Large attractive public open spaces with supportive infrastructure for PA may promote recreational walking and other forms of exercise [53, 54]. Engagement in after-school PA is enhanced if the local park contains play or sports equipment [48, 55]. Parks with supportive infrastructure are used frequently for PA in neighborhoods with low land use diversity [56]. According to some studies in rural and small communities, proximity to parks with walking and hiking trails may be positively associated with PA [57–59]. According to others, proximity to parks may not always be associated with PA for everyone living in rural areas [60, 61]. Overall, evidence suggests that access to and availability of parks and green spaces may be positively associated with lifestyle in urban areas, but studies in rural and small communities show no clear association.

Studies show that recreational activities, such as walking and biking, among children and adults increase when PA resources, including recreational destinations, are in close proximity [62, 63]. For example, increased access to and availability of sports centers increases walking among adults [64] and moderate to vigorous physical activity (MVPA) among boys and girls [48, 55, 63, 65, 66]. Residents are more likely to meet required MVPA in census blocks with a higher number of facilities relative to those with zero facilities per block group [67]. A number of studies have provided compelling evidence on the associations between access to local sporting or recreational facilities and adults' PA and sports participation in high socioeconomic status neighborhoods [68], but the evidence on similar associations for adults with access to a motor vehicle is less compelling. There is some suggestion that the convenience, rather than the proximity of PA and recreational destinations, is more important [69]. Hence, the proximity of PA and recreational destinations near or en route to work may be more pertinent to adults' PA levels than their proximity to home.

Regarding socioeconomic inequalities, Diez-Roux et al. [70] found that the density of PA resources was beneficially associated with slightly higher odds of achieving recommended PA levels among minority and low-income residents. Regarding gender differences, Norman et al. [45] reported significant associations between MVPA and the number of recreational facilities within a one-mile network catchment of each respondent's residence, except for girls. Regarding education, Pan et al. [71] found that the availability of PA facilities was more strongly associated with higher levels of PA among respondents with a university degree than those with less education. Regarding cost of services, a cross-continental study encompassing 11 countries found that higher levels of PA were reported in neighborhoods with more low-cost recreational facilities [44].

Several studies of rural and small communities report significant associations between use of, distance to, or access to recreational facilities and PA [53, 60, 72–75]. Some of these studies show that limited access to recreational resources, whether perceived or real, discourages PA in rural communities. Others show that lack of accessible walking trails is perceived to be a barrier to PA by American Indian women [76], rural African American women [77], and rural parents of children in diverse locations throughout the United States [58]. Yet others show that access to facilities in the neighborhood generally does not increase PA [78] but does increase regular walking [74]. Positive relationships were observed between use of PA facilities and regular PA among adults with diabetes [75]. When lower- and higher-income rural adults were considered separately, significant positive associations were reported between use of indoor gyms and regular PA among those with higher incomes but not among those with lower incomes [60]. Studies in rural communities also show that use of community malls was not associated with regular walking [60, 72], whereas those who reported not using malls (versus no malls reported) for PA were less likely to walk regularly [72].

It is noteworthy that individuals' perceptions of the availability of PA facilities may not be associated with objectively measured availability of PA facilities [69]. It is also noteworthy that a few studies have reported counterintuitive findings, indicating that the use of a particular sports or recreation facility might be governed by individual preferences rather than by availability and access within a defined neighborhood. In other words, the presence of a facility may not imply its usage if it is not the type of facility that an individual chooses to use. In terms of the economies of service provision and planning, this implies that these services cannot be substituted for one another and that people cannot be expected necessarily to use the nearest facility [79]. Among other counterintuitive findings reported in the literature include no significant association between the proximity (or accessibility) to and the intensity (or density) of recreation facilities and PA or body mass index [80], and between PA and proximity to PA facilities described using perceived and objectively measured predictors [81]. These counterintuitive findings indicate that confounding factors could have been present.

In summary, the literature reports many studies on the associations between the availability of key destinations and facilities and lifestyle. Most of these studies used parks and green spaces, PA facilities, and retail outlets. Studies involving parks and green spaces and PA facilities were conducted in both urban and rural areas. Studies involving rural areas generally do not identify small cities as a subject of interest, which indicates a need for studies on the associations between availability of key destinations and facilities and lifestyle in small towns.

Things We Observe in Small Cities of Kansas

According to the findings of the correlational analyses, the availability of key facilities and destinations, described as numbers per 10,000 people and square mile, shows several statistically significant associations of moderate to large effect size with work-related behaviors. In small Kansas cities, as the availability of supermarkets or grocery stores, convenience stores, convenience stores with gas, and full-service restaurants increases, the number of people who live and work in the city decreases. One way to explain this finding is that as the number of key destinations and facilities increases in small cities, the number of jobs available in these cities also increases. Since small cities have a limited supply of working population, the need for those living outside the city increases. As a result, the relative number of people who live and work in the city decreases. Another way to explain this finding is that as the number of key destinations and facilities increases in small cities, these cities get crowded, pushing a segment of working population out of the city.

In contrast, in small cities of Kansas, as the availability of supermarkets or grocery stores, convenience stores with gas, and full-service restaurants increases, the number of people who drive alone to work increases but the number of people who carpool to work decreases. One explanation may be that in a small city with more of these facilities people are richer; as a result, more people drive to work alone, which brings down the number of people who carpool to work. This is supported by a strong and statistically significant negative correlation found between people who drive alone and people who carpool in a separate analysis.

The availability of key facilities and destinations also shows several statistically significant associations of moderate to large effect size with food shopping and eating behaviors. The findings show that as the availability of super-markets, grocery stores, and convenience stores with gas increases, income spent at these stores decreases. Could this be related to the fact that more supermarkets, grocery stores, and conveniences stores with gas are generally found in more affluent areas of the city, where people spend less of their income on food? The findings also show that as the availability of full-service restaurants increases, income spent at supermarkets and grocery stores decreases. These findings indicate that if people are eating more frequently in full-service restaurants they may go to supermarkets and grocery stores less frequently. A negative correlation between the availability of full-service restaurants and the percentage of income spent at supermarkets and grocery stores seems to support this explanation. Additionally, as the availability of supermarkets, grocery stores, and full-service restaurants increases in these small cities, the percentage of people taking healthy diet increases. This makes sense because these food outlets generally provide healthy foods.

In addition, the availability of key facilities and destinations shows several statistically significant associations with different types of PA in small Kansas cities. In the small cities with more health care facilities, supermarkets or grocery stores, convenience stores with gas, and full-service restaurants, people seem to do more moderate-intensity work activities but less biking and walking. These findings can be explained by a negative correlation found in a separate analysis between moderate-intensity work-related activities and walking and biking to work, indicating that when people do more work-related PA, they may be less eager to bike or walk.

In contrast, in small cities with more business establishments, people seem to do less moderate-intensity work activities but more biking and walking. It is possible that in many business establishments, people generally do not do PA while working; therefore, they remain eager to walk and bike. This is supported by a negative correlation between moderate-intensity work-related activities and walking and biking to work, as noted, and a positive correlation between sedentary work-related activities and walking and biking to work in a separate analysis.

The associations between the availability of key facilities and destinations with sedentary activities seem to follow a similar pattern. In cities with more supermarkets or grocery stores, convenience stores with gas, and full-service restaurants, people report more sedentary activity because they walk and bike less. In contrast, in cities with more business establishments, people report less sedentary activity because they are walking and biking more.

Vigorous-intensity work and recreational activities and moderate-intensity recreational activities generally have no statistically significant association with the availability of key facilities and destinations in small cities of Kansas, indicating a need for further studies.

In summary, the findings reported in this section indicate that with several significant correlations of large effect size the availability of key destinations and facilities is important for lifestyle in small Kansas cities.

Land Use and Lifestyle

Several studies report associations between land use and lifestyle behaviors [35]. Besides promoting a range of viable economic opportunities or attractive destinations, land use diversity, where many destinations are found close to one another, may encourage multipurpose walking and bike trips, reducing dependence on cars [35]. For example, residents of neighborhoods with commercial and industrial land use mix (LUM) show significantly higher transport-related walking as compared to residents of neighborhoods with a recreational profile [82, 83]. Using measures defined based on the number of different types of businesses in a neighborhood, Boer et al. [84] reported that moving from two different business types to three types significantly improved the probability of walking. Similar improvements in walk propensity were reported when moving from three to four different business types in the neighborhood. Troped et al. [34] used four-category LUM (residential, commercial, recreational, and urban public) and reported a significant beneficial association between LUM and MVPA within a one-kilometer home buffer.

In a study of four neighborhoods in the San Francisco Bay Area, Handy [85] found that residents of traditional, mixed-use neighborhoods on average made two to four more walk and cycle trips per week to their neighborhood retail stores than those living in proximity to areas served primarily by automobile-oriented strip retail establishments. In another study of six communities of Palm Beach County in Florida, Ewing et al. [86] found that residents of sprawling suburban areas characterized by homogeneous land uses reported significantly more per capita vehicle hours traveled (VHT) than residents of mixed traditional neighborhoods served by internal community services in the form of shopping, recreation, and school facilities. In yet another study, Frank and Pivo [26] found that increases in density (both employment and population) and LUM improved transit usage and walking to work and shopping trips and reduced the use of single-occupant vehicles for work and shopping trips.

Cervero [87] found significant associations between the presence of LUM within 300 feet of a respondent's residence and increased propensity for active travel, after adjusting for residential densities and vehicle ownership levels. In contrast, the presence of LUM between 300 feet and 1 mile of residences was associated with higher levels of auto commuting. This was attributed to the relative ease of efficiently linking work and shopping trips through vehicular trips beyond the threshold of 300 feet. The researchers, however, had employed a relatively simple binary measure of LUM of 0 and 1, indicating the presence or absence of nonresidential uses within some predefined neighborhood. In another study examining how the "3Ds"—density, diversity, and design—affect trip rates and mode choice of residents in the San Francisco Bay Area, Cervero and Kockelman [88] found that, along with density and pedestrian-oriented designs, land use diversity reduces trip rates and encourage non-auto travel in statistically significant ways, though their influences appear to be fairly marginal. In contrast, Cerin et al. [89] found no significant associations between LUM and weekly minutes of walking for transport.

Overall, studies reported in the literature generally do not focus on any particular land use type. Instead, they focus on LUM and report that higher mix is generally synonymous with the presence of diverse destinations, shorter trips lengths, and hence a more permeable and walkable neighborhood and that higher mix generally promote more PA. Similar studies in small cities and rural areas do not exist. Therefore, there is a need for studies on the associations between lifestyle and LUM, which the studies of this book address.

Things We Observe in Small Cities of Kansas

According to the findings of the correlational analyses, among the land use types considered in this study, only industrial land use shows statistically significant associations with work-related travel behaviors. In these cities, as industrial areas increase, the number of people who live and work in the city also increases. A statistically significant negative correlation between industrial land use and per capita income and a statistically significant positive correlation between industrial land use and poverty found in a separate analysis seem to support that people in small cities with more industrial areas are generally poor and, therefore, do not have cars to drive to work.

Concerning land use types and food shopping and eating behaviors in small Kansas cities, the findings of the correlational analyses show that as industrial land use increases, income spent at supermarkets and grocery stores also increases. The finding can be explained by the fact that people who live in cities with more industrial land use are poorer, as indicated by a statistically significant positive correlation between industrial land use and poverty in these cities. Since people have less wealth, they probably spend a greater portion of their income in supermarkets and grocery stores. The findings also show that as industrial land use increases in a city, the percentage of people taking healthy diet decreases, again indicating that people in cities with more industrial land use may be living in poverty.

Concerning land use types and physical and sedentary activities, the findings of the study show that as open areas increase, walking and biking decrease, and as industrial land use increases, biking and walking increase and sedentary activities decrease. These findings indicate that the effects these areas have on PA in small cities may not be similar to the effects these areas have on PA in urban areas, where open areas generally increase walking and biking. That open areas do not have notable associations or have only marginal associations with lifestyle in small cities is surprising but not without reasons. In small cities, open areas may be less needed because of a lack of density. They may also be poorly maintained and unsafe for public use.

Finally, with the exception of one weak correlation with income spent on food at supermarkets or grocery stores, LUM does not show any associations with lifestyle in small cities. This is certainly surprising because LUM consistently shows statistically significant associations with lifestyle in urban areas. This and other findings reported in this section indicate a need for more studies on the association between land use types and mix and lifestyle in small cities.

Street Properties and Lifestyle

The literature reports numerous studies that show associations between street properties and lifestyle behaviors. Several use buffers. In one example, Wells and Yang [32] studied the effects of total linear length of streets, number of street intersections, and number of cul-de-sacs on walking levels within a quarter-mile street network buffer prior to and after relocation to new neighborhoods in four towns of the Southeast US states of Georgia, Alabama, and Florida. They found that relocation to neighborhoods with fewer cul-de-sacs was associated with an increase of 5,303 steps per week (or 757 more steps per day) after controlling for demographic variables. Gomez et al. [90] defined street connectivity as the number of street links divided by the number of street nodes within a 500-meter buffer of the neighborhood centroid and observed that residents in high-connectivity neighborhoods are more likely to walk for at least 60 minutes than residents in low-connectivity neighborhoods. Troped et al. [34] defined intersection density as the number of intersections within a one-kilometer network buffer divided by the total street segment length. They reported a positive significant relationship between their calculated intersection density and levels of MVPA within a one-kilometer home buffer.

Among studies conducted without buffer, Forsyth et al. [42] reported a negative association between travel and leisure walking and street patterns expressed in several terms, including intersections per unit area, number of access points per unit area, road length per unit area, intersections per unit area, ratio of four-way intersections to all intersections, four-way intersections per unit land area, ratio of three-way intersections to all intersections, and connected node ratio. In contrast, Li et al. [47] reported a positive association between the number of street intersections per unit area of a neighborhood and walking activity at the neighborhood level. Boer et al. [84] reported significant associations between the numbers of four-way intersections with observed walk propensity within a neighborhood in 10 US metropolitan areas. Li et al. [91] used the number of street intersections divided by the area of the census block in square miles as their measure of density of street connectivity and found that neighborhoods with high density of street connectivity were significantly related to higher prevalence of walking activity and meeting PA recommendations.

Some studies involving street properties and lifestyle indicate a need to consider accessibility at multiple spatial scales. For example, Handy [85] considered two components of accessibility, namely micro-level local accessibility associated with the closeness to local opportunities of activity and macro-level regional accessibility associated with the degree of connectivity to large regional service destinations. Comparing the levels of local and regional accessibility of the Santa Clara and Santa Rosa Valleys of the San Francisco Bay Area, Handy found that residents of high-local-accessibility areas generally reported significantly higher than average walking trips to local commercial destinations. She also found that in higher-regional-accessibility areas, the downtown shopping trips did not appear to substitute for trips to regional shopping centers. On the contrary, in low-regional-accessibility areas, the downtown shopping trips acted as a substitute for regional trips to some extent. In a subsequent study conducted on the San Francisco Bay Area, Handy [92] found that traditional neighborhoods with higher physical accessibility to community resources are generally associated with a higher proportion of walking trips.

Studies involving street properties and adolescent behaviors seem to indicate differences between boys and girls and between those living in urban, suburban, and rural areas. In one of the studies involving adolescents, Norman et al. [45] reported that intersection density, defined as the number of street intersections per acre of a one-mile street network buffer around participants' residences, was negatively associated with propensity for MVPA only in the case of adolescent girls, while no association was observed in the case of boys. In another study, Nelson et al. [93] used the density of three-way and four-way intersections, the ratio of observed to maximum possible route alternatives between nodes, the ratio of observed node linkages to the maximum possible links in the network, and a cyclomatic index, which is the number of route alternatives between nodes, to characterize connectivity within a three-kilometer buffer for a comparative study on the associations of street connectivity with adolescent overweight and activity in six distinct classes of neighborhoods—rural working class, exurban, newer suburban, upper-middle class and older suburban, mixed-race urban, and low-socioeconomic-status inner-city areas. They reported that adolescents in older suburban areas had higher odds of being physically active than those of newer suburbs. They also reported that adolescents in low-socioeconomic-status inner-city neighborhoods had higher odds of being more active, though the finding was not significant.

In general, connected street networks have been shown to facilitate walking for transport in most age groups [94, 95] and to promote recreational walking in adult and elderly populations [91, 96]. Similarly, for adolescents with some level of independence, having a connected street network facilitates their mobility in the same way that it does for adults. The evidence for younger children is less clear [97–99]. Neighborhoods with fewer connected streets and more cul-de-sacs provide additional spaces for young children's active play, and they are often perceived by parents as safer [100]. Yet children are more likely to walk to school [101, 102] and to be more independently mobile [103, 104] where there is high street connectivity and low traffic volume. Conversely, in neighborhoods with a combination of high street connectivity and high traffic volume, children are less likely to walk to school [101], and boys are less likely to cycle [105].

Rarely does a set of modeling techniques cover as many traffic-flow and travel-behavior related research issues as does space syntax [106, 107], even though criticisms and limitations of space syntax persist [108–111]. Space syntax techniques have been used in several more frequently cited studies describing, explaining, and theorizing the density and distribution of traffic flow [106, 112–115]. They have been also used in studies explaining wide-ranging issues related to different modalities, such as the flow of pedestrians [116–120], bicycles [121, 122], and cars [109, 123, 124]. Additionally, space syntax techniques have been used in studies explaining different behavioral outcomes related to traffic flow, such as travel time [125, 126], transit ridership [127], and wayfinding and spatial decision-making [128–131].

Furthermore, attributes of street networks measured using space syntax have been demonstrated to influence retail distribution [132, 133] and individual behaviors in shopping areas [115], both of which have the potential to impact local food environments and the food-related behaviors of consumers. Thus, developing a more nuanced and substantial understanding of local food environments requires empirical studies on the impact of street network attributes on local food environments and food-related individual behaviors. Without this understanding, it is difficult to develop comprehensive planning solutions to the problem of local food insecurity and to improve public health [134].

According to the literature, therefore, the associations between lifestyle and street properties have been studied extensively. Some of these studies report the relationships between street properties and PA involving rural areas and small cities. Among them, some use national data and therefore are not sensitive to local differences. Some that use local data have either a very narrow scope or a very small sample size and therefore do not allow within- and between-group comparisons. As a result, it is difficult to draw any general conclusions on the relationships between street properties and lifestyle in small cities, indicating a need for more studies to understand these relationships better. It is, however, important to note that the techniques of space syntax, which have been successfully used in many urban studies, have not been applied to behavioral studies in rural areas and small towns and cities at all, indicating a need to apply these techniques in studies on lifestyle behaviors in small towns and cities.

Things We Observe in Small Cities of Kansas

According to the findings of the correlational analyses, total street length shows no statistically significant association with work-related travel behaviors, one statistically significant association with food shopping and eating behaviors, and two statistically significant associations with physical and sedentary activities. Street density shows no statistically significant associations with work-related travel behaviors, food shopping and eating behaviors, and physical and sedentary activities.

Street network properties, however, have statistically significant associations of moderate to large effect size with two types of work-related travel behaviors—live and work in the city, and carpool to work—among the three considered in this study. The work-related travel behavior not associated with street properties is drive alone to work. According to these findings, as some mean integration values, mean choice values, and node counts increase, the number of people who live and work in the city and the number of people who carpool to work increase. Recall that integration measures accessibility, choice measures movement potentials, and node count measures directional choices in street systems. These findings therefore seem to indicate that more accessibility, movement potential, and directional choices may encourage more people to live and work in the city and encourage carpooling.

Almost all street properties have statistically significant positive associations of moderate to large effect size with income spent on food at supermarkets and grocery stores, indicating that more accessibility, movement potentials, and directional choices increase this behavior in small cities. Almost all street properties also have statistically significant negative associations of moderate to large effect size with people taking healthy diet, indicating that in small cities people take less-healthy diet when street systems are characterized by more accessibility, movement potentials, and directional choices. The food shopping and eating behaviors not associated with street network properties are income spent on food at other stores and income spent on eating out.

As the analyses show, street network properties have statistically significant associations of moderate to large effect size with moderate-intensity work activities, walking or biking, vigorous-intensity recreational activities, moderate-intensity recreational activities, and average hours of sedentary activities. Only vigorous-intensity work activities show no statistically significant association with street network properties, which makes sense because it is hard to see how these activities can or should be related to these properties in small cities.

More specifically, moderate-intensity work activities decrease as different types of choice values of street systems increase, indicating that in cities with more movement potentials, people do less MVPA. This makes sense because as choice values increase, vehicular movement also increases, which decreases public safety and affects PA. In contrast, walking and biking increase as some street network properties increase. In simple words, accessibility, movement potential, and directional choices all seem to have positive effects on walking and biking in small Kansas cities, confirming the findings of many previous studies reported in the literature. Likewise, vigorous- and moderate-intensity recreational activities and sedentary activities decrease as the values of most of the street properties increase, indicating that accessibility, movement potential, and directional choices all seem to have negative effects on these activities. Again, this may be related to a decreased sense of safety with increased vehicular movement in the streets.

In summary, street properties show several statistically significant associations of moderate to large effect size with work-related behaviors, food shopping and eating behaviors, and physical and sedentary activities in small Kansas cities. Except street density, every property of street systems appears to have several associations with lifestyle in these cities.

Conclusions

This chapter provides an overview of the literature on the associations between spatial factors and lifestyle and presents the findings of a correlational study looking at these associations in small Kansas cities. It is known that as cities grow, they take over arable land, create a need for long commutes, cause traffic congestion, increase energy consumption, and produce environmental pollution. In essence, there is an inevitable link between the growth of cities and lifestyle behaviors. The literature, however, generally has concentrated on commuting behaviors when considering the associations between city size and lifestyle behaviors. The associations of city size with many other work-related travel behaviors, food shopping and eating behaviors, and physical and sedentary activities therefore remain unknown for both large and small cities. In this regard, the study presented in this chapter is relevant for it considers city size in relation to different types of lifestyles in small Kansas cities.

According to the findings of the study, city size may not be associated with work-related travel behaviors but may be associated with some food shopping and eating behaviors and PA in small Kansas cities. Small cities do not provide the needed economic benefits for city size to have an impact on work-related travel behaviors, and poverty in small cities may be a factor in determining many lifestyle choices, including food shopping and eating behaviors and physical activities. Clearly, more studies are needed on the topic. The next chapter therefore studies the associations of city size with lifestyle in two subsamples of small Kansas cities defined based on population size. Even though population size is not a spatial factor, it is an important factor of rurality.

Studies on the relationships between density and lifestyle have remained focused on urban areas for good reasons: the benefits of density seem to occur only in high-density urban areas, and small cities rarely show high densities and notable variations in density. As noted in chapter 7, a variation in density can still be observed in small cities of Kansas, exemplifying a need for a study exploring the effects of these variations on lifestyle. This study reveals that among all the lifestyle behaviors considered, census block density shows only one association with work-related travel behaviors and housing density shows no association at all. The findings of the study seem to validate the concern that, unlike in urban areas, in low-density small cities, variations in densities may not have any notable associations with lifestyle. To explore this topic further, the effects of population density on the spatial associations of lifestyle behaviors will be studied in the next chapter because population density is an important factor of rurality.

The review of the literature on the relationships between the availability of key destinations and facilities and lifestyle found very few studies that were conducted in small cities and towns. Given that the availability of key destinations and facilities shows statistically significant associations with lifestyle in urban areas and in some cases in rural areas, a study on these associations in small cities was needed. According to the studies presented in this chapter, the availability of key destinations and facilities except parks and green spaces show several statistically significant associations with lifestyle in small Kansas cities. As noted, there are many reasons why parks and green space may not show any beneficial effects of lifestyle behaviors in small cities. First, parks and green spaces may not be maintained properly in small cities. Second, small-city residents may use parks and green space less for PA than do their urban counterparts. Third, small-city residents may not be as deprived of open space and green space as may be urban residents.

As reported in this chapter, the literature does not present studies on the associations between land use type and lifestyle in small towns. Instead, it presents studies that consider the relationships between LUM and lifestyle in urban areas focusing on PA. This literature generally finds positive associations between LUM and PA. We do not find studies on the associations between LUM and lifestyle in small cities because they are small and lack complexity and urbanicity. Contradicting the generally held assumptions, according to the findings of this study, both land use type and LUM seem to have some associations with lifestyle behaviors in small towns. Among the land use types, the area of industrial use shows the most associations with lifestyle. In contrast to the findings of studies in urban areas, the area of open spaces fails to show associations with lifestyle in small cities in this study. According to the findings of this study, LUM shows statistically significant associations with several work-related travel behaviors, food shopping and eating behaviors, and physical and sedentary activities in small Kansas cities. The results of this study are important because no other previous study in urban or rural areas has covered so many different lifestyle behaviors in relation to land use type and mix.

Finally, it was observed that the literature reports numerous studies on the associations between street properties and lifestyle, but these studies generally do not involve small cities. According to this study, street properties, more particularly street network properties, show numerous associations with different lifestyle behaviors, including work-related travel behaviors, food shopping and eating behaviors, and physical activities. In general, the findings of the study seem to indicate that more accessibility, movement potential, and directional options may affect people living and working in the city and people carpooling. They may also affect the amount of income spent on food at supermarkets or grocery stores and people taking healthy diet. Additionally, they may affect people doing moderate-intensity work activities, walking or biking, doing vigorous-intensity recreational activities, and doing moderate-intensity recreational activities. Only vigorous-intensity work activities show no statistically significant associations with street properties in small Kansas cities. These findings are important because street properties are among those spatial factors that can be defined and described easily for comparative studies.

In conclusion, the significance of the findings presented in this chapter must be considered in light of the fact that the associations between the built environment and lifestyle in small cities have not been explored in public and population health studies. One primary reason for this lack of explorations is that most spatial factors such as density, LUM, and parks and green spaces that show associations with lifestyle in urban areas do not appear to be important in small cities given their smallness and lack of complexity. Despite this, this study identifies several spatial factors that show frequent associations with lifestyle in small Kansas cities. In most cases, however, the underlying reasons for these observed associations remain unknown. The next chapter will explore if the factors of rurality can help explain some of the associations between spatial factors and lifestyle observed in this chapter.

NOTES

1. Batty, "The Size, Scale, and Shape of Cities."
2. Batty, "A Theory of City Size."
3. Bettencourt et al., "Growth, Innovation, Scaling, and the Pace of Life in Cities."
4. Fragkias et al., "Does Size Matter?"
5. Isalgue, Coch, and Serra, "Scaling Laws and the Modern City."
6. Kennedy et al., "Energy and Material Flows of Megacities."
7. Kühnert, Helbing, and West, "Scaling Laws in Urban Supply Networks."
8. Schläpfer et al., "The Scaling of Human Interactions with City Size."
9. Zipf, *Human Behavior and the Principle of Least Effort.*
10. Gordon, Kumar, and Richardson, "The Influence of Metropolitan Spatial Structure."
11. Gordon and Wong, "The Costs of Urban Sprawl."
12. Kim, "Commuting Time Stability."
13. Schwanen, "Urban Form and Commuting Behaviour."
14. Vandersmissen, Villeneuve, and Thériault, "Analyzing Changes in Urban Form and Commuting Time."
15. Chen et al., "Life Satisfaction in Urbanizing China."
16. Cheung, Leung, and Nguyen, "City Size Matters."
17. Ferré, Ferreira, and Lanjouw, "Is There a Metropolitan Bias?"
18. Ray and Ghosh, "City Size and Health Outcomes."
19. Zhou, Rybski, and Kropp, "The Role of City Size and Urban Form."
20. Fuguitt, "Commuting and the Rural-Urban Hierarchy."
21. WSP and Arup, *Impacts of Land Use Planning.*
22. Cutumisu and Spence, "Exploring Associations between Urban Environments and Children's Physical Activity."
23. Burgoine, Alvanides, and Lake, "Assessing the Obesogenic Environment."
24. Brown et al., "Neighborhood Design for Walking and Biking."
25. Brown et al., "Mixed Land Use and Walkability."
26. Frank and Pivo, "The Impacts of Mixed Use and Density."
27. Frank, Andresen, and Schmid, "Obesity Relationships."
28. Frank et al., "Many Pathways from Land Use to Health."
29. Lee and Moudon, "The 3Ds+ R."
30. Lee and Moudon, "Correlates of Walking."
31. Pouliou and Elliott, "Individual and Socio-Environmental Determinants."
32. Wells and Yang, "Neighborhood Design and Walking."
33. Wood, Frank, and Giles-Corti, "Sense of Community and Its Relationship."
34. Troped et al., "The Built Environment and Location-Based Physical Activity."
35. Saelens and Handy, "Built Environment Correlates of Walking."
36. Barton et al., *The Routledge Handbook of Planning for Health and Well-Being.*
37. McCann and Ewing, *Measuring the Health Effects of Sprawl.*
38. Handy, *Critical Assessment of the Literature.*
39. Campoli, *Made for Walking.*
40. Learnihan et al., "Effect of Scale on the Links between Walking and Urban Design."
41. Handy, Cao, and Mokhtarian, "Self-Selection in the Relationship between the Built Environment and Walking."

42. Forsyth et al., "Design and Destinations."
43. Nagel et al., "The Relation between Neighborhood Built Environment and Walking Activity."
44. Sallis et al., "Neighborhood Environments and Physical Activity among Adults."
45. Norman et al., "Community Design and Access to Recreational Facilities."
46. Cervero, "Land-Use Mixing and Suburban Mobility."
47. Li et al., "Neighborhood Influences on Physical Activity."
48. Cohen et al., "Public Parks and Physical Activity."
49. Coutts et al., "County-Level Effects of Green Space Access."
50. Duncan and Mummery, "Psychosocial and Environmental Factors."
51. Takano, Nakamura, and Watanabe, "Urban Residential Environments and Senior Citizens' Longevity."
52. Maas et al., "Green Space, Urbanity, and Health."
53. Giles-Corti et al., "Increasing Walking."
54. Sugiyama et al., "Associations between Recreational Walking and Attractiveness, Size, and Proximity."
55. Cohen et al., "Proximity to School and Physical Activity."
56. Kaczynski, Johnson, and Saelens, "Neighborhood Land Use Diversity and Physical Activity."
57. Sallis and Glanz, "Physical Activity and Food Environments."
58. Hennessy et al., "Active Living for Rural Children."
59. Findholt et al., "Environmental Influences on Children's Physical Activity and Eating Habits."
60. Parks, Housemann, and Brownson, "Differential Correlates of Physical Activity."
61. Wilson et al., "Socioeconomic Status and Perceptions of Access and."
62. Giles-Corti et al., "The Influence of Urban Design on Neighbourhood Walking."
63. Epstein et al., "Reducing Sedentary Behavior."
64. Rutt and Coleman, "Examining the Relationships among Built Environment, Physical Activity, and Body Mass Index."
65. McCormack, Giles-Corti, and Bulsara, "Correlates of Using Neighborhood Recreational Destinations."
66. Evenson et al., "Girls' Perception of Neighborhood Factors."
67. Gordon-Larsen et al., "Inequality in the Built Environment."
68. Michael et al., "Physical Activity Resources and Changes in."
69. Sallis et al., "Distance between Homes and Exercise Facilities."
70. Diez-Roux et al., "Availability of Recreational Resources."
71. Pan et al., "Individual, Social, Environmental, and Physical Environmental Correlates."
72. Addy et al., "Associations of Perceived Social and Physical Environmental Supports."
73. Boehmer et al., "What Constitutes an Obesogenic Environment?"
74. Brownson et al., "Promoting Physical Activity in Rural Communities."
75. Deshpande et al., "Environmental Correlates of Physical Activity."
76. Thompson et al., "Environmental, Policy, and Cultural Factors."
77. Sanderson, Littleton, and Pulley, "Environmental, Policy, and Cultural Factors."
78. Wilcox et al., "Determinants of Leisure Time Physical Activity."
79. Sarkar, Webster, and Gallacher, *Healthy Cities.*
80. Kligerman et al., "Association of Neighborhood Design and Recreation Environment Variables."
81. Jilcott et al., "Association between Physical Activity and Proximity to Physical Activity Resources."

82. Cerin, Leslie, and Owen, "Explaining Socio-Economic Status Differences."
83. Cerin and Leslie, "How Socio-Economic Status Contributes to Participation."
84. Boer et al., "Neighborhood Design and Walking Trips."
85. Handy, "Regional versus Local Accessibility."
86. Ewing, Haliyur, and Page, "Getting Around."
87. Cervero, "Mixed Land-Uses and Commuting."
88. Cervero and Kockelman, "Travel Demand and the 3Ds."
89. Cerin et al., "Measuring Perceived Neighbourhood."
90. Gomez et al., "Built Environment Attributes and Walking Patterns."
91. Li et al., "Built Environment, Adiposity, and Physical Activity."
92. Handy, "Understanding the Link between Urban Form and Nonwork Travel Behavior."
93. Nelson et al., "Built and Social Environments."
94. Frank et al., "Urban Form Relationships with Walk Trip Frequency and Distance."
95. Sugiyama et al., "Destination and Route Attributes."
96. Sugiyama, Thompson, and Alves, "Associations between Neighborhood Open Space Attributes and Quality of Life."
97. Kerr et al., "Urban Form Correlates of Pedestrian Travel in Youth."
98. Carver et al., "Are Safety-Related Features of the Road Environment Associated with Smaller Declines in Physical Activity?"
99. Veitch, Salmon, and Ball, "Individual, Social and Physical Environmental Correlates."
100. Carver, Timperio, and Crawford, "Playing It Safe."
101. Giles-Corti et al., "School Site and the Potential to Walk to School."
102. Trapp et al., "Increasing Children's Physical Activity."
103. Villanueva et al., "How Far Do Children Travel from Their Homes?"
104. Villanueva et al., "Where Do Children Travel To and What Local Opportunities Are Available?"
105. Trapp et al., "On Your Bike!"
106. Hillier, *Space Is the Machine*.
107. Hillier and Hanson, *The Social Logic of Space*.
108. Hillier and Penn, "Rejoinder to Carlo Ratti."
109. Jiang and Liu, "Street-Based Topological Representations."
110. Rashid, "On Space Syntax as a Configurational Theory."
111. Ratti, "Space Syntax."
112. Hillier and Iida, "Network and Psychological Effects in Urban Movement."
113. Hillier et al., "Natural Movement."
114. Penn et al., "Configurational Modelling of Urban Movement Networks."
115. Peponis, Ross, and Rashid, "The Structure of Urban Space."
116. Baran, Rodríguez, and Khattak, "Space Syntax and Walking."
117. Chiaradia, Moreau, and Raford. "Configurational Exploration of Public Transport Movement Networks."
118. Greene, "Housing and Community Consolidation."
119. Law, Chiaradia, and Schwander. "Towards a Multimodal Space Syntax Analysis."
120. Parvin, Ye, and Jia. "Multilevel Pedestrian Movement."
121. McCahil and Garrick, "The Applicability of Space Syntax to Bicycle Facility Planning."
122. Raford, Chiaradia, and Gil, "Space Syntax."
123. Barros et al., "Analysis of Trip Generating Developments."
124. Scoppa, French, and Peponis. "The Effects of Street Connectivity."
125. Barros, da Silva, and de Holanda. "Exploratory Study of Space Syntax as a Traffic Assignment Tool."

126. Paul, "An Integrated Approach to Modeling Vehicular Movement Networks."
127. Ozbil, Peponis, and Bafna. "The Effects of Street Configuration on Transit Ridership."
128. Kim, "The Role of Spatial Configuration in Spatial Cognition."
129. Lee and Ryu, "Multiple Path-Finding Models."
130. Long, "The Relationships between Objective and Subjective Evaluations."
131. Penn, "Space Syntax and Spatial Cognition."
132. Porta, Crucitti, and Latora, "Multiple Centrality Assessment."
133. Porta, Paolo, and Vito, "The Network Analysis of Urban Streets."
134. Raja, Ma, and Yadav, "Beyond Food Deserts."

CHAPTER NINE

Rurality and Spatial Associations of Lifestyle in Small Cities of Kansas

Comparative Correlational Analyses

"Rurality" is not a commonly used term in population or public health literature, which tends to have an urban focus. Instead, a more commonly used term is "urbanicity," which is the absence of rurality. Urbanicity allows one to discuss a city or a town in positive terms because it generally refers to progress whereas rurality refers to a lack of progress. Since this book focuses on small towns and cities that generally possess low levels of urbanicity, it uses the term "rurality," which recognizes that in most cases small cities remain more rural than urban.

As we will see, researchers commonly agree that there are significant disparities in health-related lifestyle behaviors between urban and rural America. Since small-town America is generally considered a part of rural America in the literature, it is probably safe to assume that there are disparities in lifestyle between urban and small-town America as well. If urbanicity creates urban-rural disparities as has been noted in the literature, then does rurality create similar disparities among small cities and towns by affecting spatial associations of lifestyle behaviors?

The purpose of this chapter is to explore how the associations between spatial factors and lifestyle in small cities of Kansas reported in chapter 8 vary based on the five factors of rurality, which were identified in chapter 6 based on the discussion of rurality in chapter 2. These factors include population size and density, daytime population change due to commuting, distance to the nearest city with 50,000 or more people, and mean travel time to work (commuting time). The spatial factors used in the studies of this chapter remain unchanged from those used in chapter 8. They include measures describing city size, density, availability of key destinations and facilities, land use types and mix, and several street properties. Lifestyle behaviors included in chapter 8 also remain unchanged. They include work-related travel behaviors, food shopping and eating behaviors, and physical and sedentary activities.

For the purpose of this chapter, the sample of 36 small cities from Kansas is divided into two subsamples based on each of the five factors of rurality. When possible, the cut line is determined to keep any two subsamples somewhat equal. These subsamples are used for the following purposes:

1. Cities with population between ≥5,000 and ≤9,999 people are compared to cities with population between ≥10,000 and ≤49,999 people to study the effects of population size on the associations between spatial factors and lifestyle.
2. Small cities with ≤1,834.50 people per square mile are compared to cities with 1,834.51+ people per square mile to study the effects of population density on the associations between spatial factors and lifestyle.
3. Small cities with ≤6.25% population change due to daytime travel are compared to cities with 6.26%+ population change due to daytime travel to study the effects of daytime population change on the associations between spatial factors and lifestyle.
4. Small cities ≤63.40 miles from the nearest large city with ≥50,000 people are compared to cities 63.41+ miles from the nearest large city with ≥50,000 people to study the effects of distance from the nearest city on the associations between spatial factors and lifestyle.
5. Small cities with ≤14.90 minutes of commuting time were compared to small cities with 14.91+ minutes of commuting time to study the effects of commuting time on the associations between spatial factors and lifestyle.

The summary of these comparative correlational analyses are provided in tables 9.1–9.4, where the number in a cell shows the number of statistically significant correlations of a lifestyle behavior with spatial factors. The percentages of the number of statistically significant correlations of the total number of correlations considered for a lifestyle behavior with spatial factors are shown in parentheses.

Rurality and Spatial Associations of Work-Related Travel Behaviors

Getting people physically active on a daily basis, as part of their transport to and from work, is critical for good health. On one end of the spectrum, people can drive alone to work. A convenient mode of traveling to work that takes less time, driving alone to work is harmful for health and the environment and contributes to higher levels of air and noise pollution, more traffic accidents, and lower rates of active travel. At the other end of the spectrum, people can walk to work, which is beneficial to health and the environment but often inconvenient and time consuming. Between these two extremes, people can carpool, bike, or take public transportation to work. They can also use some combination of modes to get to work.

Walking, biking, and taking public transportation to work offer an effective way of increasing physical activities by integrating activities into people's daily lives [1–4]. Often termed as active commuting (AC), these transportation modes have well-documented health benefits, such as a reduced risk of obesity, diabetes, cardiovascular disease, and all-cause mortality [5, 6]. AC also leads to a reduction of carbon dioxide emissions by reducing vehicle use and traffic congestion, generating indirect health benefits. In addition, AC provides economic benefits through savings in vehicle operating and maintenance costs [3] but also, more importantly, through a reduction in premature deaths [7]. According to the World Health Organization (2007), the economic benefits of AC attributable to health gains would be even larger than those from reductions in mortality alone if morbidity costs were included [cited in 8]. Increasing the number of local pedestrians, cyclists, and users of public transportation can increase the economic viability of cafes and corner stores, as well as improve access to jobs and services without increasing congestion or vehicle emissions. For example, in Toronto people who biked and walked to Bloor Street, a commercial area, spent more money in the area per month than those who drove there [9]. Healthier work-related travel behaviors (or commuting) underpin population health. They promote environmental sustainability, which can be a further motivation for their uptake by both the individual and the policymaker [10].

The prevalence of different work-related travel behaviors varies among urban and rural populations [11]. In a study using 2010 Census data supplemented with other datasets, Fan et al. [4] investigated rural-urban differences in participation rates for three modes of AC in 70,172 US census tracts—12,844 rural tracts and 57,328 urban. They found that the average AC rates were 3.44% rural and 2.77% urban ($p<0.01$) for walking to work, 0.40% rural and 0.58% urban ($p<0.01$) for biking to work, and 0.59% rural and 5.86% urban ($p<0.01$) for public transportation to work. In simple terms, rural tracts had a higher rate of walking to work but lower rates of biking to work or public transportation to work, with the difference in prevalence of public transportation to work being substantial. This is likely a result of the general lack of public transportation options in rural areas as low population density renders the development of public transportation infrastructure cost ineffective. These findings suggest that unless a more cost-effective method of public transportation is developed for low-population-density areas, the focus to promote AC in rural areas should be on walking and biking, while in urban areas, all three AC modes can be targeted.

The differences in AC between urban and rural areas are also evident in that while higher population density is positively associated with AC in the literature [12, 13], this relationship only holds for urban tracts. For rural tracts, population density is negatively associated with AC, recent national studies reported [4, 14]. It is not clear what the mechanism is behind such a negative association. The bottom line is, because the majority of Americans live in urban areas, our understanding of both rural and urban areas is dominated by the findings on urban relationships. Attention needs to be given to rural-urban differences in order to prevent unintended negative consequences of one-size-fits-all approaches for policies and strategies to promote AC participation.

Variations in AC may be associated with rural-urban health disparities [15–18]. In a national study, Zhang et al. [19] compared urban-rural obesity in terms of neighborhood commuting environment and found that commuting time was positively associated with obesity in large and small urban areas, as well as in rural and remote areas. In contrast, the dependence on a motor vehicle for commuting to work was strongly associated with obesity for urban areas but not for rural. It is important to know why the differences in the associations of commuting environment with obesity between urban and rural areas exist.

In a study reported above, Fan et al. [4] provided some explanations for the differences in AC between urban and rural areas in terms of the built environment. They compared the rural and urban tracts in terms of the effects of spatial factors on three modes of AC and found a negative association between tract greenness and prevalence of walking to work in rural and urban tracts. They also found significant differences in the associations between street network variables and AC between urban and rural tracts [4]. In addition, they found that tract intersection density was positively associated with AC for urban tracts—a finding supported by the majority of existing literature [12, 13, 20, 21]. The association for rural tracts, however, was negative but statistically insignificant (p=0.128). This may be because compared to urban settings, rural towns tend to be small with a limited number of streets; as such, whether these streets are well connected is less important for AC.

In another study, Kim and Heinrich [22] provided additional explanation for the differences in AC between urban and rural areas in terms of the built environment. In contrast to national studies, which do not consider local differences, Kim and Heinrich compared the associations between walking to school (WTS) and the built environment of a small city and a large city in the United States. WTS is a daily routine behavior among schoolchildren that can help establish an active lifestyle from early childhood. It generally adds more daily moderate-to-vigorous physical activity than other ways of transporting children to school [23–25]. Previous studies had shown that several environmental factors affect WTS, including distance, travel time, safety, urban form and density, land use, and street design (i.e., speed limit, traffic volume, sidewalks, crosswalks, street connectivity) [20, 26–32]. These studies focused primarily on large cities or on national and statewide cross-sectional settings using simple urban-rural classification schemes; therefore, they were unable to consider specific differences between rural and urban settings. To overcome the limitations, Kim and Heinrich [22] used fine-grain built environment data for their study and reported that, after controlling for socioeconomic and demographic variables, WTS was better associated with walking paths / trails and sidewalks with landscape buffers en route to school in the small city than it was in the large city. These associations were found despite the small city having lower perceived neighborhood social cohesion, lower school bus availability, and higher parental concerns about crime, and lacking key pedestrian infrastructure elements that the large city had.

In yet another study, Stewart et al. [33] compared the differences in the associations between spatial factors and walking among adults in urban areas of Seattle (n=464) and in nine small US towns (n=299). They used objective spatial measures around participants' residence and their walking behaviors. After adjusting for sociodemographic factors, the authors found 18 spatial features showing association with utilitarian walking (e.g., walking to work) in the Seattle area. In contrast, they found only 2 such features in small towns. Similar to prior research [34], their findings suggest that utilitarian walking may be less sensitive to home neighborhoods in less urbanized areas. Additionally, they found that the rate of utilitarian walking among small-town residents was also lower than it was among urban residents. They explained that small-town residents might find it easier to drive to and park at destinations rather than walk from their home, regardless of their home neighborhood environment. This aligns with previous research showing that small-town residents are more likely than urban residents to depend on automobiles [19], indicating the existence of a broader "car culture" in small towns.

In sum, only a very few comparative studies consider the effects of spatial factors on work-related travel behaviors in urban and rural areas. These studies often indicate that some of these behaviors are associated with spatial factors both in urban and rural areas, but the factors showing associations are different for these places. The findings presented in chapter 8 surely support that some work-related travel behaviors are associated with spatial factors in small Kansas cities. It is not known, however, if these associations vary in small cities with different levels of rurality as they do in places with different levels of urbanicity. In this regard, the findings presented next are relevant.

Things We Observe in Small Cities of Kansas
EFFECTS OF POPULATION SIZE

The subsamples defined based on *population size* are compared to determine if the spatial associations of work-related travel behaviors vary in small cities of high and low population size. As presented in table 9.1, *workers who work and live in the city* shows 12 (27.27% of the 44 correlations explored) and 10 (22.72%) statistically significant associations with spatial factors in cities with ≤9,999 and 10,000+ people. According to the findings, this behavior is somewhat sensitive to spatial factors in both subsamples of cities.

Workers drove alone to work shows 0 and 7 (15.91%) statistically significant associations with spatial factors in cities with ≤9,999 and 10,000+ people; and *workers carpool to work* shows 1 (2.27%) and 10 (22.73%). Therefore, the latter of the two work-related behaviors is more sensitive to spatial factors in cities with 10,000+ people than it is in cities with ≤9,999 people.

Overall, work-related travel behaviors show 13 (9.85% of the 132 correlations explored) and 27 (20.45%) statistically significant associations in cities with ≤9,999 and 10,000+ people, indicating that these behaviors generally are more sensitive to spatial factors in larger small cities.

EFFECTS OF POPULATION DENSITY

The differences in the correlations between spatial factors and work-related travel behaviors for the subsamples defined based on *population density* are shown in table 9.1. *Workers who work and live in the city* shows 4 (9.09% of the 44 correlations explored) and 18 (40.90%) statistically significant associations with spatial factors in cities with ≤1,834.50 and 1,834.51+ people per square mile; *workers drove alone to work* shows 0 and 12 (27.27%); and *workers carpool to work* shows 0 and 14 (31.82%). Each of these behaviors is more sensitive to spatial factors in small cities with higher densities.

Overall, work-related travel behaviors show 4 (3.03% of the 132 correlations explored) and 44 (33.33%) statistically significant associations for cities with ≤1,834.50 and 1,834.51+ people per square mile, indicating that these behaviors are far more sensitive to spatial factors in denser small cities.

EFFECTS OF DAYTIME POPULATION CHANGE

The differences in the correlations between spatial factors and work-related travel behaviors for the subsamples defined based on *daytime population change* are shown in table 9.1. *Workers who work and live in the city* shows 12 (27.27% of the 44 correlations explored) and 8 (18.18%) statistically significant associations with spatial factors in cities with ≤6.25% and 6.26%+ population change due to daytime travel. With more correlations, this behavior is slightly more sensitive to spatial factors in cities with ≤6.25% population change due to daytime travel.

Workers drove alone to work shows 14 (31.82%) and 0 statistically significant associations with spatial factors in cities with ≤6.25% and 6.26%+ population change due to daytime travel, and *workers carpool to work* shows 9 (20.45%) and 0. These behaviors are more sensitive to spatial factors only in cities with ≤6.25% population change due to daytime travel.

Overall, work-related travel behaviors show 35 (26.52% of the 132 correlations explored) and 8 (6.06%) statistically significant associations with spatial factors in cities with ≤6.25% and 6.26%+ population change due to daytime travel, indicating that these behaviors are more sensitive to spatial factors in cities with less population change due to daytime travel.

EFFECTS OF DISTANCE TO NEAREST CITY OF 50,000 OR MORE PEOPLE

The differences in the correlations between spatial factors and work-related travel behaviors for the subsamples defined based on *distance to nearest city of 50,000 or more people* are shown in table 9.1. *Workers who work and live in the city* shows 15 (34.09% of the 44 correlations explored) and 2 (4.55%) statistically significant associations with spatial factors in cities ≤63.40 and 63.41+ miles from the nearest city with 50,000 or more people. This behavior is more sensitive to spatial factors in cities ≤63.40 miles than it is in cities 63.41+ miles from the nearest large city.

Workers drove alone to work shows 8 (18.18%) and 4 (9.09%) statistically significant associations with spatial factors in cities ≤63.40 and 63.41+ miles from the nearest large city. This behavior is slightly more sensitive to spatial factors in cities ≤63.40 miles than it is in cities 63.41+ miles from the nearest large city.

Workers carpool to work shows 6 (13.64%) and 6 (13.64%) statistically significant associations with spatial factors in cities ≤63.40 and 63.41+ miles from the nearest large city. This behavior is less sensitive to spatial factors, but the effects are similar in cities regardless of distance from a larger city.

Overall, work-related travel behaviors show 29 (21.97% of the 132 correlations explored) and 12 (9.09%) statistically significant associations with spatial factors in cities ≤63.40 and 63.41+ miles from the nearest large city, indicating that these behaviors are more sensitive to spatial factors in small cities closer to cities with 50,000 or more people.

EFFECTS OF COMMUTE TIME

The differences in the correlations between spatial factors and work-related travel behaviors for the subsamples defined based on *commute time* are shown in table 9.1. *Workers who work and live in the city* shows 0 and 8 (18.18% of the 44 correlations explored) statistically significant associations with spatial factors in cities with ≤14.90 and 14.91+ minutes of commute time, indicating that this behavior may be more sensitive to spatial factors in cities with longer commute time.

Workers drove alone to work shows 3 (6.82%) and 6 (13.64%) statistically significant associations with spatial factors in cities with ≤14.90 and 14.91+ minutes of commute time, indicating that this behavior is less sensitive to spatial factors, but the sensitivity is slightly higher in cities with longer commute time.

Workers carpool to work shows 9 (20.45%) and 2 (4.55%) statistically significant associations with spatial factors in cities with ≤14.90 and 14.91+ minutes of commute time, indicating that the behavior is more sensitive to spatial factors in cities with less commute time.

Overall, work-related travel behaviors show 12 (9.09% of the 132 correlations explored) and 16 (12.12%) statistically significant associations with spatial factors in cities with ≤14.90 and 14.91+ minutes of commute time, indicating that these behaviors may be less sensitive to spatial factors, but the effects are similar in both subsamples.

TABLE 9.1.
Significant correlations between spatial factors and work-related travel behaviors

		Significant correlations, n (%)			
		Workers who live and work in this city	Drive alone to work	Carpool to work	Total
Rurality factors					
Population	≤9,999	12 (27.27)	0 (0.00)	1 (2.27)	13 (9.85)
	10,000+	10 (22.72)	7 (15.90)	10 (22.72)	27 (20.45)
Population density (per square mile)	≤1,834.50	4 (9.09)	0 (0.00)	0 (0.00)	4 (3.03)
	1,834.51+	18 (40.91)	12 (27.27)	14 (31.82)	44 (33.33)
Population change due to daytime travel (as % of total population)	≤6.25	12 (27.27)	14 (31.82)	9 (20.45)	35 (26.52)
	6.26+	8 (18.18)	0 (0.00)	0 (0.00)	8 (6.06)
Distance to nearest city of 50,000 or more people (in miles)	≤63.40	15 (34.09)	8 (18.18)	6 (13.64)	29 (21.97)
	63.41+	2 (4.55)	4 (9.09)	6 (13.64)	12 (9.09)
Commute time (in minutes)	≤14.90	0 (0.00)	3 (6.82)	9 (20.45)	12 (9.09)
	14.91+	8 (18.18)	6 (13.64)	2 (4.55)	16 (12.12)

In summary, based on the numbers shown in the last column of the table, work-related travel behaviors are more sensitive to spatial factors in cities with more people, more population density, and less population change due to daytime travel and in small cities closer to large cities. They are less sensitive to spatial factors, but the effects are similar in cities with low and high commute time. Notably, different behaviors are differently associated with spatial factors in the subsamples defined based on the factors of rurality. Spatial design and planning strategies to affect the spatial associations of work-related travel behaviors therefore should consider different factors of rurality of these small cities based on the work-related travel behavior being considered.

Rurality and Spatial Associations of Food Shopping and Eating Behaviors

Diet and food environment are among the root causes of obesity [35]. Worldwide, 2.6 million deaths a year are attributable to insufficient fruit and vegetable intake [36], and an estimated 2.1 billion people are overweight or obese [37]. In the United States, food environments and diet-related health conditions are a growing public health concern [38, 39]. The intake of healthy foods among Americans is significantly below recommendations. Because of limitations within local food environments, including economic barriers and poor physical food accessibility, only 12.2% of Americans meet the recommendation for fruit consumption, and only 9.3% meet the recommendation for vegetable consumption [40]. The US Department of Agriculture (USDA) reports that approximately 10.5% (13.8 million) of US households were food insecure at some time during 2020. These households were uncertain of having, or unable to acquire, enough food to meet the needs of all their members because they had insufficient money or other resources for food [41].

Food spending and diet are likely to be influenced by the accessibility and affordability of food, which include travel time to shopping, availability of healthy foods, and food prices. Some people and places may face greater barriers in accessing healthy and affordable food, which may negatively affect diet and food security. A growing body of literature explores food quality and availability, food affordability, and food accessibility [35]. Some of these studies explore relationships between food attributes and food access. Others focus on the attributes of food stores, such as quality, availability, and price of food items, high purchasing frequency food variables, and square footages of stores. Others use food attributes to delineate food deserts [35, 42–49]. For instance, in Jiao's research [43], "food desert" is defined by combining physical food accessibility with food availability in food stores based on food costs. Among many things, the literature indicates that adequate physical accessibility of supermarkets reduces rates of obesity [35], and that better physical/geographical accessibility to supermarkets and the provision of a wider variety of healthy foods are found in higher income areas, while the limited physical/geographical accessibility to healthy foods are found in more socially disadvantaged areas [39, 45].

While research on neighborhood food environments has taken advantage of more technically sophisticated ways to assess distance and density, in general, it has not thoroughly considered how individual or neighborhood conditions and transportation characteristics might modify physical distance and thereby affect patterns of spatial accessibility. In one rare example, Dutko et al. [50] examine the socioeconomic and demographic characteristics of more than 6,500 food desert tracts in the United States to see how they differ from other census tracts and the extent to which these differences influence food desert status. Relative to all other census tracts, they find, food desert tracts tend to have smaller populations, higher rates of abandoned or vacant homes, and residents who have lower levels of education, lower incomes, and higher rates of unemployment. Census tracts with higher poverty rates are more likely to be food deserts than otherwise similar low-income census tracts in rural and in very dense (highly populated) urban areas. For less dense urban areas, census tracts with higher concentrations of minority populations are more likely to be food deserts, while tracts with substantial decreases in minority populations between 1990 and 2000 were less likely to be identified as food deserts in 2000.

In another rare example, Bader and colleagues [51] carry out a series of sensitivity analyses to illustrate the effects on the measurement of disparities in food environments of adjusting for cross-neighborhood variations in vehicle ownership rates, public transit access, and impediments to pedestrian travel, such as crime and poor traffic safety. They find that adjusting for vehicle ownership and crime tended to increase measured disparities in access to supermarkets by neighborhood race/ethnicity and income, while adjusting for public transit and traffic safety tended to narrow these disparities.

In yet another rare example, McKenzie [52] uses five-year American Community Survey data for the 2006–2010 period to compare a travel time and distance measure of supermarket access for neighborhoods of concentrated poverty relative to other neighborhoods, taking into account their distance to the city center. The findings of the research demonstrate the potential for variation in results across methods measuring access to neighborhood amenities and suggest that more nuanced methodology will be required for us to understand socio-spatial disparities in access.

In general, the literature seems to show that studies involving spatial factors mostly consider physical accessibility measures and their effects on behaviors and health in urban areas with disparity [35] and that the most common approaches to determining physical accessibility are the measurement of distances to food resources and the density of food stores [42, 45, 53]. While these measures help researchers understand spatial inequalities in food access, other spatial factors, including land use type and mix and street properties that also shape local food environments, are less reported in the literature.

The effects of spatial factors on food environments, food shopping behaviors, and population health are by no means limited to accessibility and availability of healthy foods. According to the literature, they can affect food environment and population health through affecting food shopping and eating behaviors as well. Most studies involving spatial factors generally consider food shopping patterns in relation to daily healthy diet. The research finds that the proximity to food stores is associated with fruit consumption by house-holds; that the use of farmers' markets is not associated with health; that there is no association between proximity to farmers' markets and body mass index (BMI); and that the price of healthy food items, the proximity to the nearest supermarket, and the three potential difficulties—non–car ownership, diffi-culties with walking, and being reliant on public transport—are not signifi-cantly associated with fruit and vegetable consumption [54–56]. These find-ings suggest that, besides spatial factors defining accessibility and availability, there may be other factors influencing healthy food consumption. Since the results from existing research are inconclusive, more empirical studies are needed to explore the relationships between spatial factors and food shopping and eating behaviors.

Existing literature provides very little evidence on the relationships be-tween spatial factors and food shopping and eating behaviors in small towns and cities and on the effects of rurality on these relationships. The lack of evidence is significant because rural people generally consume significantly higher fat because of the culture of their eating patterns (e.g., "country cook-ing") [57–59]. They also have less access to healthy foods due to a lack of healthy food outlets or conventional grocery stores [60, 61]. As a result, rural residents shop in smaller local stores with limited variety, poorer quality, and higher prices, compromising health and potentially widening inequities [62, 63]. The situation is made worse by farms that avoid specialty farming for financial reasons. In the absence of specialty farming, access to a wide variety of fruits and vegetables is limited in rural areas. It is not surprising that rural adults have lower intake of fiber and fruits and higher intake of sweetened beverages than their urban counterparts [64].

Without doubt, the lack of studies on most aspects of food shopping and eating behaviors in small US cities is significant. Therefore, a study on the effects of rurality on the relationships between food shopping and eating be-haviors and the conventional physical food accessibility measures (such as density and proximity) and the expanded measures of food environments (such as land use type and mix and metric and network properties of street systems) is necessary. Understanding how spatial factors affect food-related behaviors in small cities based on rurality may offer important insights into strategies for improving population health and nutrition. In this regard, the findings on the effects of various dimensions of rurality on spatial associa-tions of food shopping and eating behaviors in small Kansas cities presented below may be relevant.

Things We Observe in Small Cities of Kansas
EFFECTS OF POPULATION SIZE

According to a comparison of the correlations between spatial factors and food shopping and eating behaviors for the two subsamples defined based on *population size* (table 9.2), *income spent on food at supermarkets or grocery stores* shows 11 (25% of the 44 correlations explored) and 13 (29.22%) statistically significant associations with spatial factors in cities with ≤9,999 and 10,000+ people, indicating that this behavior may be almost equally sensitive to spatial factors in both subsamples of cities.

Income spent on food at other stores shows 4 (9.09%) and 2 (4.55%) statistically significant associations with spatial factors in cities with ≤9,999 and 10,000+ people, indicating that spatial factors may be less important for this food shopping behavior in small cities.

Income spent on eating out shows 9 (20.45%) and 1 (2.27%) statistically significant associations with spatial factors in cities with ≤9,999 and 10,000+ people, indicating that spatial factors may be important for the subsample of cities with ≤9,999 people.

People taking healthy diet shows 8 (18.18%) and 19 (43.18%) statistically significant associations with spatial factors in cities with ≤9,999 and 10,000+ people, indicating that while spatial factors are important for this behavior in both samples, they are more important in cities with 10,000+ people.

Overall, food shopping and eating behaviors show 32 (18.18% of the 176 correlations explored) and 35 (19.89%) statistically significant associations with spatial factors in cities with ≤9,999 and 10,000+ people, indicating that these behaviors are almost equally sensitive to spatial factors in both the subsamples.

EFFECTS OF POPULATION DENSITY

According to a comparison of the correlations between spatial factors and food shopping and eating behaviors for the two subsamples defined based on *population density* (table 9.2), *income spent on food at supermarkets or grocery stores* shows 8 (18.18% of the 44 correlations explored) and 24 (54.55%) statistically significant associations with spatial factors in cities with ≤1,834.50 and 1,834.51+ people per square mile. According to these findings, this behavior may be quite sensitive to spatial factors in cities with higher densities.

Income spent on food at other stores shows 0 and 4 (9.09%) statistically significant associations with spatial factors in cities with ≤1,834.50 and 1,834.51+

people per square mile. This behavior may not be sensitive to spatial factors in cities with ≤1,834.50 people per square mile, but it may be slightly sensitive to some of these factors in cities with 1,834.51+ people per square mile.

Income spent on eating out shows 6 (13.64%) and 0 statistically significant associations with spatial factors in cities with ≤1,834.50 and 1,834.51+ people per square mile. This behavior may be slightly sensitive to spatial factors in cities with ≤1,834.50 people per square mile but may not be sensitive to these factors in cities with 1,834.51+ people per square mile.

People taking healthy diet shows 9 (20.45%) and 22 (50%) statistically significant associations with spatial factors in cities with ≤1,834.50 and 1,834.51+ people per square mile. The findings indicate that the behavior is significantly more sensitive to spatial factors in cities with higher densities.

Overall, food shopping and eating behaviors show 23 (13.07% of the 176 correlations explored) and 50 (28.41%) statistically significant associations with spatial factors in cities with ≤1,834.50 and 1,834.51+ people per square mile, indicating that these behaviors are more sensitive to spatial factors in small cities with higher densities.

EFFECTS OF DAYTIME POPULATION CHANGE

According to a comparison of the correlations between spatial factors and food shopping and eating behaviors for the two subsamples defined based on *daytime population change* (table 9.2), *income spent on food at supermarkets or grocery stores* shows 12 (27.27% of the 44 correlations explored) and 6 (13.64%) statistically significant associations with spatial factors in cities with ≤6.25% and 6.26%+ population change due to daytime travel; *income spent on food at other stores* shows 4 (9.09%) and 0; *income spent on eating out* shows 9 (20.45%) and 7 (15.91%); and *people taking healthy diet* shows 11 (25%) and 7 (15.91%).

Overall, food shopping and eating behaviors show 36 (20.45% of the 176 correlations explored) and 20 (11.36% of all correlations) statistically significant associations with spatial factors in cities with ≤6.25% and 6.26%+ population change due to daytime travel, indicating that these behaviors may be more sensitive to spatial factors in cities with less population change due to daytime travel.

EFFECTS OF DISTANCE TO NEAREST CITY OF 50,000 OR MORE PEOPLE

According to a comparison of the correlations between spatial factors and food shopping and eating behaviors for the two subsamples defined based on *distance to nearest city of 50,000 or more people* (table 9.2), *income spent on food at supermarkets or grocery stores* shows 17 (38.64% of the 44 correlations explored) and 9 (20.45%) statistically significant associations with spatial factors for cities ≤63.40 and 63.41+ miles from the nearest large city. According to the findings, this behavior is more sensitive to spatial factors in cities closer to large cities.

Income spent on food at other stores shows 2 (4.55%) statistically significant associations with spatial factors for each subsample of cities. *Income spent on eating out* shows 1 (2.27%) and 0 statistically significant associations with spatial factors for cities ≤63.40 and 63.41+ miles from the nearest large city. These two behaviors may not be sensitive to spatial factors in these subsamples of cities.

People taking healthy diet shows 12 (27.27%) and 12 (27.27%) statistically significant associations with spatial factors for cities ≤63.40 and 63.41+ miles from the nearest large city. Spatial factors are equally important for this behavior in both subsamples.

Overall, food shopping and eating behaviors show 32 (18.18% of the 176 correlations explored) and 23 (13.07%) statistically significant associations with spatial factors in cities ≤63.40 and 63.41+ miles from the nearest large city, indicating that these behaviors may be more sensitive to spatial factors in cities with less distance from the nearest large city.

EFFECTS OF COMMUTE TIME

Finally, according to a comparison of the two subsamples defined based on *commuting time* (table 9.2), *income spent on food at supermarkets or grocery stores* shows 1 (2.27% of the 44 correlations explored) and 14 (31.82%) statistically significant association with spatial factors in cities with ≤14.90 and 14.91+ minutes of commute time, indicating that this behavior is far more sensitive to spatial factors in small cities with longer commute time.

Income spent on food at other stores shows no statistically significant associations with spatial factors in cities with ≤14.90 and 14.91+ minutes of commute time. This behavior may not be sensitive to spatial factors in either of the subsamples of cities.

Income spent on eating out shows 2 (4.55%) and 6 (13.64%) statistically significant associations with spatial factors in cities with ≤14.90 and 14.91+ minutes of commute time. According to these findings, though this behavior in general is less sensitive to spatial factors in these subsamples of cities, it may be somewhat more sensitive to spatial factors in cities with longer commute time.

TABLE 9.2.

Significant correlations between spatial factors and food shopping and eating behaviors

		Significant correlations, n (%)				
		Income spent on food at supermarkets / grocery stores	Income spent on food at other stores	Income spent on eating out	Healthy diet rate	Total
Rurality factors						
Population	≤9,999	11 (25.00)	4 (9.09)	9 (20.45)	8 (18.18)	32 (18.18)
	10,000+	13 (29.55)	2 (4.55)	1 (2.27)	19 (43.18)	35 (19.89)
Population density (per square mile)	≤1,834.50	8 (18.18)	0 (0.00)	6 (13.64)	9 (20.45)	23 (13.07)
	1,834.51+	24 (54.55)	4 (9.09)	0 (0.00)	22 (50.00)	50 (28.41)
Population change due to daytime travel (as percentage of total population)	≤6.25	12 (27.27)	4 (9.09)	9 (20.45)	11 (25.00)	36 (20.45)
	6.26+	6 (13.64)	0 (0.00)	7 (15.91)	7 (15.91)	20 (11.36)
Distance to nearest city of 50,000 or more people (in miles)	≤63.40	17 (38.64)	2 (4.55)	1 (2.27)	12 (27.27)	32 (18.18)
	63.41+	9 (20.45)	2 (4.55)	0 (0.00)	12 (27.27)	23 (13.07)
Commute time (in minutes)	≤14.90	1 (2.27)	0 (0.00)	2 (4.55)	7 (15.91)	10 (5.68)
	14.91+	14 (31.82)	0 (0.00)	6 (13.64)	8 (18.18)	28 (15.91)

People taking healthy diet shows 7 (15.91%) and 8 (18.18%) statistically significant associations with spatial factors in cities with ≤14.90 and 14.91+ minutes of commute time. This behavior may be less sensitive to spatial factors, but the effects are similar in both subsamples.

Overall, food shopping and eating behaviors show 10 (5.68% of the 176 correlations explored) and 28 (15.91%) statistically significant associations with spatial factors in cities with ≤14.90 and 14.91+ minutes of commute time, indicating that these behaviors in general are less sensitive to spatial factors in these subsamples. In relative terms, they are less sensitive to spatial factors in cities with ≤14.90 minutes of commute time than in cities with 14.91+ minutes of commute time.

In summary, based on the total numbers of statistically significant associations shown in the last column of the table, spatial factors may be equally important for food shopping and eating behaviors in cities with high and low population size. But they may be more important in cities with higher density, less population change due to daytime travel, less distance to large cities with 50,000 or more people, and longer commute time.

Rurality and Spatial Associations of Physical and Sedentary Activities

The health benefits of physical activities have been extensively studied since the 1950s. These studies show, among other things, that adults with physically active lifestyles suffer fewer than half the coronary events of those with sedentary lifestyles, while controlling for lifestyle factors such as smoking and alcohol consumption [65, 66]. Today, it is a well-established fact that physical activity reduces overweight, obesity, stroke, type 2 diabetes, colon cancer, breast cancer, depression, and anxiety, in addition to increasing life expectancy [67–71].

Conversely, sedentary behaviors—that is, too much sitting, as distinct from too little physical activity—are associated with increased risk of type 2 diabetes, cardiovascular disease, some cancers, and all-cause mortality [72–76]. Prolonged sitting, including time spent in cars, watching TV, and using a computer, is a risk factor for cardiovascular disease [77, 78] and poor mental health [79–81]. The risk associated with poor physical fitness resulting from physical inactivity and sedentary activities is comparable to, and in some studies greater than, the risk associated with hypertension, high cholesterol, diabetes, and even smoking [70, 82]. Overweight people die at as much as 2.5 times the rate of non-obese people [82–86].

Several studies report differences in physical and sedentary activities between rural and urban areas in the United States. According to *The 2014 Update of the Rural-Urban Chartbook* [87], nationwide, physical activity during leisure time varied with level of urbanization, but the patterns differed by US region. Inactivity during leisure time was most common for men and women in the most rural counties (41% for both sexes in 2010–2011) and was highest in nonmetropolitan counties for residents of all regions, except for men and women in the Northeast and women in the West. In a study using data provided by 14,039 participants in the 1999–2006 National Health and Nutrition Examination Survey (NHANES), Trivedi et al. [64] found that compared to urban adults, more rural adults reported no leisure-time physical activity (38.8% vs. 31.8%, p<0.01), and fewer rural adults met or exceeded physical activity recommendations (41.5% vs. 47.2%, p<0.01). In another study using NHANES data, Fan et al. [88] found that compared to urban residents, rural residents reported more physical activity but spent less time in higher-intensity physical activity, and they spent more time in lower-intensity physical activity, especially household physical activity. Other studies report similar findings for young adults [14, 89]. Studies also show that rural adults, both men and women, are less likely to meet public health recommendations for physical activity compared to their urban counterparts [90, 91].

Reporting on the differences in physical and sedentary activities, like other lifestyle behaviors, between rural and urban residents is not straightforward. Evidence regarding rural-urban differences in physical activity generally is mixed depending on whether physical activity was subjectively or objectively measured and what intensity threshold was used in objectively measured physical activity [14]. Evidence also conflicts on whether rural residents are less physically active than urban residents, and findings vary by age and type of activity. For instance, recent national data show no overall urban-rural differences in the frequency of children meeting physical activity recommendations [92, 93].

Still, several researchers have focused on the differences in the built environment to address rural-urban differences in physical and sedentary activities. The evidence remains underdeveloped when compared to urban-suburban efforts, however. Included among these researchers are a few who study how the spatial associations of physical and sedentary activities may depend on the rurality or urbanicity of a place. In one such instance reported above, Stewart et al. [33] found positive association between the number of neighborhood restaurants and walking in Seattle but negative association in small towns. They explained the difference as a function of site design related to the density of development. On average, restaurants in small towns were located in large retail areas characterized by huge setbacks from the street, large parking lots, and insufficient pedestrian infrastructure, discouraging pedestrian travel. In contrast, Seattle had more restaurants in pedestrian-friendly areas, encouraging pedestrian travel. This is in line with previous research [94] that showed more destinations might induce more walking in denser metropolitan areas with pedestrian-supportive urban designs.

Stewart et al. [33] also found that the perception of slow traffic on nearby streets was positively associated with recreational walking in small towns, but not in Seattle. It is possible that recreational walks occurred in the home neighborhood of these small towns more than they occurred in the neighborhoods of Seattle. People in small towns, therefore, were more sensitive to the perceived comfort and safety of their home neighborhood pedestrian environment than were people in Seattle areas. The perceived speed of traffic also could have been particularly important in small towns, where relatively lower traffic volumes and a greater range of traffic speeds could make speeding cars seem especially dangerous to pedestrians.

More recently, Stowe et al. [95] studied the association between neighborhood walkability and youth obesity in relation to urbanicity and found that neighborhood Walk Score was positively associated with BMI among urban youth and negatively associated with BMI among rural youth. However, they observed no relationship between Walk Score and youth in urban-rural mixed areas. Based on the findings, the authors concluded that neighborhood walkability might affect youth differently across geographic areas.

Other comparative studies report that spatial factors affect the relationship between physical activities and healthy weight in rural and urban areas differently [96]; that the likelihood of meeting physical activity recommendations increased with the number of places available for exercise for urban residents and not for rural residents [97]; that urban residents have better accessibility to physical activity resources than have rural residents [91, 97, 98]; that the availability of safe parks promotes physical activity for adolescents in urban areas but not in rural areas [99]; that rural areas possess fewer physical activity resources, negatively affecting physical activity [100]; and that active travel to school predicted physical activity for urban but not for rural youth [101].

According to the literature, many spatial factors may help reduce sedentary behaviors and sitting time [102, 103]. A recent review of 17 studies identified 89 associations between environmental attributes and sedentary behaviors; the most consistent finding was that residents in large urban areas spend less sedentary time than do residents in smaller towns or cities [104]. That is because large urban areas often have more extensive public transport infrastructure, which allows more residents to spend less time sitting in private vehicles.

Based on the findings reported in the literature, it can be suggested that evidence on spatial correlates of physical activity in US rural areas and small towns is weak and that the degree of rurality or urbanicity should be considered an important moderator in the physical activity and built environment relationships. Very little evidence is found on spatial correlates of sedentary activities in US rural areas and small towns. Again, the findings of any reported studies are not straightforward. Often, they report null or even opposite relationships [21, 105, 106]. One potentially confounding variable that may help explain these mixed results is how the rural-urban status of the areas is defined in these studies. Since the relationships between physical activity and the built environment or between sedentary activities and built environment may differ due to differences between rural versus urban settings [107], a simple demography or distance-based definition of rurality or urbanicity may be insufficient in studies exploring spatial associations of physical and sedentary activities. In this regard, the findings reported below may be important because they show how different aspects of rurality may affect spatial associations of physical and sedentary activities in small cities of rural Kansas.

Things We Observe in Small Cities of Kansas
EFFECTS OF POPULATION SIZE

As reported in table 9.3, according to a comparison of the two subsamples defined based on *population size, people doing vigorous-intensity work activities* shows 2 (4.55% of the 44 correlations explored) and 6 (13.64%) statistically significant associations with spatial factors in cities with ≤9,999 and 10,000+ people. Spatial factors may be less important for this behavior in both these subsamples of cities.

People doing moderate-intensity work activities shows 22 (50%) and 6 (13.64%) statistically significant associations with spatial factors in cities with ≤9,999 and 10,000+ people. Spatial factors may be more important for this behavior in cities with ≤9,999 people.

People walking or bicycling shows 0 and 6 (13.64%) statistically significant associations with spatial factors in cities with ≤9,999 and 10,000+ people. Spatial factors may be less important for this behavior in both these subsamples of cities.

People doing vigorous-intensity recreational activities shows 10 (22.73%) and 5 (11.36%) statistically significant associations with spatial factors in cities with ≤9,999 and 10,000+ people, indicating that the behavior may be more sensitive to this behavior in small cities with lower population size.

People doing moderate-intensity recreational activities shows 12 (27.27%) and 11 (25%) statistically significant associations with spatial factors in cities with ≤9,999 and 10,000+ people, indicating that the behavior may be equally sensitive to spatial factors in these subsamples.

Average hours a day doing sedentary activities shows 8 (18.18%) and 20 (45.45% statistically significant associations with spatial factors in cities with ≤9,999 and 10,000+ people, indicating that this behavior is particularly sensitive to spatial factors in cities with 10,000+ people.

Overall, physical and sedentary activities show 54 (20.45% of the 264 correlations explored) statistically significant associations with spatial factors in both subsamples of cities with ≤9,999 and 10,000+ people, indicating that they may be equally sensitive to spatial factors.

EFFECTS OF POPULATION DENSITY

As reported in table 9.3, according to a comparison of the two subsamples defined based on *population density, people doing vigorous-intensity work activities* shows 0 and 13 (29.55% of the 44 correlations explored) statistically significant associations with spatial factors in cities with ≤1,834.50 and 1,834.51+ people per square mile; *people doing moderate-intensity work activities* shows 4 (9.09%) and 20 (45.45%); *people walking or bicycling* shows 8 (18.18%) and 23 (52.27%). For these behaviors, spatial factors may be more important in small cities with higher population density.

In contrast, *people doing vigorous-intensity recreational activities* shows 10 (22.73%) and 0 statistically significant associations with spatial factors for cities with ≤1,834.50 and 1,834.51+ people per square mile. In other words, spatial factors may be important for this behavior in small cities with lower population density only.

People doing moderate-intensity recreational activities shows 14 (31.82%) and 18 (40.91%) statistically significant associations with spatial factors for cities with ≤1,834.50 and 1,834.51+ people per square mile, indicating that this behavior may be a bit more sensitive to spatial factors in small cities with higher population density.

Average hours a day doing sedentary activities shows 8 (18.18%) and 20 (45.45%) statistically significant associations with spatial factors in cities with ≤1,834.50 and 1,834.51+ people per square mile. This behavior may be more sensitive to spatial factors in the subsample with higher population density.

Overall, physical and sedentary activities show 44 (16.67% of the 264 correlations explored) and 94 (35.61%) statistically significant associations with spatial factors in cities with ≤1,834.50 and 1,834.51+ people per square mile, indicating that these behaviors are far more sensitive to spatial factors in cities with higher population density.

EFFECTS OF DAYTIME POPULATION CHANGE

As reported in table 9.3, according to a comparison of the two subsamples defined based on *daytime population change, people doing vigorous-intensity work activities* does not show any statistically significant association with spatial factors in the subsamples. Therefore, spatial factors may not be important for this behavior in these subsamples.

People doing moderate-intensity work activities shows 7 (15.91% of the 44 correlations explored) and 2 (4.55% of the total) statistically significant associations with spatial factors in cities with ≤6.25% and 6.26%+ population change due to daytime travel; *people walking or bicycling* shows 17 (38.64%) and 10 (22.73%); *people doing vigorous-intensity recreational activities* shows 15 (34.09%) and 9 (20.45%); *people doing moderate-intensity recreational activities* shows 15 (34.09%) and 7 (15.91%). The importance of spatial factors appears to vary for these behaviors as population change due to daytime travel varies in small cities.

Average hours a day doing sedentary activities shows 7 (15.91%) and 6 (13.64%) statistically significant associations with spatial factors in cities with ≤6.25% and 6.26%+ population change due to daytime travel, indicating that this behavior may be less but almost equally sensitive to spatial factors in these subsamples of cities.

Overall, physical and sedentary activities show 61 (23.11% of the 264 correlations explored) and 34 (12.88%) statistically significant associations with spatial factors in cities with ≤6.25% and 6.26%+ population change due to daytime travel, indicating that these behaviors may be more sensitive to spatial factors in cities with less population change due to daytime travel.

EFFECTS OF DISTANCE TO NEAREST CITY OF 50,000 OR MORE PEOPLE

As reported in table 9.3, according to a comparison of the two subsamples defined based on *distance to nearest city of 50,000 or more people, people doing vigorous-intensity work activities* shows 8 (18.18% of the 44 correlations explored) and 0 statistically significant associations with spatial factors in cities ≤63.40 and 63.41+ miles from the nearest large city; *people doing moderate-intensity work activities* shows 16 (36.36%) and 7 (15.91%); *people walking or bicycling* shows 17 (38.64%) and 7 (15.91%); *people doing vigorous-intensity recreational activities* shows 5 (11.36%) and 2 (4.55%); and *people doing moderate-intensity recreational activities* shows 9 (20.45%) and 1 (2.27%). Therefore, spatial factors appear less important for these behaviors in small cities farther away from the nearest large city.

In contrast to the above behaviors, *average hours a day doing sedentary activities* shows 8 (18.18%) and 13 (29.55%) statistically significant associations with spatial factors for cities ≤63.40 and 63.41+ miles from the nearest large city. This behavior appears more sensitive to spatial factors in cities farther away from the nearest large city.

Overall, physical and sedentary activities show 63 (23.86% of the 264 correlations explored) and 30 (11.36%) statistically significant associations with spatial factors in cities ≤63.40 and 63.41+ miles from the nearest large city, indicating that these behaviors may be more sensitive to spatial factors in cities closer to the nearest large city.

EFFECTS OF COMMUTE TIME

As reported in table 9.3, according to a comparison of the two subsamples defined based on *commuting time, people doing vigorous-intensity work activities* shows 0 and 12 (27.27% of the 44 correlations explored) statistically significant associations with spatial factors for cities with ≤14.90 and 14.91+ minutes of commute time; *people doing moderate-intensity work activities* shows 6 (13.64%) and 14 (31.82%); *people walking or bicycling* shows 6 (13.64%) and 11 (25%); *people doing vigorous-intensity recreational activities* shows 2 (4.55%) and 14 (31.82%); and *people doing moderate-intensity recreational activities* shows 2 (4.55%) and 14 (31.82%). Spatial factors appear more important for these behaviors in cities with longer commute time.

In contrast, *average hours a day doing sedentary activities* shows 10 (22.73%) and 6 (13.64%) statistically significant associations with spatial factors for cities with ≤14.90 and 14.91+ minutes of commute time. Spatial factors appear less important for these behaviors in cities with longer commute time.

Overall, physical and sedentary activities show 26 (9.85% of the 264 correlations explored) and 71 (26.89%) statistically significant associations with spatial factors in cities with ≤14.90 and 14.91+ minutes of commute time, indicating that these behaviors may be more sensitive to spatial factors in cities with longer commute time.

In summary, based on the numbers shown in the last column of the table, spatial factors may be equally important for physical and sedentary activities in both the subsamples defined based on population size. They may be more important for these behaviors in cities with higher densities, less daytime population change, at closer distance from the nearest large city with 50,000 or more people, and with longer commute time.

Conclusions
Concerning the Effects of Population Size

According to the findings of the study (table 9.4), with 99 (17.31% of all the correlations considered) and 116 (20.28%) associations between spatial factors

TABLE 9.3.

Significant correlations between spatial factors and physical and sedentary activities

	Significant correlations, n (%)						
	People doing vigorous-intensity work activities	People doing moderate-intensity work activities	People walking or bicycling	People doing vigorous-intensity recreational activities	People doing moderate-intensity recreational activities	Average hours a day doing sedentary activities	Total
Rurality factors							
Population							
≤9,999	2 (4.55)	22 (50.00)	0 (0.00)	10 (22.73)	12 (27.27)	8 (18.18)	54 (20.45)
10,000+	6 (13.64)	6 (13.64)	6 (13.64)	5 (11.36)	11 (25.00)	20 (45.45)	54 (20.45)
Population density (per square mile)							
≤1,834.50	0 (0.00)	4 (9.09)	8 (18.18)	10 (22.73)	14 (31.82)	8 (18.18)	44 (16.67)
1,834.51+	13 (29.55)	20 (45.45)	23 (52.27)	0 (0.00)	18 (40.91)	20 (45.45)	94 (35.61)
Population change due to daytime travel (as percentage of total population)							
≤6.25	0 (0.00)	7 (15.91)	17 (38.64)	15 (34.09)	15 (34.09)	7 (15.91)	61 (23.11)
6.26+	0 (0.00)	2 (4.55)	10 (22.73)	9 (20.45)	7 (15.91)	6 (13.64)	34 (12.88)
Distance to nearest city of 50,000 or more people (in miles)							
≤63.40	8 (18.18)	16 (36.36)	17 (38.64)	5 (11.36)	9 (20.45)	8 (18.18)	63 (23.86)
63.41+	0 (0.00)	7 (15.91)	7 (15.91)	2 (4.55)	1 (2.27)	13 (29.55)	30 (11.36)
Commute time (in minutes)							
≤14.90	0 (0.00)	6 (13.64)	6 (13.64)	2 (4.55)	2 (4.55)	10 (22.73)	26 (9.85)
14.91+	12 (27.27)	14 (31.82)	11 (25.00)	14 (31.82)	14 (31.82)	6 (13.64)	71 (26.89)

and lifestyle for cities with ≤9,999 and 10,000+ people, lifestyle behaviors appear more sensitive to spatial factors in small cities with more population.

Among the three work-related travel behaviors considered, *workers who live and work in the city* appears most sensitive to spatial factors in both subsamples defined based on population size, indicating that spatial strategies may be most effective to change this behavior in these small cities.

At least two of the four food shopping and eating behaviors show very high numbers of associations with spatial factors in both the subsamples defined based on population size: *income spent on food at supermarkets or grocery stores* and *people taking healthy diet*. The latter appears to be most sensitive to spatial factors in cities with 10,000+ people.

At least three out of six physical and sedentary activities show very high numbers of associations with spatial factors in both subsamples defined based on population size. Among them, *people doing moderate-intensity work activities* shows the highest number of associations with spatial factors in cities with ≤9,999 people. From the spatial planning and design perspective, the findings of the study indicate that it may be wise to focus on small cities with ≤9,999 to have the most impact on this and other physical activities.

In contrast, *average hours a day doing sedentary activities* shows the highest number of associations with spatial factors in cities with 10,000+ people, indicating that it may be wise to focus on spatial strategies in this subsample of small cities to have the most impact on sedentary activities.

Concerning the Effects of Population Density

The findings of the study (table 9.4) show that lifestyle and spatial factors have 71 (12.41% of all the correlations considered) and 188 (32.87%) statistically significant associations in cities with ≤1,834.50 and 1,834.51+ people per square mile. These findings indicate that spatial factors may be more important for lifestyle in small cities with higher population density than in cities with lower densities.

Clearly, all three work-related behaviors—*workers who live and work at home, workers who drove alone to work*, and *workers who carpooled to work*—show high numbers of associations with spatial factors in cities with 1,834.51+ people per square mile, indicating that in this subsample spatial strategies may be an effective way to modify these behaviors.

At least two food-shopping and eating behaviors, *income spent on food at supermarkets or grocery stores* and *people taking healthy diet*, show high numbers of associations with spatial factors in cities with 1,834.51+ people per square mile, again indicating that in this subsample spatial strategies may be an effective way to modify these behaviors.

Interestingly, all of the physical activities but one—*people doing vigorous-intensity recreational activities*—show frequent associations with spatial factors in cities with 1,834.51+ people per square mile, suggesting a close link between them. *Average hours a day doing sedentary activities* also shows a higher number of associations with spatial factors in cities with 1,834.5+ people per square mile. These findings indicate that spatial strategies may be more effective in changing physical and sedentary activities in denser small cities.

Based on the findings reported here, it may be wise to focus on small cities with 1,834.51+ people per square mile to make an impact on lifestyle through spatial planning and design strategies. If conceived well, these strategies could affect significant changes in several work-related travel behaviors, food shopping and eating behaviors, and physical and sedentary activities in these cities. In many other cases, spatial strategies could also be effective for lifestyle changes in small cities with ≤1,834.50 people per square mile.

Concerning the Effects of Daytime Population Change

Altogether there are 132 (23.08% of all the correlations considered) and 62 (10.84%) statistically significant associations in cities with ≤6.25% and 6.26%+ population change due to daytime travel (table 9.4). Based on these findings, spatial factors are clearly more important for lifestyle in small cities with less daytime population change.

All three work-related travel behaviors, all four food shopping and eating behaviors, and five out of six physical and sedentary activities show higher numbers of statistically significant associations with spatial factors in cities with ≤6.25% population change due to daytime travel, indicating that it may be possible to affect significant changes to lifestyle in this subsample of cities through spatial planning strategies. The findings of the study, however, also indicate that spatial planning and design strategies could affect several behaviors in cities with 6.26%+ population change due to daytime travel but to a lesser extent.

Concerning the Effects of Distance from the Nearest Large City

According to the findings (table 9.4), there are 124 (21.68% of all the correlations considered) and 65 (11.36%) statistically significant associations in cities ≤63.40 and 63.41+ miles from the nearest city of 50,000 or more people, indicating that spatial factors are more important for lifestyle in small cities closer to big cities.

The total numbers of associations between spatial factors and work-related travel behaviors, between spatial factors and food shopping and eating behaviors, and between spatial factors and physical and sedentary activities are over 1.5 to 2 times more in cities ≤63.40 miles than in cities 63.41+ miles from the nearest big city. Spatial design and planning strategies therefore should focus on small cities ≤63.40 miles from the nearest big city to affect most changes to lifestyle.

Concerning the Effects of Commute Time

The findings show 48 (8.39% of all the correlations considered) and 115 (20.10%) statistically significant associations for cities with ≤14.90 and 14.91+ minutes of commute time (table 9.4). Spatial factors may be more important for lifestyle in cities with longer commute time.

The findings also show that spatial factors are generally more important for work-related travel behaviors, food shopping and eating behaviors, and physical and sedentary activities in cities with 14.91+ minutes of commute time. For some of these behaviors, the numbers of associations with spatial factors are several times higher in cities with 14.91+ minutes of commute time. It may therefore be wise to consider small cities with 14.91+ minutes of commute time for the most impact on food shopping and eating behaviors and physical and sedentary activities through spatial design and planning interventions, guidelines, and policies.

Exceptions to the above exist, however. *Carpooled to work* and *average hours of sedentary activities a day* are more sensitive to spatial factors in cities with less commute time. It may therefore be necessary to target small cities with less commute time to effectively change these behaviors through spatial strategies.

Concerning the Effects of Rurality

Spatial associations of lifestyle may increase in small cities with more population, higher population density, less daytime population changes, less distance to large cities, and more commute time. Each of the lifestyle behaviors appears to have some number of statistically significant associations with spatial factors in either or both subsamples of small cities defined based on the high and low values of the factors of rurality, which include population size and density, population change due to daytime travel, distance to the nearest city, and commute time.

Among the subsamples of small cities defined based on the factors of ru-

TABLE 9.4.
Ranking of significant correlations between spatial factors and lifestyle

		Lifestyle	Rank
Rurality factors			
		n (%)	
Population	≤9,999	99 (17.31)	6
	10,000+	116 (20.28)	4
Population density (per square mile)	≤1,834.50	71 (12.41)	7
	1,834.51+	188 (32.87)	1
Population change due to daytime travel (as percentage of total population)	≤6.25	132 (23.08)	2
	6.26+	62 (10.84)	9
Distance to nearest city of 50,000 or more people (in miles)	≤63.40	124 (21.68)	3
	63.41+	65 (11.36)	8
Commute time (in minutes)	≤14.90	48 (8.39)	10
	14.91+	115 (20.1)	5

rality, small cities with 1,851+ people per square mile show the most numbers of associations between lifestyle and spatial factors. This subsample is followed by the subsamples of cities with ≤6.25% population change due to daytime travel, cities ≤63.40 miles from the nearest large city, cities with 10,000+ people, and cities with 14.91+ minutes of commute time in a descending order. The numbers of spatial associations for these categories of small cities vary between 114 and 188. The numbers for the remaining subsample of small cities vary between 48 and 99 (table 9.4).

Clearly, different factors of rurality affect spatial associations of lifestyle differently in small cities of Kansas. Therefore, instead of focusing on the whole sample, it may be wise to focus on different subsamples of cities defined based on different factors of rurality to have the most impact on lifestyle through spatial design and planning interventions, policies, and guidelines.

NOTES

1. Bopp, Kaczynski, and Besenyi, "Active Commuting Influences."
2. Bopp, Kaczynski, and Campbell, "Social Ecological Influences."
3. Shephard, "Is Active Commuting the Answer to Population Health?"
4. Fan, Wen, and Wan, "Built Environment and Active Commuting."
5. Andersen et al., "All-Cause Mortality Associated With Physical Activity."
6. Hamer and Chida, "Active Commuting and Cardiovascular Risk."

7. Cavill et al., "Economic Analyses of Transport Infrastructure and."
8. Davis and Parkin, "Active Travel."
9. Clean Air Partnership, *Bike Lanes, On-Street Parking and Business.*
10. Thompson, "The Human Experience."
11. Fuguitt, "Commuting and the Rural-Urban Hierarchy."
12. Ewing et al., "Identifying and Measuring Urban Design Qualities."
13. Frank et al., "Many Pathways from Land Use to Health."
14. Fan, Wen, and Kowaleski-Jones, "Rural-Urban Differences."
15. Bennett, Olatosi, and Probst, *Health Disparities.*
16. Martin et al., "Urban, Rural, and Regional Variations in Physical Activity."
17. Patterson et al., "Obesity and Physical Inactivity."
18. Weaver et al., "Rural-Urban Differences in Health Behaviors."
19. Zhang et al., "Neighborhood Commuting Environment and Obesity."
20. Berrigan, Pickle, and Dill, "Associations between Street Connectivity and Active Transportation."
21. Panter and Jones, "Attitudes and the Environment as Determinants."
22. Kim and Heinrich, "Built Environment Factors Influencing Walking to School Behaviors."
23. Alexander et al., "The Broader Impact of Walking to School."
24. Cooper et al., "Physical Activity Levels of Children."
25. Fulton et al., "Active Transportation to School."
26. Ewing, Schroeer, and Greene, "School Location and Student Travel Analysis."
27. Sallis and Glanz, "The Role of Built Environments."
28. Chillón et al., "A Systematic Review of Interventions."
29. Giles-Corti et al., "School Site and the Potential to Walk to School."
30. Salmon et al., "Associations among Individual, Social, and Environmental Barriers."
31. Ewing, Forinash, and Schroeer, "Neighborhood Schools and Sidewalk Connections."
32. Zhu and Lee, "Ethnic Disparity in the Multi-Level Walkability and Safety."
33. Stewart et al., "Comparing Associations between the Built Environment and Walking."
34. Hirsch et al., "Discrete Land Uses and Transportation Walking."
35. Caspi et al., "The Local Food Environment and Diet."
36. Lock et al., "The Global Burden of Disease."
37. Ng et al., "Global, Regional, and National Prevalence."
38. Auchincloss et al., "Improving Retrospective Characterization."
39. Morland et al., "Neighborhood Characteristics."
40. Centers for Disease Control and Prevention, "Only 1 in 10 Adults Get Enough Fruits or Vegetables."
41. US Department of Agriculture, "Key Statistics and Graphics."
42. Charreire et al., "Measuring the Food Environment."
43. Jiao et al., "How to Identify Food Deserts."
44. Usher, "Exploring the Effects of Formalised, Targeted Municipal Food Planning Initiatives."
45. Kelly, Flood, and Yeatman, "Measuring Local Food Environments."
46. Liese et al., "Food Store Types, Availability, and Cost of Foods."
47. Christian, "Using Geospatial Technologies."
48. Hillier et al., "A Discrete Choice Approach."
49. Križan et al., "Potential Food Deserts and Food Oases."
50. Dutko, Ver Ploeg, and Farrigan, *Characteristics and Influential Factors.*
51. Bader et al., "Disparities in Neighborhood Food Environments."
52. McKenzie, "Access to Supermarkets among Poorer Neighborhoods."

53. McKinnon et al., "Measures of the Food Environment."
54. Pearson et al., "Do 'Food Deserts' Influence Fruit and Vegetable Consumption?"
55. Pitts et al., "Associations between Access to Farmers' Markets and Supermarkets."
56. Rose and Richards, "Food Store Access and Household Fruit and Vegetable Use."
57. Befort, Nazir, and Perri, "Prevalence of Obesity among Adults."
58. Ely et al., "A Qualitative Assessment of Weight Control."
59. Nothwehr and Peterson, "Healthy Eating and Exercise."
60. Pitts et al., "Formative Evaluation for a Healthy Corner Store Initiative."
61. Larson, Story, and Nelson, "Neighborhood Environments."
62. Coveney and O'Dwyer, "Effects of Mobility and Location."
63. Winkler, Turrell, and Patterson, "Does Living in a Disadvantaged Area Mean Fewer Opportunities?"
64. Trivedi et al., "Obesity and Obesity-Related Behaviors."
65. Morris et al., "Coronary Heart-Disease and Physical Activity of Work."
66. Paffenbarger, Wing, and Hyde, "Physical Activity as an Index of Heart Attack Risk."
67. Lee and Paffenbarger, "Associations of Light, Moderate, and Vigorous Intensity Physical Activity."
68. Sesso, Paffenbarger, and Lee, "Physical Activity and Coronary Heart Disease."
69. Wannamethee, Shaper, and Walker, "Changes in Physical Activity, Mortality, and Incidence of Coronary Heart Disease."
70. Wei et al., "Relationship between Low Cardiorespiratory Fitness and Mortality."
71. Sesso et al., "Physical Activity and Cardiovascular Disease Risk."
72. Owen, "Sedentary Behavior."
73. Owen et al., "Too Much Sitting."
74. Dunstan et al., "Too Much Sitting."
75. Dunstan et al., "Television Viewing Time and Mortality."
76. Thorp et al., "Sedentary Behaviors and Subsequent Health Outcomes."
77. Sugiyama, Ding, and Owen, "Commuting by Car."
78. Sugiyama, Neuhaus, and Owen, "Active Transport, the Built Environment, and Human Health."
79. Vallance et al., "Accelerometer-Assessed Physical Activity and Sedentary Time."
80. Pengpid and Peltzer, "High Sedentary Behaviour and Low Physical Activity."
81. Wang, Li, and Fan, "The Associations between Screen Time–Based Sedentary Behavior and Depression."
82. Blair et al., "Influences of Cardiorespiratory Fitness and Other Precursors."
83. Must et al., "The Disease Burden Associated with Overweight and Obesity."
84. Willett, Dietz, and Colditz, "Guidelines for Healthy Weight."
85. Sesso, Lee, and Paffenbarger, "Physical Activity and Breast Cancer Risk."
86. Shaper, Wannamethee, and Walker, "Body Weight."
87. Meit et al., *The 2014 Update of the Rural-Urban Chartbook.*
88. Fan, Wen, and Kowaleski-Jones, "An Ecological Analysis of Environmental Correlates."
89. Moore et al., "Association of the Built Environment with Physical Activity and Adiposity."
90. Blackwell, Lucas, and Clarke, "Summary Health Statistics for US Adults."
91. Wilcox et al., "Determinants of Leisure Time Physical Activity."
92. Davis et al., "Obesity and Related Health Behaviors."
93. Kenney, Wang, and Iannotti, "Residency and Racial/Ethnic Differences."
94. Glazier et al., "Density, Destinations or Both?"
95. Stowe et al., "Associations between Walkability and Youth Obesity."

96. Hansen et al., "Built Environments and Active Living."
97. Parks, Housemann, and Brownson, "Differential Correlates of Physical Activity."
98. Jilcott et al., "Association between Physical Activity and Proximity."
99. Babey et al., "Physical Activity among Adolescents."
100. Badland, Duncan, and Mummery, "Travel Perceptions, Behaviors, and Environment."
101. Loucaides, Plotnikoff, and Bercovitz, "Differences in the Correlates of Physical Activity."
102. Owen et al., "Sedentary Behaviour and Health."
103. Owen et al., "Adults' Sedentary Behaviur."
104. Koohsari et al., "Neighborhood Environmental Attributes."
105. Bassett, "Encouraging Physical Activity and Health."
106. Bauman et al., "Correlates of Physical Activity."
107. Frost et al., "Effects of the Built Environment on Physical Activity."

PART FIVE

RURALITY, SPATIAL FACTORS, AND HEALTH STATUS IN SMALL CITIES OF KANSAS

Spatial Associations of Health in Small Cities of Kansas

Correlational Analyses

In this chapter, the associations of spatial (planning and design) factors with health indicators in small Kansas cities are studied using correlational analyses. As presented in the previous chapters, the categories of health indicators include those related to mortality and morbidity and physical, mental, and social health; the categories of spatial factors include city size and density defined in spatial terms, availability of key destinations and facilities, land use types and mix, and various street properties. These spatial factors, according to studies reported in the literature, generally show frequent associations with health indicators in studies involving urban areas within big cities. Similar studies involving rural counties and small towns, however, are hard to find. A brief review of the studies reported in the literature is provided here along with the findings of correlational analyses involving spatial factors and health indicators for the sample of small cities selected from Kansas. The correlation coefficient (Spearman's rho) and the significance level (p-value) of the correlations are given in tables 10.1 and 10.2 (available online at https://hdl.handle.net/1808/34227).

There are 44 spatial factors and 23 health indicators in the analysis, producing 1,012 correlations to report. Following the strategy used in chapter 8, the correlations of each spatial factor are reported by the categories of health indicators. Again, these categories are mortality and morbidity, physical health, mental health, and social health. As in chapter 8, only significant correlations and their effect size and level of significance are considered. The numbers of significant correlations of a spatial factor with different categories of health indicators are used to determine how important the spatial factor is for these health indicators. Spatial factors with higher numbers of significant correlations are considered to have broader associations with health indicators than spatial factors with fewer numbers of correlations. To put it differently, health indicators are considered to be more sensitive to spatial factors when there are higher numbers of significant associations between them.

City Size and Health

Evidence presented in the literature seems to support that health varies systematically with city size. For example, using 2001 National Health Interview Survey data for the adult US population living in urban areas, Ray and Ghosh [1] showed that individual health is better in bigger cities compared to small or medium cities. They also showed that this result holds after controlling for potentially confounding variables, including age, gender, education, marital status, smoking, income, asset ownership, and race. Evidence supporting a health gradient for city size is also presented by Cheung et al. [2]. In a cross-national study involving 691 Vietnamese immigrants to the United States, they showed that residing in a large city was one of the factors significantly related to mental health.

Studies conducted in other countries also report associations between city size and health. For example, using a representative survey conducted in 2011 of adults living in urban China, Chen et al. [3] found that, after controlling for individual sociodemographic characteristics, health status, and household wealth, new urbanites (rural-to-urban migrants and in situ urbanized rural residents) who settle in cities with urban populations between 200,000 and 500,000 are more satisfied with their lives than those who settle in either larger or smaller cities. Zhou et al. [4] studied urban heat island (UHI) effects, which are important health risk factors, in relation to city size. They found that the UHI intensity increases with the logarithm of city size among the largest 5,000 cities in Europe. Typically, the size has the strongest influence, followed by the compactness, and the smallest is the influence of the degree to which the cities stretch on UHI.

Ferré et al. [5] studied poverty, which is also an important health risk factor, in relation to city size. Using evidence from eight developing countries, their study shows an inverse relationship between poverty and city size. It shows that poverty is both more widespread and deeper in very small and small towns than in large or very large cities in these countries. This pattern is particularly pronounced in the larger, more urbanized countries in their sample. In these countries, poverty in the very small cities is up to six times greater than in the metropolitan areas and often only slightly lower than in rural areas. This basic pattern generally remains stable regardless of how poverty is defined. Their study also shows that for all eight countries, a majority of the poor live in medium, small, or very small towns. Additionally, the study shows that the greater incidence and severity of consumption poverty in smaller towns are generally compounded by similarly greater deprivation in terms of access to basic infrastructure services, such as electricity, heating gas, sewerage, and solid waste disposal.

These and other similar findings reported in the literature on the relationships between city size and health and health risk factors indicate a need for a study on the health effects of the size of small cities. It is possible, however, that any associations between city size and health may not be as noticeable in small cities as the ones presented in the literature involving big cities or urban areas within big cities.

Things We Observe in Small Cities of Kansas

In small Kansas cities, city size measured using land area shows a significant negative association with death rate, indicating that as the size of small cities increases, death rate decreases. Though any reason for the association remains unknown, it is possible that as small cities increase in size, they are able to acquire more resources to protect lives. This issue is further explored in relation to rurality in the next chapter. It should be noted that the analysis does not show any association with the other three mortality and morbidity indicators included in this study.

Among the four physical health indicators, city size shows a significant weak negative correlation with the percentage of people with adult diabetes and a significant strong negative correlation with the percentage of overweight people. In simple words, as the size of the small cities increases both diabetes and overweight rates decrease. Again, it is possible that larger small cities have more health resources for their residents to deal with diabetes and overweight than smaller small cities.

City size does not show any significant associations with any one of the five indicators of mental health, which include people feeling badly about themselves, having little interest in doing things, having thoughts that they would be better off dead, and having ever used marijuana or hashish. This is despite size possibly being an independent factor affecting mental health in large cities.

Notably, city size shows significant weak to strong positive correlations with several indicators of social health. They include two violent crimes (murder and robbery) and two property crimes (theft and auto theft). City size also shows positive correlations with violent and property crime rates. The findings indicate that as city size increases, crimes in these small cities increase. The finding may be related to small cities with larger areas having more people, hence more crimes.

In summary, according to the findings of this study, *city size* as measured by land area may be an important health factor in small Kansas cities. More studies are needed, however, to understand why city size is associated with health in these small cities.

Density and Health

Though it is often suggested that urban areas with high density support high demographic heterogeneity and cultural integration, leading to a heightened sense of community, greater community participation, and greater social capital, the evidence is mixed and sometimes contradictory regarding their effects on mental and community health [6]. In general, access to services and facilities is better in higher-density environments, increasing walking trips with benefits to physical and mental health and well-being [7]. With higher density, however, privacy is sometimes compromised and social engagement reduced. Higher-density environments also tend to be associated with restricted access to nature. Higher densities coupled with the spatial concentration of facilities can create traffic congestion, which increases fuel consumption, air pollution, and CO_2 emissions. They worsen conditions for non-car trips and health. This has been termed the "paradox of intensification" [8].

Notably, several studies have linked density with crime in urban areas. In these studies, higher density areas show higher crime rates than areas with lower densities [9, 10]. High densities also show high rates of violent crime [11]. In dense, mixed-use locations, informal social controls are found to be more difficult to maintain; offenders are more anonymous; and increased opportunities for crime are observed [12]. Specific types of nonviolent crime, such as pickpocketing, are reported in crowded locations [13]. A large number of residents sharing a common entrance is linked with increased crime [14], but a large number of onlookers ("eyes on the street") is linked with reduced crime [15].

In practice, therefore, delivery of health benefits offered by high-density developments may be dependent on complementary policies concerning the location of facilities and, at a larger scale, on policies and forms of traffic demand management to limit car use. They may also depend on ensuring safety through spatial design and planning, as well as on policies and practices related to safety and policing.

It is important to note that the density of an urban area within a metropolitan region and the density of small cities in rural areas may not be comparable. While density may vary from one small city to another, it is unlikely that the density of a small city would be as high as that of an urban area within a metropolitan region, which generally has been the focus of most studies reported in the literature. Therefore, it would be interesting to see if variations in low-density small cities produce noticeable differences in health in small cities.

Things We Observe in Small Cities of Kansas

The four indicators of mortality and morbidity, the four indicators of physical health, and the five indicators of mental health do not show any correlation with census block density and housing density. The nine indicators of crime and one indicator of social isolation also do not show any correlation with census block density. Housing density, however, shows a significant weak negative association with burglaries, indicating that burglaries may decrease with increasing housing density.

That density does not show significant associations with health indicators in small cities despite showing numerous associations with the same in urban areas can be explained in several ways. First, as dictated by spatial and social structures, any spatial dependency of health may simply be different in urban areas from small cities. Second, the density of any small city is unlikely to be as high as it is in urban areas; therefore, it may not affect health in small cities in the way it may in urban areas. Finally, high social integration in small cities may work as a deterrent to any negative effects of density in small cities.

Overall, census block density and housing density may not be important health factors in small Kansas cities.

Availability of Key Destinations and Facilities and Health

Public open spaces or *green spaces* are among the key choice destinations. They often include a variety of spaces such as green spaces, parks, playgrounds, open sports fields, and urban squares. Many studies generally show that improved perception of and access to parks and green space provide numerous community and health benefits, including improved physical and mental health, social support, and local sense of community [16–25]. In some cases, these benefits are seen even after adjusting for age, sex, and socioeconomic status [26]. Even acute short-term exposures to green space during facilitated exercise have been associated with improved self-esteem and mood, independent of duration, intensity, location, gender, age, and health status [27]. Urban areas providing easy access to parks and green space have also been associated with reduced all-cause mortality in low-income communities [28]. In contrast, reduced access to parks and green space has been associated with increased risk of anxiety and depression, feelings of loneliness, and perceived shortage of social support [29]. Health inequalities related to income deprivation have been shown to be lower in populations living in the greenest areas [28]. For instance, in England, some affluent neighborhoods contain several times the amount of green space than deprived neighborhoods [30].

Benefits of green space are not limited to healthy people. Easy access to parks and green space has been shown to provide positive benefits for vulnerable populations. Contact with nature has been linked with reduced stress, anxiety, and severity of attention-deficit/hyperactivity disorder (ADHD) symptoms in children [31]; with preventive, psychological, physical, and social benefits among people suffering from mental illness and dementia [32]; with reduced hospital admissions for mental illness, even after controlling for deprivation and population density [31]; and with positive benefits among other patient groups, including those who underwent surgeries [33]. Living in areas with walkable green space is associated with increased longevity over a five-year period among older population [34]. Both park space (in acres) within a 500-meter buffer and the number of recreation programs within a 10-kilometer buffer of homes are beneficially associated with weight outcomes among children [35]. Playgrounds are essential resources in helping to combat the childhood obesity epidemic [36, 37].

Various types of physical activity (PA) facilities are also among the destinations shown to influence health. It is generally assumed that improved availability of and access to PA facilities, whether within public open spaces and parks or not, improve PA, which leads to better health outcomes. Supporting this assumption, Giles-Corti et al. [38] report associations between decreased access to recreational facilities and increased odds of being obese. Mobley et al. [39] report associations between higher number of fitness facilities per 1,000 residents and lower odds of body mass index (BMI) and coronary heart disease risk outcomes. In contrast to studies supporting the benefits of PA facilities, Boehmer et al. [40] found no significant association between the availability of recreational facilities and obesity.

Studies of rural and small communities that examined park access found lack of access to be positively associated with obesity and inactivity [41] but not among older adults [42]. Rural residents did not feel comfortable in health clubs outside their home communities, where people of other backgrounds might be present [43]. Obesity among adults was associated with perceived distance to the nearest recreation facility in 13 rural communities of Arkansas, Missouri, and Tennessee [41]. Rural recreational facilities located more than a 10-minute walk from home were associated with increased odds of obesity and inactivity [41]. When walking trails were viewed as isolated or primarily used by snowmobilers, rural walkers reported feeling unsafe [43].

Food environments, especially the availability of and the ease of access to healthy food outlets, are important for health. Unhealthy, high-calorie food has been associated with overweight and obesity. In many studies, obesity outcomes have been associated with the availability of and the ease of access to supermarkets, grocery stores, convenience stores, beverage and snack stores, full-service restaurants, franchised fast food and other limited-service restaurants, and emergency food providers [44]. In general, these studies report that healthy food environments with high densities of supermarkets and grocery stores may reduce the risk of obesity for both adults and children [45–48]. In one of these studies, Morland et al. [47] considered all types of food stores and food service places per census tract and found that an increase in the availability of supermarkets was associated with a decrease in the prevalence of overweight and obesity and that an increase in the availability of convenience stores was associated with an increase in the prevalence of overweight and obesity. In another study, Dengel et al. [49] reported that longer distance to convenience stores was significantly associated with a lower metabolic syndrome (METS) score (indicating lower odds of METS development) in adolescents. Yet another study found that people living in metropolitan counties with better supermarket accessibility were more likely to eat fruits and vegetables and less likely to be obese [50].

Other studies indicate the significance of different types of restaurants for population health. The quality of food served in fast food versus full-service restaurants differs, which may affect obesity outcomes. Full-service restaurants often provide a variety of healthier food options [51]. People who use full-service restaurants frequently are therefore more likely to eat healthy foods [52, 53], and proximity to restaurants providing fast food, but not full service, is correlated with weight gain [54]. In a large-scale study using the data from the 2002–06 Behavioral Risk Factor Surveillance System (BRFSS), Mehta and Chang [55] reported that a higher density of fast food restaurants (i.e., the number of restaurants per 10,000 residents) and a higher ratio of fast food to full-service restaurants were associated with higher BMI and obesity among adults and that a higher density of full-service restaurants was associated with reduced odds of obesity among adults. In a 2008 article, Li et al. [56] reported increased overweight and obesity with increasing density of fast food restaurants. In a subsequent short-term longitudinal study conducted over a period of one year, another group led by Li [57] reported that the density of fast food outlets in a neighborhood was positively associated with the frequency of use of these facilities and the amount of gains in weight and waist circumference by residents of the neighborhood.

Yet other studies highlight the significance of socioeconomic differences for the effects of food environments on population health. Low income and area deprivation are both barriers to purchasing fresh and nutritious foods [58]. This combination of economic and spatial barriers means that people living in areas of deprivation are less likely to have access to healthy diets [59–61]. Fast food restaurants are more available in lower- to middle-income and predominantly Black communities compared to high-income and white communities in urban areas [62, 63]. Those living in areas with the lowest socioeconomic status (SES) often have access to more fast food restaurants than those in the highest SES neighborhoods [64, 65]. Residents in socially deprived areas and residents shopping from grocery stores located in deprived areas often exhibit higher BMI levels. Car owners traveling farther to shop in grocery stores also show higher BMI levels [66].

In contrast to the studies reported above, Mobley et al. [39] found that no food environment feature was significantly associated with BMI and coronary heart disease risks in a study that used the number of full-sized grocery stores, fast food establishments, restaurants, and mini-marts per 1,000 residents for each residential zip code. Similarly, Burgoine et al. [67] did not find any significant relationship between BMI levels and food availability measured as the number of food outlets in a census area.

Since retail functions, such as shops and commercial facilities, are also among key choice destinations, it is expected that they would be associated with health and community benefits. The literature reports a positive association between obesity and the perception of having no shop within walking distance [38] and a beneficial association between high commercial floor area ratio and a sense of community [68]. Contrary to these and many other studies reporting positive health and well-being outcomes in relation to retail functions, at least one study in one metropolitan area reported that retail functions negatively affect the psychological health of older adults [69].

According to the studies reported in the literature, increased availability of parks and green space, PA resources, food outlets, and retail outlets generally show positive health benefits. Notably, an overwhelming body of evidence indicates beneficial health effects of public open space and green space. Such effects exist for healthy as well as vulnerable populations. They also exist for people of different socioeconomic classes. According to the literature, health disparities are reduced among different socioeconomic classes living close to green space, and differences in the availability of public open space or green space among residential areas may indicate health disparities. Though some of these studies pertain to rural areas, they rarely focus on small cities within rural areas. There is therefore a need for studies looking at the associations between the availability of key destinations and facilities and health outcomes in small cities.

Things We Observe in Small Cities of Kansas

Concerning *mortality* and *morbidity*, the findings of the study show several significant positive correlations between death rate and the availability of health care facilities, supermarkets or grocery stores, convenience stores with gas, and full-service restaurants. In contrast, the availability of business establishments shows significant negative correlation with death rate in these cities. Weak but significant positive correlations are found between availability of convenience stores with gas and full-service restaurants and general health conditions. Again, the availability of business establishments shows significant negative correlation with general health conditions in these cities. Weak but significant correlation is also found between availability of convenience stores with gas and suicide rate. It is not clear why these associations are found in small Kansas cities.

Concerning *physical health*, the findings of the study show that as the availability of health care facilities, supermarkets or grocery stores, convenience stores with gas, and full-service restaurants increases, so do adult diabetes and overweight. While the associations are significant for both diabetes and overweight, they are generally stronger for overweight than diabetes. In contrast, as the availability of supermarkets or grocery stores, convenience stores with gas, and business establishments increases, obesity decreases. The reason for these contrasting findings concerning obesity and overweight is that they are negatively associated—that is, as obesity increases, overweight decreases in small Kansas cities because obese people come from the same pool of overweight people.

Concerning *mental health*, the findings of the study show that the availability of key destinations and facilities does not have any significant associations with *people feeling badly about themselves, people feeling down, depressed, or hopeless*, or *people having thoughts that they would be better off dead*. *People having little interest in doing things* shows significant negative correlations with the availability of convenience stores with gas; and *people having ever used marijuana or hashish* shows positive correlations with parks per 10,000 people and businesses per 10,000 people. Overall, mental health indicators are not sensitive to the availability of key destinations and facilities, with few exceptions.

Concerning *social health*, the availability of key destinations and facilities shows several significant negative associations with crime, including murder, rape, robbery, assault, and burglary. The availability of key destinations and facilities also shows several significant negative weak to strong correlations with violent crime but only one significant negative correlation with property crime. In simple words, as the availability of key destinations and facilities increases, crime decreases, probably indicating better social health. Only *businesses per square mile* shows several positive correlations with violent crimes. It is not immediately clear why these correlations are found.

The availability of key destinations and facilities also shows several significant positive associations with the percentage of people over 65 years living alone, probably indicating less social support in cities with more key destinations and facilities. The reason for this may be that in cities with more key destinations and facilities more adults go to work, leaving older people alone at home. This is generally supported by very strong positive correlations between income and all available key destinations and facilities per square mile of these cities found in a separate analysis.

Overall, of the 46 possible associations with health indicators, the availability of health care facilities shows 7 associations; the availability of parks and green space shows 4 associations; the availability of supermarkets and grocery stores shows 17 associations; the availability of convenience stores shows 12 associations; the availability of convenience stores with gas shows 19 associations; the availability of business establishments shows 12 associations; and the availability of full-service restaurants shows 16 associations. In general, these findings support the literature, but with one significant difference—

parks and green spaces do not show as many associations with health indicators in small Kansas cities as they show in urban areas of large cities.

Land Use and Health

A comprehensive literature review by Ramirez et al. [70] found land use mix (LUM) as one of the 10 promising indicators of activity-friendly communities that can promote health. Strongly supporting Ramirez et al. [70], a more recent review by Mackenbach et al. [71] found that LUM was one of the two factors consistently associated with weight, although only in North America. Examples of the literature they reviewed include Frank et al. [72], which measured a four-category LUM, using the proportion of estimated square footage of residential, commercial, office, and institutional functions within a one-kilometer network buffer from each participant's household. Later, Frank et al. [73] employed a similar approach to evaluating a six-category LUM (single-family residential, multifamily residential, education, entertainment, retail, and office uses). They reported that LUM had a strong association with obesity, suggesting a reduction in the likelihood of obesity across gender and ethnicity with increase in LUM. Mobley et al. [39] used an additional category for rural land in their LUM calculations and reported that BMI was lower by 2.60 kg/m² and cardiac heart disease risk was lower by 20% in women living in an environment of maximum LUM as compared to those living in single-use uniform environments. Li et al. [56] reported a reduction in the prevalence of overweight and obesity with increases in LUM. In a study that used two-, three-, and six-category LUM, Brown et al. [74] reported that the six-category LUM was the best predictor of BMI, overweight, and obesity outcomes. In a study exploring whether parks were more likely to be used for PA if surrounded by greater LUM, Kaczynski et al. [75] found that greater LUM within a park's buffer of 500 meters was related to a lesser likelihood of the park being used for PA. Parks with a high number of facilities in low LUM areas were most likely to be used for PA.

Among other reported studies, Norman et al. [76] did not find any significant association between LUM and adolescent PA or BMI. They defined LUM as the geometric mean of residential, institutional, entertainment, retail, and office acreage within each one-mile street network buffer. Rundle et al. [77] found that LUM shows inverse and statistically significant association with BMI after adjustment for individual- and neighborhood-level sociodemographic characteristics. Using a five-category LUM for the two metropolitan cities of Toronto and Vancouver, Canada, Pouliou and Elliott [78] found that residents of areas with higher LUM exhibited improved weight outcomes compared to those living in areas with single or fewer land use types in Vancouver. No significant association could be established in the case of Toronto, however.

Concerning the relationships of LUM with mental and social health, it is suggested that compact neighborhoods with considerable heterogeneity are able to combine diverse uses, including dwellings, shops, supermarkets and food stores, offices, recreational facilities, green or open spaces, schools, places of worship, and other uses. They therefore encourage walking, which in turn promotes casual social contacts and a sense of community. Nasar and Julian [79] conducted a series of 25 interviews in four neighborhoods of Upper Arlington, Ohio, each of which differs with respect to LUM (having one, two, three, and four categories of land uses). They concluded that single-use residential neighborhoods were associated with a reduced sense of community as compared with multiuse neighborhoods. In another study, Lund [80] reported a similar trend, wherein increased sense of community was observed in traditional neighborhoods, manifested by a distinctively accessible road network and an enhanced mix of diverse land use categories. Leslie and Cerin [81] reported that a more heterogeneous LUM was beneficially associated with four of the five domains of neighborhood satisfaction, namely safety and walkability, access to destinations, social network, and travel network, which in turn acted as independent predictors of mental health. Wood et al. [68] considered measures of a three-category LUM of residential, commercial, and office land uses within a one-kilometer network buffer and reported significant associations with the sense of community score. Contrary to the general trend, however, in their study, LUM was inversely associated with sense of community—those living in low mixed land use areas were more likely to have a higher sense of community score than those in a high mixed land use area. In another study, Saarloos et al. [69] reported similar results. A higher LUM was associated with higher odds of depression among older men independent of other factors, including street connectivity and residential density.

Extensive research from the field of environmental criminology reveals that specific types of environmental settings (for example, mixed-use areas) are more criminogenic than other settings [82]. In general, informal social controls are more difficult to maintain in mixed-use locations [12]. In mixed-use locations, it is easy for offenders to remain anonymous [12]. Mixed-use communities exhibit weaker social cohesion and higher crime rates [83–85] than single-use residential environments [86, 87]. In mixed-use environments, increased vehicular and pedestrian flows may reduce the potential for inter-action and for recognizing strangers [88, 89]. Proximity to a range of mixed land uses may generate crime [90, 91]. Burglary is more frequent in proper-ties close to commercial areas and in properties located in mixed-use sites [92, 93]. Businesses in residential areas exhibit increased burglary rates [94]. Different land use types are associated with varying types of crime. For ex-ample, burglary is associated with industrial, commercial, and residential settings, while hospitals and bars are often linked to increased incidents of assaults.

LUM in urban areas appears to be positive for physical, mental, and social health and well-being in most cases. The mix of uses has to be right, however, to be positive [68]. Certain uses, such as industrial areas, nightclubs, or late-night bars, may cause stress through noise annoyance. Having too many commercial properties in a residential area can cause concern for safety when they are shut up at night and there are no eyes on the street. Perceived safety is lower in more mixed neighborhoods [95]. So, again, a mix of uses is good, but land use compatibility is important.

It is not surprising that studies involving LUM and health in rural areas and small cities are absent. First, it may be a part of the general neglect of the health in small cities by researchers. Second, LUM in small cities has never been an issue, because these cities often do not have an urban life in the ways urban areas in big cities do. Finally, small cities probably are not complex enough to present LUM as an interesting health issue. It is nevertheless a fact that small cities possess LUM. They are small, but they serve some of the several functions that urban cores of large cities serve. Therefore, a need to understand the associations between health and LUM in small cities exists.

Things We Observe in Small Cities of Kansas

According to the findings of the study, in small Kansas cities, land use types (expressed as percentages of total area given to different land uses) show no correlation with the *mortality* and *morbidity* indicators. LUM shows statisti-cally significant negative correlations with general health conditions and sui-cide rate, however, indicating that as LUM increases, the value of each of these two indicators declines. It is not clear why these correlations exist. Unem-ployment, which contributes to depression and anxiety, may be a reason. In general, there is more unemployment in small cities with more LUM because many establishments serving retail and commercial functions may be doing poorly due to various economic changes.

The land use types and mix of small Kansas cities also do not show any association with the *physical health* indicators, with two exceptions involving industrial land use. This land use type shows statistically significant negative correlations with average BMI and the percentage of overweight people. Again, it is not clear why these correlations exist.

According to this study, land use types and mix do not have significant associations with the indicators of *mental health*, with one exception that shows that the percentage of industrial areas shows statistically significant positive association with *people who have little interest in doing things*. In other words, as the percentage of industrial areas increases, *people who have little interest in doing things* also increases. It may be that people in cities with more industrial areas are poorer and therefore lack interest in anything. This is supported by a significant correlation between the percentage of industrial areas and poverty.

Regarding *social health*, land use types and mix do not have significant associations with different types of violent crime, with the exception of rape. According to the findings, as residential area increases, rape decreases; and as institutional area and LUM increase, rape increases. Land use types and mix also do not have significant associations with different types of property crime, with the exception of auto theft. As open area increases in the city, auto theft decreases. More studies are necessary to find some explanations for these findings.

Overall, land use factors show only a few significant associations with health indicators in small Kansas cities, and these associations are not consistent within and across different categories of health indicators. For some of these associations, there are no easy explanations.

Street Properties and Health

In studies assessing the effects of route accessibility on health, researchers use many objectively measured variables, including intersection density, percentage of four-way intersections, and number of intersections per unit length of streets. Generally, they report nonsignificant associations between these measures and population health outcomes. Frank et al. [72] quantified connectivity in their study as the density of intersections with more than three legs within a one-kilometer buffer around respondents' residences but reported nonsignificant associations with BMI outcomes. Rutt and Coleman [96] measured intersection density in terms of the total number of intersections within a quarter-mile buffer around respondents' residences. They also included the percentage of cul-de-sacs and four-way intersections in their analysis. They found no significant association of these measures with BMI or PA outcomes. Rundle et al. [77] considered intersection density, which they defined as the number of street intersections per census tract, and reported no significant association between intersection density and individual BMI. Brown et al. [74] considered intersection density within a one-kilometer network buffer (excluding street intersections involving interstate highways) in their study, and reported nonsignificant associations with BMI, overweight, and obesity outcomes. Similar findings were also reported by Burgoine et al. [67] and Ball et al. [97].

Other studies have assessed the effects of route accessibility on crime [93]. Increased street connectivity was repeatedly found to increase crime [98–100]. Properties on cul-de-sacs exhibited lower crime levels than those on grid streets [101–103]. Corner houses were more vulnerable to burglary [104, 105]. In contrast, lower rates were reported for properties located on less permeable layouts [106]. Modifying grids into cul-de-sacs using road closures reduced crime [107, 108], whereas new pathways connecting the ends of cul-de-sacs led to increases in crime [109]. Crime was more frequent in accessible areas with commercial land uses [110].

On a different topic, Wood et al. [68] considered density of intersections with more than three legs contained within the household buffer as the measure of street connectivity and reported nonsignificant association with the sense of community. Additionally, space syntax's street network analysis techniques have been used in many studies explaining different social health outcomes related to traffic flow, such as pedestrian safety [111, 112], and antisocial behavior, crime, fear, safety, and other issues related to environmental perception [113–119].

Based on the literature, it is possible to argue the associations between health and properties of street systems have been studied extensively. The evidence for associations between street properties and physical health outcomes is mixed, however, and offers no general conclusions. According to some of these studies, high intersection density may cause congestion, increasing levels of pollution and overcrowding, and reduced perception of street-level safety, thereby reducing health benefits. The directions of these associations are difficult to explain and may depend on the overall structure and function of a study area. Notably, studies exploring associations between street properties and mental health are absent. Studies that show consistent results are those exploring associations between street properties and social health focusing on crimes. Most of these studies involve urban areas. Though there are some studies linking street properties to lifestyle in rural areas and small towns and cities (see chapters 7 and 8), studies linking street properties to health in small cities in rural areas are absent. The following findings serve to fill this gap.

Things We Observe in Small Cities of Kansas

The findings of the correlational analysis between street properties with the indicators of *mortality* and *morbidity* show that *people reporting general health conditions* has significant negative associations with mean integration, choice, and node counts, indicating that more accessibility, movement potential, and directional choices of street systems may worsen general health conditions in small Kansas cities. Similarly, death rate shows significant negative associations with total street length, mean axial choice, axial node counts, and mean segment choice, indicating that more accessibility, movement potential, and directional choices of street systems may reduce death rates. These findings may be related to those reported in previous studies, where some street properties have been shown to reduce adult obesity and improve mental and social health.

Among the other *morbidity* and *mortality* indicators, *people under 65 years with disability* shows a significant negative correlation with axial connectivity, indicating that small cities with more connected streets may have more people with disabilities; and suicide rates show no association with street properties. More studies are needed to find out why these correlations are found.

Among the indicators of *physical health*, the percentage of people with adult diabetes, obesity, and overweight has significant associations with several street network properties, but average BMI has no association with properties of street systems. According to these findings, adult diabetes decreases as total street length and some of the other properties of street systems decrease, indicating that more accessibility, movement potential, and directional choices of street systems may reduce adult diabetes, maybe through enhancing movement and physical activities. There is, however, one street property—mean axial connectivity—that shows significant positive association with adult diabetes. The reason for this may be that axial connectivity shows significant negative associations with the percentage of people doing vigorous- and moderate-intensity recreational activities.

Among the other indicators of *physical health*, the percentage of obese people has positive correlations with several street properties. In contrast, the percentage of overweight people has negative correlations with several street properties. These contrasting findings can be explained by a significant negative association between obesity and overweight—as obesity increases, overweight decreases in small Kansas cities. BMI has no association with properties of street systems. BMI includes everyone, not just those who are obese or overweight, and how everyone within a population distributes themselves throughout a place may be more random than how people who are obese or overweight distribute themselves within a population.

Among the indicators of *mental health, people feeling badly about themselves* and *people having ever used marijuana or hashish* have no significant associations with street properties. In contrast, *people who have little interest in doing things, people feeling down, depressed, or hopeless,* and *people having thoughts that they would be better off dead* show several significant positive associations with street network properties. In other words, better accessibility, movement potential, and directional choices of street systems may increase some mental health issues. It is difficult to explain why these associations are found without more studies.

Among the indicators of *social health,* murder, rape, robbery, assault, burglary, and auto theft are positively associated with several street properties, indicating that more accessibility, movement potential, and directional choices of street systems may increase crime in these cities. The associations of these properties are strong and significant with robbery, weak and somewhat significant with rape and assaults, and strong and significant in some cases and weak and somewhat significant in other cases with thefts. It is important to note that while violent crime rates show associations with accessibility as measured by segment integration, no such associations exist between property crime rate and street properties, indicating that violent crime is more sensitive to some street properties than property crime is.

Overall, street properties are important health factors in small Kansas cities. They show several significant associations with the indicators of mortality and morbidity, physical health, mental health, and social health. Some of these findings are more easily explainable than others. Therefore, more studies are needed to explain any links between street properties and health.

Conclusions

This chapter provides a review of the literature on the associations between spatial factors and health indicators and reports the findings of a study looking at the same in small Kansas cities. According to the literature, health varies systematically with city size in large samples of small to large cities, but it is not known how health varies with city size in a sample of small cities. The findings of this study indicate that city size may be an important health factor in small Kansas cities; however, more studies are needed before any conclusion can be drawn.

Despite some contradictory findings, the literature generally indicates that density measured in various ways is a significant factor affecting physical, mental, and social health and that careful spatial strategies are necessary to ensure that density produces desired health benefits. According to the results of this study, however, density does not seem to affect health in any significant way in small cities of Kansas. It is quite possible that these cities do not have enough density to affect health outcomes. Since density varies from one small city to another, one wonders if cities with higher densities would be different from the ones with lower densities in terms of health—an issue that will be considered in the next chapter.

As reported in the literature, the availability of key destinations and facilities is an important health factor in urban areas. Some studies have found this to be true in rural areas and small cities as well. Among the destinations and facilities, the literature on parks and green space, physical activity facilities, food outlets, and retail outlets was reviewed. While the availability of each of these facilities shows some health effects, the availability of parks and green space seems to show the most beneficial health effects in the literature. This study examined the associations between health and the availability of parks and green space, health care facilities, supermarkets or grocery stores, convenience stores, convenience stores with gas, business establishments, and full-service restaurants in small Kansas cities.

The study reports predictable associations between health and the availability of every key destination or facility except parks and green space. In contrast to the findings reported in the literature, parks and green spaces are the only key destinations that do not seem to have statistically significant associations with health in small Kansas cities. As noted in previous chapters, there may be many reasons why parks and green space show only a few beneficial health effects in small cities. First, parks and green spaces may not be maintained properly in small cities. Second, small-city residents may use parks and green spaces for health benefits less than their urban counterparts. Third, parks and green spaces may be less attractive destinations for small-city residents than urban residents because rural residents may not be as deprived of open spaces and green spaces as may be urban residents.

The associations of land use types and LUM with health indicators were also explored. To recap, according to the studies reported in the literature, LUM shows beneficial effects on physical and mental health, but these effects seem to vary based on how LUM is defined. For the same study areas, a LUM value defined based on a higher number of land use categories appears to show better associations with health outcomes than a LUM value defined using a lower number of land use categories. In contrast, the effects of LUM on social health remain equivocal and vary depending on the type of use included in the mix: some types of mix tend to encourage crime, while others do the opposite. According to the findings of this study, among land use types, the percentage of industrial areas seems to have some associations with health in small cities of Kansas. LUM also seems to have some associations with health in small cities of Kansas, but these associations are more sporadic and less frequent than they are in urban areas. The percentage of open areas and green space does not seem to be associated with health in small Kansas cities.

Finally, like the associations between street properties and lifestyle reported in chapter 8, the associations between street properties and health were frequent in small cities of Kansas. It was noted that many previous studies did not find significant associations between street properties and physical health but that many others found significant associations between street properties and mental and social health in urban areas. More particularly, several of these studies report significant associations between street network properties measured using space syntax techniques and crime, safety, and social equity. Confirming some of the findings reported in previous studies as well as going beyond these studies, this study reports many significant associations between street network properties and indicators of mortality and morbidity and physical, mental, and social health.

In conclusion, the associations between spatial factors and health in small cities have remained understudied. We do not always have the data we need for this kind of studies; more importantly, the public and population health research community assumes that density, land use mix, or parks and green spaces—factors that show associations with health in urban areas—are not relevant for small cities. Small cities are too small to be affected by these spatial factors. This mindset likens to impose the urban models of population health on rural and small-town population health. Dismissing this mindset, according to the findings of the studies presented in this chapter, several spatial factors that show frequent associations with health indicators in urban areas also showed frequent associations with health indicators in small cities of Kansas.

Some factors showed more frequent associations with health indicators than did others. Some showed frequent associations with some but not with other health indicators. Among the spatial factors considered, street network properties stood out for showing the most frequent associations with different health indicators.

The next chapter will explore the effects of rurality on the spatial associations of health observed in this chapter to find out if more rural small cities are different from less rural small cities in terms of these associations.

NOTES

1. Ray and Ghosh, "City Size and Health Outcomes."
2. Cheung, Leung, and Nguyen, "City Size Matters."
3. Chen et al., "Life Satisfaction in Urbanizing China."
4. Zhou, Rybski, and Kropp, "The Role of City Size and Urban Form."
5. Ferré, Ferreira, and Lanjouw, "Is There a Metropolitan Bias?"
6. Dempsey, Brown, and Bramley, "The Key to Sustainable Urban Development."
7. Burton, "Mental Well-Being and the Influence of Place."
8. Melia, Parkhurst, and Barton, "The Paradox of Intensification."
9. Harries, "Property Crimes and Violence in United States."
10. Lachapelle and Noland, "Inconsistencies in Associations between Crime and Walking."
11. Calhoun, "Population Density and Social Pathology."
12. Stark, "Deviant Places."
13. Loukaitou-Sideris, "Hot Spots of Bus Stop Crime."
14. Newman, *Defensible Space: People and Design in the Violent City.*
15. Banyard, "Measurement and Correlates of Prosocial Bystander Behavior."
16. Sugiyama et al., "Associations of Neighborhood Greenness."
17. Sugiyama and Thompson, "Associations between Characteristics of Neighbourhood Open Space."
18. Coutts et al., "County-Level Effects."
19. De Vries et al., "Natural Environments—Healthy Environments?"
20. Giles-Corti et al., "The Influence of Urban Design and Planning on Physical Activity."
21. Croucher, Myers, and Bretherton, *The Links between Greenspace and Health.*
22. Pretty et al., "Green Exercise in the UK Countryside."
23. White et al., "Would You Be Happier Living in a Greener Urban Area?"
24. Hartig et al., "Tracking Restoration."
25. Kuo, "How Might Contact with Nature Promote Human Health?"
26. Grahn and Stigsdotter, "Landscape Planning and Stress."
27. Barton and Pretty, "What Is the Best Dose of Nature and Green Exercise?"
28. Mitchell and Popham, "Effect of Exposure to Natural Environment."
29. Maas et al., "Morbidity Is Related to a Green Living Environment."
30. Brown, Bramley, and Watkins, *Urban Green Nation.*
31. Allen and Allen, "Health Inequalities and the Role of the Physical and Social Environment."
32. Clark et al., *Greening Dementia.*

33. Ulrich, "View through a Window May Influence Recovery."
34. Takano, Nakamura, and Watanabe, "Urban Residential Environments and Senior Citizens' Longevity."
35. Wolch et al., "Childhood Obesity and Proximity to Urban Parks."
36. Center on the Developing Child at Harvard University, *The Foundations of Lifelong Health.*
37. Farley et al., "Safe Play Spaces to Promote Physical Activity."
38. Giles-Corti et al., "Environmental and Lifestyle Factors Associated with Overweight and Obesity."
39. Mobley et al., "Environment, Obesity, and Cardiovascular Disease Risk."
40. Boehmer et al., "Perceived and Observed Neighborhood Indicators."
41. Boehmer et al., "What Constitutes an Obesogenic Environment."
42. Wilcox et al., "Psychosocial and Perceived Environmental Correlates."
43. Maley, Warren, and Devine, "Perceptions of the Environment for Eating and Exercise."
44. Black et al., "Neighborhoods and Obesity."
45. Larsen et al., "Food Access and Children's BMI."
46. Rundle et al., "Neighborhood Food Environment and Walkability."
47. Morland, Diez-Roux, and Wing, "Supermarkets, Other Food Stores, and Obesity."
48. Morland and Evenson, "Obesity Prevalence and the Local Food Environment."
49. Dengel et al., "Does the Built Environment Relate to the Metabolic Syndrome in Adolescents?"
50. Michimi and Wimberly, "Associations of Supermarket Accessibility."
51. Glanz et al., "How Major Restaurant Chains Plan Their Menus."
52. Larson et al., "Young Adults and Eating Away from Home."
53. Duffey et al., "Differential Associations of Fast Food and Restaurant Food Consumption."
54. Currie et al., "The Effect of Fast Food Restaurants."
55. Mehta and Chang, "Weight Status and Restaurant Availability."
56. Li et al., "Built Environment, Adiposity, and Physical Activity."
57. Li et al., "Built Environment and Changes in Blood Pressure."
58. Dowler and Dobson, "Nutrition and Poverty in Europe."
59. Cummins and Macintyre, "Food Environments and Obesity."
60. Friel, Walsh, and McCarthy, "The Irony of a Rich Country."
61. Kent, Thompson, and Jalaludin, *Healthy Built Environments.*
62. Block, Scribner, and DeSalvo, "Fast Food, Race/Ethnicity, and Income."
63. Powell, Chaloupka, and Bao, "The Availability of Fast-Food and Full-Service Restaurants."
64. Cummins, McKay, and MacIntyre, "McDonald's Restaurants and Neighborhood Deprivation."
65. Reidpath et al., "An Ecological Study of the Relationship."
66. Inagami et al., "You Are Where You Shop."
67. Burgoine, Alvanides, and Lake, "Assessing the Obesogenic Environment."
68. Wood, Frank, and Giles-Corti, "Sense of Community and Its Relationship."
69. Saarloos et al., "The Built Environment and Depression in Later Life."
70. Ramirez et al., "Indicators of Activity-Friendly Communities."
71. Mackenbach et al., "Obesogenic Environments."
72. Frank, Andresen, and Schmid, "Obesity Relationships."
73. Frank et al., "Many Pathways from Land Use to Health."
74. Brown et al., "Mixed Land Use and Walkability."

75. Kaczynski, Johnson, and Saelens, "Neighborhood Land Use Diversity and Physical Activity."
76. Norman et al., "Community Design and Access to Recreational Facilities."
77. Rundle et al., "The Urban Built Environment and Obesity."
78. Pouliou and Elliott, "Individual and Socio-Environmental Determinants."
79. Nasar and Julian, "The Psychological Sense of Community."
80. Lund, "Pedestrian Environments and Sense of Community."
81. Leslie and Cerin, "Are Perceptions of the Local Environment Related to Neighbourhood Satisfaction?"
82. Felson and Boba, *Crime and Everyday Life.*
83. Roncek, "Schools and Crime."
84. Sampson, Morenoff, and Gannon-Rowley, "Assessing 'Neighborhood Effects.' "
85. Sampson and Raudenbush, "Systematic Social Observation of Public Spaces."
86. Greenberg and Rohe, "Neighborhood Design and Crime."
87. Greenberg, Rohe, and Williams, "Safety in Urban Neighborhoods."
88. Appleyard, *Livable Streets, Protected Neighborhoods.*
89. Taylor and Harrell, *Physical Environment and Crime.*
90. Luedtke, *Crime and the Physical City.*
91. Buck, Hakim, and Spiegel, "Endogenous Crime Victimization."
92. Taylor, Shumaker, and Gottfredson, "Neighborhood-Level Links."
93. Cozens, "Crime and Community Safety."
94. Wilcox et al., "Busy Places and Broken Windows?"
95. Foster et al., "Planning Safer Suburbs."
96. Rutt and Coleman, "Examining the Relationships among Built Environment, Physical Activity, and Body Mass Index."
97. Ball et al., "Street Connectivity and Obesity."
98. Bevis and Nutter, *Changing Street Layouts to Reduce Residential Burglary.*
99. Bowers, Johnson, and Hirschfield, "Closing-Off Opportunities for Crime."
100. Johnson and Bowers, "Permeability and Burglary Risk."
101. Beavon, Brantingham, and Brantingham, "The Influence of Street Networks."
102. Town, Davey, and Wooton, *Design against Crime.*
103. Teedon et al., "Evaluating Secured by Design Door and Window Installations."
104. Taylor and Nee, "The Role of Cues in Simulated Residential Burglary."
105. Hakim, Rengert, and Shachmurove, "Target Search of Burglars."
106. Yang, *Exploring the Influence of Environmental Features.*
107. Newman, "Defensible Space: A New Physical Planning Tool."
108. Lasley, *Designing Out Gang Homicides and Street Assaults.*
109. Sheard, *Report on Burglary Patterns.*
110. Davison and Smith, "Exploring Accessibility versus Opportunity Crime Factors."
111. Raford, "*Looking Both Ways.*"
112. Raford and Ragland, "Space Syntax."
113. Hillier, "Can Streets Be Made Safe?"
114. Listerborn, "Women's Fear and Space Configurations."
115. Long, "The Relationships between Objective and Subjective Evaluations."
116. Nubani and Wineman. "The Role of Space Syntax."
117. Ortega-Andeane et al., "Space Syntax as a Determinant."
118. Friedrich, Hillier, and Chiaradia. "Anti-Social Behaviour and Urban Configuration."
119. Hillier and Sahbaz, "Safety in Numbers."

CHAPTER ELEVEN

Rurality and Spatial Associations of Health in Small Cities of Kansas

Comparative Correlational Analyses

This chapter explores the effects of rurality (or lack thereof) on the associations between spatial factors and health in small Kansas cities reported in chapter 10. It also reviews the literature reporting how urbanicity or rurality affects the spatial associations of health in national and regional samples. In general, the literature shows that there is a lack of studies on the effects of urbanicity or rurality on spatial associations of health in small cities and towns. As in the previous chapters, the rurality factors used in this chapter include population size and density, daytime population change due to commuting, distance to the nearest large city with 50,000 or more people, and mean travel time to work (commuting time). The spatial factors used in this chapter include measures describing city size, density, availability of key destinations and facilities, land use types and mix, and several street properties. They remain unchanged from those used in chapters 8, 9, and 10. Health outcomes and indicators include mortality and morbidity indicators and physical, mental, and social health indicators and outcomes. The same health outcomes and indicators were also used in the studies of chapter 10. All the spatial, health, and rurality factors included in this chapter were defined and described in chapter 6.

As in chapter 9, the sample of small cities included in the studies of this chapter is divided into two subsamples based on each of the five factors of rurality. When possible, the cut line is determined to keep any two subsamples somewhat equal. These subsamples are used for the following purposes:

1. Cities with population between ≥5,000 and ≤9,999 people are compared to cities with population between ≥10,000 and ≤49,999 people to

study the effects of population size on the associations between spatial factors and health.

2. Small cities with ≤1,834.50 people per square mile are compared to cities with 1,834.51+ people per square mile to study the effects of population density on the associations between spatial factors and health.

3. Small cities with ≤6.25% population change due to daytime travel are compared to cities with 6.26%+ population change due to daytime travel to study the effects of daytime population change on the associations between spatial factors and health.

4. Small cities ≤63.40 miles from the nearest large city with ≥50,000 people are compared to cities 63.41+ miles from the nearest large city with ≥50,000 people to study the effects of distance from the nearest large city on the associations between spatial factors and health.

5. Small cities with ≤14.90 minutes of commuting time are compared to small cities with 14.91+ minutes of commuting time to study the effects of commuting time on the associations between spatial factors and health.

The findings of these comparative correlational studies are presented in tables 11.1–11.5, where the number in a cell is the number of statistically significant correlations between spatial factors and a health indicator or outcome. The percentages of the number of statistically significant correlations of the total number of observed correlations are shown in the parentheses.

Rurality and Spatial Associations of Mortality and Morbidity

In the United States, the *mortality rate* for rural residents has been higher than for urban residents since at least 1968, although recent numbers indicate improvement [1]. The motor vehicle fatality rate for rural residents is almost double that of urban residents [2, 3]. The number of work-related accidents is higher for rural than urban residents, partly because rural residents often have more hazardous occupations, a fact interconnected with social and economic factors. Rural accident victims also have access to fewer health care professionals, services, and facilities, reducing their survival rate from accidental injuries. Deaths caused by unintentional injuries, such as poisoning, suffocation, and falls, are more likely to occur in rural areas partly due to poor health care access, including longer prehospital times and delays in emergency response [4, 5].

Increases in mortality in rural areas of the United States can also be attributed to a lack of healthy eating habits and healthy low-cost eating options among rural residents [6]. With fewer transportation options and high travel costs, rural residents are more likely to buy food at convenience stores rather than at conventional grocery stores. As a result, food deserts, areas where residents do not have access to affordable and healthful food, are frequently present in rural areas, although they can also be present in the cores of highly urbanized areas [7, 8]. A lack of healthy foods often leads to increased chronic diseases, leading to more deaths among rural populations.

A higher suicide rate adds to increasing mortality in rural areas as well. Suicide rates, which affect the number of years of potential life lost (YPLL), are generally higher for both males and females living in rural areas than their urban counterparts. Rural youth are twice as likely to commit suicide than their urban counterparts [9]. Studies that explore the association between population density and suicide rates taking into account the level of urbanicity [10–13] have found that living in more sparsely populated areas was associated with higher rates of suicide in males when controlling for variations such as divorce rate and ethnicity [11]. The evidence for the association between population density and suicide among females was equivocal, with some finding no association and some, which provided analysis stratified by age group, finding an association. One of the studies reported that women aged 30–44 living in areas of medium population density had a higher rate of suicide compared with their counterparts in rural and urban areas [12]. Another study reported that rates of suicide were higher for women aged 15–24 living in the least populated areas [11]. Again, the precise mechanisms linking rurality or urbanicity with suicide rates remain unclear, but poor mental health and increased social isolation associated with rural living cannot be ruled out as factors.

The *morbidity* outcomes, which are related to quality of life and birth issues, including mental health and physical and mental disabilities, are generally poor among rural residents. For example, rural residents provide poorer overall self-ratings for individual health than do urban residents [14], although the exact reasons remain unknown. At least one European study [15] investigated the strength of the relationship between the amount of green space in people's living environment and their perceived general health as an indicator of morbidity, taking into account urbanicity. According to the findings of the study, the amount of green space in people's living environment is important for perceived general health regardless of the urbanicity of a city. However, other problems, such as lack of transportation, lack of reporting health issues, and frequent self-reliance for health care, often limit access to health care more in rural areas than in urban areas [16, 17]. Doubts about the importance of clinical care for health generally are also high among rural population. Taken together, these problems probably make morbidity more harmful in rural areas than in urban areas of the country.

Differences in mortality and morbidity between rural and urban population are indicative of the fact that these outcomes are affected by the quality of a place. Since small-town America is different from rural as well as urban America, we may expect to find mortality and morbidity in small towns to be different from rural and urban America. The findings reported next may be interesting in this regard.

Things We Observe in Small Cities of Kansas
EFFECTS OF POPULATION SIZE

As reported in table 11.1, *people reporting general health conditions* shows 11 (25% of 44 total correlations) and 11 (25%) statistically significant associations with spatial factors in cities with ≤9,999 and 10,000+ people; *people under 65 with disability* shows 6 (13.64%) and 4 (9.09%); *death rate per 100,000 people* shows 2 (4.55%) and 7 (15.91%); and *suicide rate per 100,000 people* shows 1 (2.27%) and 2 (4.55%). Based on these findings, it may be suggested that *people reporting general health conditions* appears equally sensitive to spatial factors in cities with ≤9,999 and 10,000+ people; *people under 65 with disability* appears somewhat equally sensitive to spatial factors in cities with ≤9,999 and 10,000+ people; and *death rate per 100,000 people* appears more sensitive to spatial factors in cities with 10,000+ people. For *suicide rate per 100,000 people*, the numbers of statistically significant associations are generally very low, indicating that spatial factors may be less important for this indicator in both subsamples of small cities.

Overall, mortality and morbidity indicators show 20 (11.36% of 176 total correlations) and 24 (13.64%) statistically significant associations with spatial factors in cities with ≤9,999 and 10,000+ people, indicating that they may be less but somewhat equally sensitive to spatial factors in these subsamples.

EFFECTS OF POPULATION DENSITY

As shown in table 11.1, *people reporting general health conditions* shows 9 (20.45% of 44 total correlations) and 21 (47.73%) statistically significant associations with spatial factors in cities with ≤1,834.50 and 1,834.51+ people per square mile; *people under 65 with disability* shows 0 and 0; *death rate per*

100,000 people shows 7 (15.91%) and 10 (22.73%); and *suicide rate per 100,000 people* shows 1 (2.27%) and 0. These findings indicate that spatial factors are more important for *people reporting general health conditions* in cities with 1,834.51+ people per square mile. They are somewhat equally important for *death rate per 100,000* in both subsamples of cities. They are not important for *people under 65 with disability* or *suicide rate per 100,000 people* in either of the subsamples.

Overall, mortality and morbidity indicators show 17 (9.66% of 176 total correlations) and 31 (17.61%) statistically significant associations with spatial factors in cities with ≤1,834.50 and 1,834.51+ people per square mile. Therefore, spatial factors may be more important for mortality and morbidity in denser small cities.

EFFECTS OF DAYTIME POPULATION CHANGE

As displayed in table 11.1, *people reporting general health conditions* shows 15 (34.09% of 44 total correlations) and 7 (15.91%) statistically significant associations with spatial factors for cities with ≤6.25% and 6.26%+ population change due to daytime travel; *people under 65 with disability* shows 0 and 2 (4.55%); *death rate per 100,000 people* shows 11 (25%) and 11 (25%); and *suicide rate per 100,000 people* shows 0 and 0. Therefore, according to our findings, spatial factors are more important for *people reporting general health conditions* in cities that observe less population change due to daytime travel. They are equally important for *death rate per 100,000* in cities with ≤6.25% and 6.26%+ population change due to daytime travel. They are not important for *people under 65 with disability* or *suicide rate per 100,000 people* in either subsample.

Overall, mortality and morbidity indicators show 26 (14.77% of 176 total correlations) and 20 (11.36%) statistically significant associations with spatial factors in cities with ≤6.25% and 6.26%+ population change due to daytime travel. These findings indicate that spatial factors may be slightly more important for mortality and morbidity in small cities with less population change due to daytime travel.

EFFECTS OF DISTANCE TO NEAREST CITY OF 50,000 OR MORE PEOPLE

As displayed in table 11.1, *people reporting general health conditions* shows 10 (22.73% of 44 total correlations) and 2 (4.55%) statistically significant associations with spatial factors for cities ≤63.40 and 63.41+ miles from the nearest large city; *people under 65 with disability* shows 12 (27.27%) and 4 (9.09%);

death rate per 100,000 people shows 0 and 7 (15.91%); and *suicide rate per 100,000 people* shows 2 (4.55%) and 5 (11.36%). According to these findings, spatial factors are more important for *people reporting general health conditions* and *people under 65 with disability* in cities ≤63.40 miles from the nearest large city. In contrast, spatial factors are less important for *death rate per 100,000* and *suicide rate per 100,000 people* in cities ≤63.40 miles from the nearest large city.

Overall, mortality and morbidity indicators show 24 (13.64% of 176 total correlations) and 18 (10.23%) statistically significant associations with spatial factors in cities ≤63.40 and 63.41+ miles from the nearest large city. Between the two subsamples, mortality and morbidity may be a bit more sensitive to spatial factors in small cities closer to large cities.

EFFECTS OF COMMUTE TIME

As shown in table 11.1, *people reporting general health conditions* shows 1 (2.27% of 44 total correlations) and 13 (29.55%) statistically significant associations with spatial factors for cities with ≤14.90 and 14.91+ minutes of commute time; *people under 65 with disability* shows 1 (2.27%) and 13 (29.55%); *death rate per 100,000 people* shows 11 (25%) and 0; and *suicide rate per 100,000 people* shows 4 (9.09%) and 7 (15.91%). Based on these findings, it can be concluded that spatial factors are more important for *people reporting general health conditions* and *people under 65 with disability* in cities with 14.91+ minutes of commute time. They are important for *death rate per 100,000* in cities with ≤14.91 minutes of commute time but not important for the same in cities with 14.91+ minutes of commute time. Finally, spatial factors are less important for *suicide rate per 100,000 people* in both subsamples.

Overall, mortality and morbidity indicators show 17 (9.66% of 176 total correlations) and 33 (18.75%) statistically significant associations with spatial factors in cities with ≤14.90 and 14.91+ minutes of commute time. Therefore, spatial factors may be more important for mortality and morbidity in small cities with more commute time.

Rurality and Spatial Associations of Physical Health

The physical health of a population includes much more than obesity, but obesity has become a national epidemic in recent decades. Being overweight or obese is itself a well-established risk factor for a number of diseases, including diabetes, coronary heart disease, hypertension, and stroke. Indeed,

TABLE 11.1.
Significant correlations between spatial factors and mortality and morbidity indicators

		General health condition	Percentage of people with disability under 65 years	Death rate	Suicide rate	Total
			Significant correlations, n (%)			
Rurality factors						
Population	≤9,999	11 (25.00)	6 (13.64)	2 (4.55)	1 (2.27)	20 (11.36)
	10,000+	11 (25.00)	4 (9.09)	7 (15.91)	2 (4.55)	24 (13.64)
Population density (per square mile)	≤1,834.50	9 (20.45)	0 (0.00)	7 (15.91)	1 (2.27)	17 (9.66)
	1,834.51+	21 (47.73)	0 (0.00)	10 (22.73)	0 (0.00)	31 (17.61)
Population change due to daytime travel (as percentage of total population)	≤6.25	15 (34.09)	0 (0.00)	11 (25.00)	0 (0.00)	26 (14.77)
	6.26+	7 (15.91)	2 (4.55)	11 (25.00)	0 (0.00)	20 (11.36)
Distance to nearest city (in miles)	≤63.40	10 (22.73)	12 (27.27)	0 (0.00)	2 (4.55)	24 (13.64)
	63.41+	2 (4.55)	4 (9.09)	7 (15.91)	5 (11.36)	18 (10.23)
Commute time (in minutes)	≤14.90	1 (2.27)	1 (2.27)	11 (25.00)	4 (9.09)	17 (9.66)
	14.91+	13 (29.55)	13 (29.55)	0 (0.00)	7 (15.91)	33 (18.75)

the risk associated with overweight and obesity is comparable to, and in some studies greater than, the risk associated with hypertension, high cholesterol, diabetes, and even smoking. Overweight people die at as much as two and a half times the rate of non-obese people. Obese people are generally more vulnerable than are non-obese people to inhibiting aspects of the built environment, such as inaccessible or nonexistent sidewalks, walking paths, and bicycle paths. Such inhibiting influence can force them into physical inactivity and sedentary lifestyles and, consequently, can increase their health risks [18–26].

Physical inactivity and sedentary lifestyles are not limited to only obese people. They are also common among the rising elderly population. The obesity prevalence in older adults has tripled since the early 1980s [27]. In 2012, the prevalence of overweight and obesity was 71.3% in the population aged 60+, nearly 20% higher than the population aged between 20 and 39 [28]. As physical activities are gradually taken out of our everyday lives with the help of technology, we all become susceptible to more physical inactivity and sedentary lifestyles. This may partly explain the rapid increase in the prevalence of overweight and obesity in recent years [21–24, 29]. Also contributing to the recent overweight and obesity trends are changes in dietary behaviors, particularly among people living in poverty. A lack of access and availability of healthy foods along with greater availability and demand for unhealthy foods, particularly fast foods, in poor areas have increased obesity among many [30]. The link between energy-dense fast food intake and the epidemic of obesity has been widely reported in the literature [31, 32].

Representing more than 15% of the US population [33], the rural population is a "priority population" in the fight to reduce obesity and improve population health [34]. In a review of the literature published between 2000 and 2015 on built environments and active living in rural and remote areas, Hansen [35] reported that rural residents—children and adults, and men and women—are significantly more likely to be obese than their urban counterparts [18, 19, 36–42], even after accounting for socioeconomic factors, eating behaviors, and physical activity [18, 39, 40]. Prevalence of obesity is greater for rural children (22%) than urban children (17%) [39]. Rural minority children are at highest risk for obesity [43]. More rural adults (40%) than urban adults (33%) are obese [18].

According to *The 2014 Update of the Rural-Urban Chartbook* [44], self-reported obesity varied by urbanization level and increased with increasing levels of rurality in the United States. In 2010–2011, women living in central counties of large metro areas nationwide had the lowest age-adjusted prevalence of obesity, while women in the most rural counties had the highest. The pattern for men was the same as for women, with self-reported obesity rates higher in more rural areas.

Significantly higher prevalence of overweight and obesity in rural America may be why diabetes, coronary heart disease, hypertension, stroke, cancers, and all-cause mortality are higher in rural than urban areas [18–20, 45–50]. Some studies have observed notable rural-urban disparities in obesity-related health care services utilization [51]. Studies focused specifically on rural-urban disparities in obesity among older adults are rare, but rural older adults may be especially vulnerable due to functional limitations, geographic isolation, limited resources and income, and other factors.

In a study exploring the effects of urbanicity on spatial associations of physical health outcomes, Zhang et al. [52] used the 1997–2005 National Health Interview Survey (NHIS) data with the 2000 US Census data to assess the effects of neighborhood commuting environment—census tract–level automobile dependency and commuting time—on individual obesity status in regions with different urbanicity levels. They reported that higher neighbor-hood automobile dependency was associated with increased obesity risk in urbanized, large fringe metro, medium metro, small metro, and micropolitan areas but not in non-core rural areas. Longer neighborhood commuting time was associated with increased obesity risk in large central metro areas, as well as in less urbanized, micropolitan, and non-core rural areas, but not in large fringe metro or medium metro areas. Based on their findings, they concluded that the link between commuting environment and obesity differed across the regional urbanicity levels.

In another study, Wang et al. [53] used the Behavioral Risk Factor Surveil-lance System (BRFSS) data to analyze the association of street connectivity with physical activity and obesity while controlling for various individual-and county-level variables, including urbanicity. They found that the positive influence of street connectivity on obesity was limited to the more urbanized areas but not the mostly urbanized areas. Xu and Wang [54] also used the BRFSS data to examine the association of neighborhood built environments with individual obesity in the United States based on urbanicity at the county level. They found that among the built environment variables, poor street con-nectivity and increased presence of fast food restaurants are associated with higher obesity risk, especially for areas of certain urbanicity levels.

Higher prevalence of overweight and obesity even after controlling for individual-level factors suggests that rural built environments may be "obe-sogenic" in ways that stretch beyond individual factors [36, 41, 55, 56]. Iden-tifying these obesogenic factors is a necessary first step in the fight to reduce obesity and improve population health in rural America. Most studies on rural-urban health disparities do not distinguish between rural and small-town America. Instead, they consider small-town America as an integral part of rural America. In this sense, it is probably safe to assume that small-town America is obesogenic as well.

Things We Observe in Small Cities of Kansas
EFFECTS OF POPULATION SIZE

According to our study (table 11.2), *adult diabetes rate* shows 2 (4.55% of 44 total correlations) and 6 (13.64%) statistically significant correlations with spatial factors in cities with ≤9,999 and 10,000+ people; *average BMI* shows 1 (2.27%) and 1 (2.27%); *overweight people* shows 10 (22.73%) and 11 (25%); *adult obesity rate* shows 5 (11.36%) and 11 (25%). According to these findings, spatial factors are not important for *average BMI* in either of the two subsamples of cities defined using population size. They are equally important for *overweight people* in cities with ≤9,999 and 10,000+ people. They are more important for *adult obesity rate* and slightly more important for *adult diabetes rate* in cities with 10,000+ people than they are in cities with ≤9,999.

Overall, physical health outcomes and indicators show 18 (10.23% of 176 total correlations) and 29 (16.48%) statistically significant associations with spatial factors in cities with ≤9,999 and 10,000+ people, indicating that they may be more sensitive to spatial factors in cities with 10,000+ people.

EFFECTS OF POPULATION DENSITY

As reported in table 11.2, *adult diabetes rate* shows 5 (11.36% of 44 total correlations) and 22 (50%) statistically significant associations with spatial factors in cities with ≤1,834.50 and 1,834.51+ people per square mile; *average BMI* shows 5 (11.36%) and 3 (6.82%); *overweight people* shows 6 (13.64%) and 22 (50%); and *adult obesity rate* shows 0 and 12 (27.27%). These findings suggest that spatial factors are more important for *adult diabetes, overweight people,* and *adult obesity rate* in cities with 1,834.51+ people per square mile. They are comparatively less important for *average BMI* in both subsamples.

Overall, physical health outcomes and indicators show 16 (9.09% of 176 total correlations) and 59 (33.52%) statistically significant associations with spatial factors in cities with ≤1,834.50 and 1,834.51+ people per square mile. Therefore, spatial factors may be more important for physical health in denser small cities.

EFFECTS OF DAYTIME POPULATION CHANGE

As displayed in table 11.2, *adult diabetes rate* shows 12 (27.27% of 44 total correlations) and 12 (27.27%) statistically significant associations with spatial factor in cities with ≤6.25% and 6.26%+ population change due to daytime travel; *average BMI* shows 6 (13.64%) and 3 (6.82%); *overweight people* shows 11 (25%) and 11 (25%); and *adult obesity rate* shows 10 (22.73%) and 1 (2.27%). According to these findings, spatial factors are equally important for *adult diabetes* and *overweight people* in cities with ≤6.25% and 6.26%+ population change due to daytime travel. They are more important for *adult obesity rate* in cities with ≤6.25% population change due to daytime travel. They are comparatively less important for *average BMI* in both subsamples.

Overall, physical health outcomes and indicators show 39 (22.16% of 176 total correlations) and 27 (15.34%) statistically significant associations with spatial factors in cities with ≤6.25% and 6.26%+ population change due to daytime travel. Therefore, spatial factors may be more important for physical health in small cities with less population change due to daytime travel.

EFFECTS OF DISTANCE TO NEAREST CITY OF 50,000 OR MORE PEOPLE

As shown in table 11.2, *adult diabetes rate* shows 9 (20.45% of 44 total correlations) and 13 (29.55%) statistically significant associations with spatial factors for cities ≤63.40 and 63.41+ miles from the nearest large city; *average BMI* shows 1 (2.27%) and 1 (2.27%); *overweight people* shows 18 (40.91%) and 7 (15.91%); and *adult obesity rate* shows 6 (13.64%) and 2 (4.55%). These findings indicate that spatial factors are more important for *adult diabetes* in cities 63.41+ miles from the nearest large city; and for *overweight people* in cities ≤63.40 miles from the nearest large city. They are comparatively less important for *adult obesity* and *average BMI* in both subsamples.

Overall, physical health outcomes and indicators show 34 (19.32% of 176 total correlations) and 23 (13.07%) statistically significant associations with spatial factors in cities ≤63.40 and 63.41+ miles from the nearest large city with 50,000 or more people. Spatial factors therefore may be more important for physical health in small cities closer to large cities.

EFFECTS OF COMMUTE TIME

As presented in table 11.2, *adult diabetes rate* shows 14 (31.82% of 44 total correlations) and 7 (15.91%) statistically significant associations with spatial factors in cities with ≤14.90 and 14.91+ minutes of commute time; *average BMI* shows 3 (6.82%) and 0; *overweight people* shows 8 (18.18%) and 10 (22.73%); and *adult obesity rate* shows 3 (6.82%) and 4 (9.09%). These findings suggest that spatial factors are less important for *adult diabetes* in cities with 14.91+ minutes of commute time. They may be equally important for *overweight people* in both subsamples of cities. They may be less important for *adult obesity rate*, and *average BMI* in both subsamples.

Overall, physical health outcomes and indicators show 28 (15.91% of 176 total correlations) and 21 (11.93%) statistically significant associations with spatial factors in cities with ≤14.90 and 14.91+ minutes of commute time, indicating that spatial factors are generally less important for physical health in these subsamples of cities. In relative terms, however, they may be slightly more important for physical health in small cities with shorter commute time.

TABLE 11.2.
Significant correlations between spatial factors and physical health indicators

		Significant correlations, n (%)				
		Adult diabetes rate	Average BMI	Overweight people	Adult obesity rate	Total
Rurality factors						
Population	≤9,999	2 (4.55)	1 (2.27)	10 (22.73)	5 (11.36)	18 (10.23)
	10,000 +	6 (13.64)	1 (2.27)	11 (25.00)	11 (25.00)	29 (16.48)
Population density (per square mile)	≤1,834.50	5 (11.36)	5 (11.36)	6 (13.64)	0 (0.00)	16 (9.09)
	1,834.51+	22 (50.00)	3 (6.82)	22 (50.00)	12 (27.27)	59 (33.52)
Population change due to daytime travel (as percentage of total population)	≤6.25	12 (27.27)	6 (13.64)	11 (25.00)	10 (22.73)	39 (22.16)
	6.26+	12 (27.27)	3 (6.82)	11 (25.00)	1 (2.27)	27 (15.34)
Distance to nearest city (in miles)	≤63.40	9 (20.45)	1 (2.27)	18 (40.91)	6 (13.64)	34 (19.32)
	63.41+	13 (29.55)	1 (2.27)	7 (15.91)	2 (4.55)	23 (13.07)
Commute time (in minutes)	≤14.90	14 (31.82)	3 (6.82)	8 (18.18)	3 (6.82)	28 (15.91)
	14.91+	7 (15.91)	0 (0.00)	10 (22.73)	4 (9.09)	21 (11.93)

Rurality and Spatial Associations of Mental Health

Evidence suggests that mental health and well-being can influence physical health and vice versa [57]. Since significant urban-rural disparities exist for physical health, it can be expected that significant rural-urban disparities also exist for mental health and general well-being [36, 37, 41, 58]. This is supported by the proportion of adults who reported having any mental illness (AMI) in the past year differing by urbanization level. Differences across urbanization levels were more common for women than men [44].

Nationally, the percentage of adult men and women who reported having a serious mental illness (SMI) in the past year increased with increasing rurality. Across all regions, the largest urban-rural disparity—measured by percentage difference—was found in the West for men and in the Northeast for women [44].

The highest percentages of adult major depressive episodes (MDE) were found in the middle segments of the urban-rural continuum. For both sexes, the largest percentage of MDE was reported in micropolitan counties. Across all regions, the largest percentages of men and women who reported MDE in the past year were found in micropolitan counties in the West [44].

Rural children generally have more behavioral and mental health problems than urban children [59]. Adolescents reporting MDE in the past year ranged from 4–5% across urbanization levels for males and 11–13% among females. The highest percentages were found in nonmetropolitan counties. Across all regions, the largest percentage of adolescent males reporting MDE in the past year resided in nonmetro counties with a city, while the largest percentage of females resided in the most rural counties in the West [44].

Nationwide, the percentage of adults with serious psychological distress (SPD) in the past 30 days was lowest in fringe counties of large metro areas and highest in nonmetro counties. Regionally, no clear patterns emerged by urbanization level except in the South, where the percentage of adults who had SPD was higher in nonmetro counties than in metro counties. The highest percentage of men and women who had SPD within the past 30 days was found in the most rural counties of the South [44].

Tobacco use is a significant problem among rural youth. Rural youth over the age of 12 are more likely to smoke cigarettes (26.6% versus 19% in large metro areas). They are also far more likely to use smokeless tobacco, with usage rates of 6.7% in rural areas and 2.1% in metropolitan areas [60].

A lack of access to and availability of mental health services and a lack of acceptability of mental health create more challenges in rural areas than in urban areas. Rural residents often travel long distances to receive mental health services, they are less likely to be insured for mental health services, and they are less likely to recognize mental illnesses. Chronic shortages of mental health professionals exist in rural areas, as mental health providers are more likely to live in urban centers. A lack of choices of trained professionals creates barriers to mental health care in rural areas. The stigma of needing or receiving mental health care is stronger is rural areas than it is urban areas, often due to smaller community size and religious beliefs [60].

Concerning the effects of rurality or urbanicity on spatial associations of mental health, several studies explored the association between population density at birthplaces and the development of schizophrenia in adulthood, taking into account level of urbanicity [61–71]. These studies found that higher population density was associated with increased rates of schizophrenia and that an urban-rural difference may exist in incidence rates for schizophrenia but not for prevalence rates. Though the precise mechanisms linking rurality or urbanicity with schizophrenia remain unclear, high stress associated with urban living can be a factor.

Penkalla and Kohler [72] systematically reviewed 11 quantitative studies, published in English between January 2002 and October 2012, on the relationship between urbanicity and prevalent mental disorders in Europe. They found that these studies used different measures of urbanicity. The types of mental disorders most often examined were mood and anxiety disorders, psychosis, and substance use disorders. Seven out of nine studies reported more mood and anxiety disorders in areas with more urbanicity. Two out of three studies indicated higher rates of psychosis in areas with more urbanicity. Four out of six studies found more substance abuse, again, in areas with more urbanicity. The same studies found no evidence for a relationship between urbanicity and mental disorders in several instances, and a lower prevalence of anxiety disorders in medium-sized cities compared to rural areas. Based on their review, the authors concluded that the levels of urbanicity of European cities could be a risk factor for mood and anxiety disorders, psychotic disorders, and substance abuse.

The significance of rural-urban differences in mental illnesses cannot be overstated for small-town America because a majority of the rural population indeed lives in small towns and cities across America. These rural-urban differences point to the fact that rurality and, its obverse, urbanicity are important factors for mental health and general well-being and that the problems of mental health and general well-being of a small town or city are likely to vary depending on its urbanicity or rurality level.

Things We Observe in Small Cities of Kansas
EFFECTS OF POPULATION SIZE

As shown in table 11.3, *people feeling badly about themselves* shows 0 and 5 (11.36% of 44 total correlations); *people who have little interest in doing things* shows 0 and 11 (25%); *people feeling down, depressed, or hopeless* shows 3 (6.82%) and 11 (25%); *people having thoughts they would be better off dead* shows 4 (9.09%) and 5 (11.36%); and *people having ever used marijuana or hashish* shows 3 (6.82%) and 6 (13.64%) statistically significant associations with spatial factors for cities with ≤9,999 and 10,000+ people. Therefore, for *people who have little interest in doing things* and *people feeling down, depressed, or hopeless*, spatial factors are more important in cities with 10,000+ people. Spatial factors are generally less important for the other mental health outcomes and indicators.

Overall, mental health outcomes and indicators show 10 (4.55% of 220 total correlations) and 38 (17.27%) statistically significant associations with spatial factors for cities with ≤9,999 and 10,000+ people. Based on the findings, spatial factors are more important for mental health in cities with 10,000+ people.

EFFECTS OF POPULATION DENSITY

According to our findings (table 11.3), *people feeling badly about themselves* shows 1 (2.27% of 44 total correlations) and 1 (2.27%) statistically significant associations with spatial factors in cities with ≤1,834.50 and 1,834.51+ people per square mile; *people who have little interest in doing things* shows 14 (31.82%) and 7 (15.91%); *people feeling down, depressed, or hopeless* shows 7 (15.91%) and 3 (6.82%); *people having thoughts they would be better off dead* shows 6 (13.64%) and 2 (4.55%); and *people having ever used marijuana or hashish* shows 3 (6.82%) and 1 (2.27%). These findings indicate that spatial factors are important for *people who have little interest in doing things*, particularly in cities with ≤1,834.51 people per square mile, and they are less important for the other mental health outcomes and indicators.

Overall, mental health outcomes and indicators show 31 (14.09% of 220 total correlations) and 14 (6.36%) statistically significant associations with spatial factors in cities with ≤1,834.50 and 1,834.51+ people per square mile. Spatial factors therefore may be relatively more important for mental health in less dense small cities.

EFFECTS OF DAYTIME POPULATION CHANGE

As presented in table 11.3, *people feeling badly about themselves* shows 1 (2.27% of 44 total correlations) and 9 (20.45%) statistically significant associations with spatial factors in cities with ≤6.25% and 6.26%+ population change due to daytime travel; *people who have little interest in doing things* shows 10 (22.73%) and 6 (13.64%); *people feeling down, depressed, or hopeless* shows 3 (6.82%) and 6 (13.64%); *people having thoughts they would be better off dead* shows 2 (4.55%) and 6 (13.64%); and *people having ever used marijuana or hashish* shows 0 and 0. These findings indicate that spatial factors are important for *people feeling badly about themselves*, particularly in cities with 6.26%+ population change due to daytime travel, and for *people who have little interest in doing things*, particularly in cities with ≤6.25% population change due to daytime travel. For the other mental health outcomes and indicators, spatial factors are less important or not important in either subsample.

Overall, mental health outcomes and indicators show 16 (7.27% of 220 total correlations) and 27 (12.27%) statistically significant associations with spatial factors in cities with ≤6.25% and 6.26%+ population change due to daytime travel. Spatial factors therefore may be relatively more important for mental health in small cities with more population change due to daytime travel.

EFFECTS OF DISTANCE TO NEAREST CITY OF 50,000
OR MORE PEOPLE

As reported in table 11.3, *people feeling badly about themselves* shows 4 (9.09% of 44 total correlations) and 1 (2.27%) statistically significant associations with spatial factors in cities ≤63.40 and 63.41+ miles from the nearest large city; *people who have little interest in doing things* shows 1 (2.27%) and 12 (27.27%); *people feeling down, depressed, or hopeless* shows 0 and 4 (9.09%); *people having thoughts they would be better off dead* shows 2 (4.55%) and 0; and *people having ever used marijuana or hashish* shows 0 and 1 (2.27%). Based on these findings, it seems that spatial factors are important for *people who have little interest in doing things*, particularly in cities 63.41+ miles from the nearest large city. They are less important or not important for the other mental health outcomes and indicators.

Overall, mental health outcomes and indicators show 7 (3.18% of 220 total correlations) and 18 (8.18%) statistically significant associations with spatial factors for cities ≤63.40 and 63.41+ miles from the nearest large city. Spatial factors in general are therefore not important for mental health in the subsamples of small cities defined based on distance from the nearest city with 50,000 or more people.

EFFECTS OF COMMUTE TIME

As reported in table 11.3, *people feeling badly about themselves* shows 2 (4.55% of 44 total correlations) and 4 (9.09%) statistically significant associations with spatial factors for cities with ≤14.90 and 14.91+ minutes of commute time; *people who have little interest in doing things* shows 3 (6.82%) and 7 (15.91%); *people feeling down, depressed, or hopeless* shows 5 (11.36%) and 5 (11.36%); *people having thoughts they would be better off dead* shows 0 and 0; and *people having ever used marijuana or hashish* shows 0 and 1 (2.27%).

Overall, mental health outcomes and indicators show 10 (4.55% of 220 total correlations) and 17 (7.73%) statistically significant associations with spatial factors in cities with ≤14.90 and 14.91+ minutes of commute time. Spatial factors generally are not very important for mental health in these subsamples of small cities defined based on commute time.

Rurality and Spatial Associations of Social Health

It is generally assumed that the social health of rural communities is better than that of urban communities. In contrast to negative physical and mental

TABLE 11.3.
Significant correlations between spatial factors and mental health indicators

Rurality factors		Significant correlations, n (%)					
		People feeling badly about themselves	People who have little interest in doing things	People feeling down, depressed, or hopeless	People having thoughts that they would be better off dead	People having ever used marijuana or hashish	Total
Population	≤9,999	0 (0.00)	0 (0.00)	3 (6.82)	4 (9.09)	3 (6.82)	10 (4.55)
	10,000 +	5 (11.36)	11 (25.00)	11 (25.00)	5 (11.36)	6 (13.64)	38 (17.27)
Population density (per square mile)	≤1,834.50	1 (2.27)	14 (31.82)	7 (15.91)	6 (13.64)	3 (6.82)	31 (14.09)
	1,834.51+	1 (2.27)	7 (15.91)	3 (6.82)	2 (4.55)	1 (2.27)	14 (6.36)
Population change due to daytime travel (as percentage of total population)	≤6.25	1 (2.27)	10 (22.73)	3 (6.82)	2 (4.55)	0 (0.00)	16 (7.27)
	6.26+	9 (20.45)	6 (13.64)	6 (13.64)	6 (13.64)	0 (0.00)	27 (12.27)
Distance to nearest city (in miles)	≤63.40	4 (9.09)	1 (2.27)	0 (0.00)	2 (4.55)	0 (0.00)	7 (3.18)
	63.41+	1 (2.27)	12 (27.27)	4 (9.09)	0 (0.00)	1 (2.27)	18 (8.18)
Commute time (in minutes)	≤14.90	2 (4.55)	3 (6.82)	5 (11.36)	0 (0.00)	0 (0.00)	10 (4.55)
	14.91+	4 (9.09)	7 (15.91)	5 (11.36)	0 (0.00)	1 (2.27)	17 (7.73)

health and sociodemographic characteristics, the social health of rural communities exhibits positive characteristics and can be utilized to improve physical and mental health outcomes [73–75].

Crime is an important indicator of social health. It is the result of complex interactions among social, socio-ecological, and structural factors of a place. Crime is also an interesting social health topic because of its widespread physical and mental health effects. Crime, perceptions of crime, and antisocial behavior, such as drunkenness and burglary, can discourage walking and other outdoor activities, thereby contributing to obesity. Fear of crime can cause anxiety and concerns affecting mental health, [76–79] but there is less clarity on the causal direction [80]. Poor upkeep of houses and neighborhoods can signal a breakdown of social control and has been associated with increased crime and a fear of crime [81]. Although evidence is mixed, the associations of crime-related safety and physical inactivity with increased obesity levels are more consistent for groups who perceive themselves to be physically vulnerable to crime (e.g., women and older adults) or who are economically vulnerable to crime (e.g., low-income and minority populations) [76, 82]. Low-income groups are exposed to more neighborhood crime and disorder and are typically more fearful but often have no alternative to walking for transport [76], which might partly explain mixed research findings [76]. Although more eyes on the street are generally interpreted as a source of safety, any benefit depends on who these people are [83]. For eyes to be effective, they must belong to people who care about the space being watched. This may explain why shopping centers, transport nodes, and street connectivity bring in more people, but they have also been associated with more opportunistic crimes.

Research has consistently found large differences in crime rates between rural and urban areas, indicating possible differences in social health between these places. Based on a study using official police data in the United States for 1966 through 1997, Weisheit and Donnermeyer [84] conclude that in comparison with rural counties, violent crime rates are between 5 and 10 times higher, and property crime rates are between 4 and 5 times higher in the largest cities. Similarly, an analysis of victimization data reveals that victimization rates for violent crimes are consistently higher in urban areas [84, 85]. Although rural crime rates are often lower than the rates for large cities, it would be a mistake to assume that patterns of crime are completely homogeneous across rural areas with uniformly low crime rates. One study notes that of the 30 counties with the highest homicide rates, 17 are nonmetropolitan. Of these 17 nonmetropolitan counties, nine are completely rural; that is, the county contains no municipality of 2,500 or more. Of the remaining eight nonmetropolitan counties, seven have no municipality over 20,000 [86].

Similarly, it would be a mistake to assume that factors that are known to influence urban crime will invariably have the same pattern of influence in rural areas [87]. Several authors have noted that the impact of poverty and unemployment on crime may be different in rural and urban areas [85, 88]. For example, it has been suggested that declining urban crime rates during the late 1990s were the result of economic growth [89, 90], but others have found that in rural areas economic growth is often accompanied by a substantial increase in crime rates [91, 92]. A few studies that have focused on differential crime patterns in rural communities using geographically limited convenience samples suggest that social factors are more important predictors of crime than are economic conditions in nonurban communities [88, 93]. This is very different from that seen in urban communities, in which Agnew writes that "economic deprivation, in fact, is perhaps the most distinguishing characteristic of high-crime communities" [94].

Using national county-level data from various sources, Wells and Weisheit [95] studied whether variables commonly used to predict urban crime patterns could be applied similarly to rural crime patterns. The dependent variables of their study included average yearly violent and property crime rates. The independent ecological variables included indices for urban density, housing instability, family instability, population changes, and economic change. The independent structural variables included indices for economic resources, racial heterogeneity, and cultural capital. The results showed that although ecological and structural variables did a good job of predicting urban patterns of crime, they were less predictive of crime rates in more rural counties. Further, the set of variables that best predicted urban crime rates was not identical to the set that best predicted rural crime rates.

Like crime, *loneliness and social isolation* have widespread effects, and their effects vary based on urbanicity or rurality. They are associated with poor mental health, adverse health behaviors (e.g., physical inactivity and smoking), and detrimental biological processes (e.g., high blood pressure and C-reactive protein and poor immune functioning) compared with regular social contact [96, 97]. Social isolation can cause depression and stress, particularly in the elderly population [98]. In contrast, social connections and engagement can create safe, happy, and healthy places [99]. Bringing people together in social settings can improve mental and physical health [100]. Health benefits from social connections include reduced risks for health issues such as depression, high blood pressure, and cardiovascular problems [97]. Social connec-tions appear to act as a protective factor against memory loss in people over 65 years of age [101]. They also appear to aid recovery after periods of illness [102]. A 2015 meta-analysis concluded that the impact of social isolation on premature mortality was comparable to other established health risk factors (e.g., obesity), highlighting its importance as a population health issue [97]. Those who are socially isolated are between two and five times more likely to die prematurely compared to those who have strong social ties [103].

It would appear that social isolation and loneliness are a bigger problem in small towns and cities than they are in urban areas. Most often, small towns and cities are not big enough to have sufficient density and local amenities promoting social, economic, and demographic diversity necessary for liveli-ness. Many people, including older adults, remain physically and socially dis-connected in these places. Because of isolation, problems such as domestic violence remain hidden and unaddressed. Mortality rates may increase due to the long response times to medical emergencies or fires [104]. It should be noted that as small cities grow and densify, a challenge is to protect residents from social ills that density produces in the absence of community safety and policing resources. We observe such phenomena frequently in small towns and cities that have grown overnight to accommodate amenity seekers. There is little understanding about the optimum density to promote social contact and interactions with outsiders while mitigating other unwanted exposures, particularly among more vulnerable and low-income populations in these small towns and cities.

Evidence suggests that spatial design and planning can decrease social isolation by encouraging social connections, interactions, and cohesion [105]; subsequently, it can provide physical and mental health benefits [96]. For ex-ample, well-designed streets and public open spaces can encourage residents to stop, linger, and interact [105]. Accessible and diverse destinations and transport options can increase walking trips, which in turn can increase un-planned social encounters and sense of community [105]. Neighborhood destinations can provide settings for cultural and informal social activities to enhance community connections and sense of belonging [105]. It is notewor-thy, however, that spatial design interventions and policies are insufficient to reduce social isolation if the neighborhood is regarded as undesirable (i.e., if it is unsafe or poorly maintained) [81].

In general, the literature makes it clear that crimes vary in rural and urban areas, and they have different spatial correlates in rural and urban areas. However, the literature does not provide evidence on how any spatial associations of crimes might vary across places with different levels of urbanicity or rurality, more particularly in small US cities. Likewise, in the absence of any knowledge on how the urbanicity or rurality of a place affects any spatial associations of social isolation, we need more attention on this topic as well, which the findings reported below seek to address.

Things We Observe in Small Cities of Kansas
EFFECTS OF POPULATION SIZE

As presented in table 11.4, in the violent crime category, *murders per 100,000* shows 0 and 4 (9.09% of 44 total correlations) statistically significant associations with spatial factors in cities with ≤9,999 and 10,000+ people; *rapes per 100,000* shows 3 (6.82%) and 13 (29.55%); *robberies per 100,000* shows 5 (11.36%) and 11 (25%); *assaults per 100,000* shows 9 (20.45%) and 6 (13.64%); and *violent crimes per 100,000* shows 8 (18.18%) and 6 (13.64%).

In the property crime category, *burglaries per 100,000* shows 10 (22.73%) and 3 (6.82%) statistically significant associations with spatial factors in cities with ≤9,999 and 10,000+ people; *thefts per 100,000* shows 1 (2.27%) and 6 (13.64%); *auto thefts per 100,000* shows 12 (27.27%) and 2 (4.55%); and *property crimes per 100,000* shows 0 and 4 (9.09%).

Regarding social isolation, *people over 65 living alone* shows 2 (4.55%) and 0 statistically significant associations with spatial factors in cities with ≤9,999 and 10,000+ people.

Spatial factors may be more important in cities with 10,000+ people than in cities with ≤9,999 for murder, rape, robbery, and theft; and they may be less important in cities with 10,000+ people than in cities with ≤9,999 for assault, burglary, and auto theft. Spatial factors are not important, however, for *people over 65 living alone* in either subsample of cities defined based on population size.

Overall, social health indicators show 50 (11.36% of 440 total correlations) and 55 (12.50%) statistically significant associations with spatial factors in cities with ≤9,999 and 10,000+ people. Spatial factors therefore are less important but show similar effects on social health in small cities with both high and low population size.

EFFECTS OF POPULATION DENSITY

As presented in table 11.4, in the violent crime category, *murders per 100,000* shows 2 (4.55% of 44 total correlations) and 19 (43.18%) statistically significant associations with spatial factors in cities with ≤1,834.50 and 1,834.51+ people per square mile; *rapes per 100,000* shows 2 (4.55%) and 18 (40.91%); *robberies per 100,000* shows 7 (15.91%) and 14 (31.82%); *assaults per 100,000* shows 0 and 14 (31.82%); and *violent crimes per 100,000* shows 0 and 15 (34.09%).

In the property crime category, *burglaries per 100,000* shows 3 (6.82%) and 2 (4.55%) statistically significant associations with spatial factors in cities ≤1,834.50 and 1,834.51+ people per square mile; *theft per 100,000* shows 2 (4.55%) and 2 (4.55%); *auto theft per 100,000* shows 7 (15.91%) and 2 (4.55%); and *property crimes per 100,000* shows 2 (4.55%) and 2 (4.55%).

Regarding social isolation, *people over 65 living alone* shows 8 (18.18% of 44 total correlations) and 1 (2.27%) statistically significant associations with spatial factors in cities with ≤1,834.50 and 1,834.51+ people per square mile.

According to these findings, violent crimes are far more sensitive to spatial factors in small cities with higher population density. In contrast, except auto theft, property crimes are generally not sensitive to spatial factors in either subsample. Notably, *people over 65 living alone* are more sensitive to spatial factors in small cities with less population density, which aligns with the existing literature.

Overall, social health indicators show 33 (7.50% of 440 total correlations) and 89 (20.23%) statistically significant associations with spatial factors in cities with ≤1,834.50 and 1,834.51+ people per square mile. Spatial factors therefore are generally more important for social health in small cities with higher population densities.

EFFECTS OF DAYTIME POPULATION CHANGE

As presented in table 11.4, in the violent crime category, *murders per 100,000* shows 2 (4.55% of 44 total correlations) and 7 (15.91%) statistically significant associations with spatial factors in cities with ≤6.25% and 6.26%+ population change due to daytime travel; *rapes per 100,000* shows 10 (22.73%) and 2 (4.55%); *robberies per 100,000* shows 15 (34.09%) and 5 (11.36%); *assaults per 100,000* shows 6 (13.64%) and 0; and *violent crimes per 100,000* shows 10 (22.73%) and 1 (2.27%).

In the property crime category, *burglaries per 100,000* shows 7 (15.91%) and 1 (2.27%) statistically significant associations with spatial factors in cities with ≤6.25% and 6.26%+ population change due to daytime travel; *thefts per 100,000* shows 0 and 0; *auto thefts per 100,000* shows 2 (4.55%) and 5 (11.36%); and *property crimes per 100,000* shows 0 and 2 (4.55%).

Regarding social isolation, *people over 65 living alone* shows 6 (13.64%) and 0 statistically significant associations with spatial factors in cities with ≤6.25% and 6.26%+ population change due to daytime travel.

These findings indicate that spatial factors are generally more important for violent crimes in small cities with less population change due to daytime travel. They are generally less important for property crimes in both subsamples of small cities defined based on population change due to daytime travel. They also indicate that spatial factors are relatively more important for *people over 65 living alone* in small cities with less population change due to daytime travel.

Overall, social health indicators show 58 (13.18% of 440 total correlations) and 23 (5.23%) statistically significant associations with spatial factors in cities with ≤6.25% and 6.26%+ population change due to daytime travel, indicating that spatial factors are relatively more important for social health in small cities with less population change due to daytime travel.

EFFECTS OF DISTANCE TO NEAREST CITY OF 50,000 OR MORE PEOPLE

As presented in table 11.4, in the violent crime category, *murders per 100,000* shows 4 (9.09% of 44 total correlations) and 8 (18.18%) statistically significant associations with spatial factors in cities ≤63.40 and 63.41+ miles from the nearest city with 50,000 or more people; *rapes per 100,000* shows 13 (29.55%) and 7 (15.91%); *robberies per 100,000* shows 11 (15%) and 9 (20.45%); *assaults per 100,000* shows 11 (25%) and 8 (18.18%); and *violent crimes per 100,000* shows 12 (27.27%) and 6 (13.64%).

In the property crime category, *burglaries per 100,000* shows 5 (11.36%) and 2 (4.55%) statistically significant associations with spatial factors in cities ≤63.40 and 63.41+ miles from the nearest city with 50,000 or more people; *theft per 100,000* shows 0 and 0; *auto theft per 100,000* shows 1 (2.27%) and 4 (9.09%); and *property crimes per 100,000* shows 0 and 0.

Regarding social isolation, *people over 65 living alone* shows 0 and 16 (36.36%) statistically significant associations with spatial factors in cities ≤63.40 and 63.41+ miles from the nearest city with 50,000 or more people.

These findings indicate that, with more correlations for each violent crime in both subsamples of small cities, spatial factors appear more important for violent crimes than property crimes. They also indicate that *people over 65 living alone* appears far more sensitive to spatial factors in small cities 63.41+ miles from the nearest city with 50,000 or more people.

Overall, social health indicators show 57 (12.95% of 440 total correlations) and 60 (13.64%) statistically significant associations with spatial factors in cities ≤63.40 and 63.41+ miles from the nearest city with 50,000 or more people. Therefore, according to the findings of this study, spatial factors are less important and show somewhat similar effects in cities ≤63.40 and 63.41+ miles from the nearest city with 50,000 or more people for social health as indicated by crime and social isolation.

EFFECTS OF COMMUTE TIME

As presented in table 11.4, in the violent crime category, *murders per 100,000* shows 10 (22.73% of 44 total correlations) and 3 (6.82%) statistically significant associations with spatial factors in cities with ≤14.90 and 14.91+ minutes of commute time; *rapes per 100,000* shows 7 (15.91%) and 12 (27.27%); *robberies per 100,000* shows 8 (18.18%) and 9 (20.45%); *assaults per 100,000* shows 0 and 13 (29.55%); and *violent crimes per 100,000* shows 0 and 13 (29.55%).

In the property crime category, *burglaries per 100,000* shows 3 (6.82%) and 6 (13.64%) statistically significant associations with spatial factors in cities with ≤14.90 and 14.91+ minutes of commute time; *thefts per 100,000* shows 0 and 0; *auto thefts per 100,000* shows 2 (4.55%) and 0; and *property crimes per 100,000* shows 1 (2.27%) and 0.

Regarding social isolation, *people over 65 living alone* shows 6 (13.64% of the total) and 0 statistically significant associations with spatial factors in cities with ≤14.90 and 14.91+ minutes of commute time.

According to the findings reported here, several violent crimes, including *violent crimes per 100,000*, are more sensitive to spatial factors in cities with 14.91+ minutes of commute time. In contrast, with very few correlations, individual property crimes and *property crimes per 100,000* do not seem to be sensitive to spatial factors in these subsamples of cities. Finally, *people over 65 living alone* shows very little sensitivity to spatial factors in cities with ≤14.90 minutes of commute time, but no sensitivity in cities with 14.91+ minutes of commute time.

Overall, social health indicators show 37 (8.41% of 440 total correlations) and 56 (12.73%) statistically significant associations with spatial factors in cities with ≤14.90 and 14.91+ minutes of commute time. Even though the total numbers of correlations between spatial factors and indicators of social health are low in both subsamples, with more correlations, spatial factors may be relatively more important for social health in small cities with longer commute time.

TABLE 11.4.
Significant correlations between spatial factors and social health indicators

| | Crime | | | | | | | | | Social Isolation | |
| | Significant correlations, n (%) | | | | | | | | | Significant correlations, n (%) | |
Rurality factors	Murders per 100,000	Rapes per 100,000	Robberies per 100,000	Assaults per 100,000	Violent crimes per 100,000	Burglaries per 100,000	Thefts per 100,000	Auto thefts per 100,000	Property crimes per 100,000	People 65+ living alone	Total
Population											
≤9,999	0 (0.00)	3 (6.82)	5 (11.36)	9 (20.45)	8 (18.18)	10 (22.73)	1 (2.27)	12 (27.27)	0 (0.00)	2 (4.55)	50 (11.36)
10,000 +	4 (9.09)	13 (29.55)	11 (25.00)	6 (13.64)	6 (13.64)	3 (6.82)	6 (13.64)	2 (4.55)	4 (5.09)	0 (0.00)	55 (12.50)
Population density (per square mile)											
≤1,834.50	2 (4.55)	2 (4.55)	7 (15.91)	0 (0.00)	0 (0.00)	3 (6.82)	2 (4.55)	7 (15.91)	2 (4.55)	8 (18.18)	33 (7.50)
1,834.51+	19 (43.18)	18 (40.91)	14 (31.82)	14 (31.82)	15 (34.09)	2 (4.55)	2 (4.55)	2 (4.55)	2 (4.55)	1 (2.27)	89 (20.23)
Population change due to daytime travel (as percentage of total population)											
≤6.25	2 (4.55)	10 (22.73)	15 (34.09)	6 (13.64)	10 (22.73)	7 (15.91)	0 (0.00)	2 (4.55)	0 (0.00)	6 (13.64)	58 (13.18)
6.26+	7 (15.91)	2 (4.55)	5 (11.36)	0 (0.00)	1 (2.27)	1 (2.27)	0 (0.00)	5 (11.36)	2 (4.55)	0 (0.00)	23 (5.23)
Distance to nearest city (in miles)											
≤63.40	4 (9.09)	13 (29.55)	11 (25.00)	11 (25.00)	12 (27.27)	5 (11.36)	0 (0.00)	1 (2.27)	0 (0.00)	0 (0.00)	57 (12.95)
63.41+	8 (18.18)	7 (15.91)	9 (20.45)	8 (18.18)	6 (13.64)	2 (4.55)	0 (0.00)	4 (9.09)	0 (0.00)	16 (0.00)	60 (13.64)
Commute time (in minutes)											
≤14.90	10 (22.73)	7 (15.91)	8 (18.18)	0 (0.00)	0 (0.00)	3 (6.82)	0 (0.00)	2 (4.55)	1 (2.27)	6 (0.00)	37 (8.41)
14.91+	3 (6.82)	12 (27.27)	9 (20.45)	13 (29.55)	13 (29.55)	6 (13.64)	0 (0.00)	0 (0.00)	0 (2.27)	0 (0.00)	56 (12.73)

Conclusions

Based on the findings of this comparative correlational study, it may be suggested that, like spatial associations of lifestyle reported in chapter 8, spatial associations of different health outcomes and indicators are also affected by various dimensions of rurality. According to the findings of the study (table 11.5), health outcomes and indicators show 98 (9.68%) and 146 (14.43%) statistically significant associations with spatial factors in cities with ≤9,999 and 10,000+ people, indicating that spatial associations of health outcomes and indicators may be more frequent in cities with more people. From the spatial planning and design perspective, these findings indicate that it may be wise to focus on cities with 10,000+ people to have the most impact on health through design interventions and planning policies and guidelines. Based on the numbers of spatial associations observed, if conceived properly, such interventions and policies could have more impact on people reporting general health conditions, people with disability under 65 years, overweight, assaults, violent crime rate, burglaries, and auto theft in cities with ≤9,999 people.

The findings of the study also show that health outcomes and indicators show 97 (9.58%) and 193 (19.07%) statistically significant associations with spatial factors for cities with ≤1,834.50 and 1,834.51+ people per square mile (table 11.5), indicating that spatial associations of health outcomes and indicators are more frequent in cities with higher population density. Therefore, from the spatial planning and design perspective, it may be wise to focus on cities with 1,834.51+ people per square mile to have the most impact on health through design interventions and planning policies and guidelines. Based on the numbers of spatial associations, these interventions and policies could have more impact on some of the mental health outcomes and indicators than the other health outcomes and indicators in cities with ≤1,834.50 people per square mile. In contrast, they could have more impact on people reporting general health conditions, death rate, adult diabetes, overweight, adult obesity, murders, rapes, robberies, and assaults than the other health outcomes and indicators in cities with 1,834.51+ people per square mile.

Health outcomes and indicators show 139 (13.74%) and 97 (9.58%) statistically significant associations with spatial factors in cities with ≤6.25% and 6.26%+ population change due to daytime travel (table 11.5), indicating that spatial associations of health outcomes and indicators are more frequent in cities with less daytime population change. These findings suggest that spatial interventions and planning policies and guidelines could be more effective in cities with ≤6.25% population change than in cities with 6.26%+ population change due to daytime travel. These spatial interventions and planning policies and guidelines could have more impact on people reporting general health conditions, death rate, adult diabetes, overweight, adult obesity, people with little interest in doing things, rapes, robberies, assaults, burglaries, and people 65+ living alone more than the other health outcomes and indicators in cities with ≤6.25% population change due to daytime travel. In contrast, they could have more impact on death rate, adult diabetes, overweight, and several mental health outcomes and indicators than the other indicators in cities with 6.26%+ population change due to daytime travel.

According to the findings of the study, health outcomes and indicators show 122 (12.06%) and 119 (11.76%) statistically significant associations with spatial factors in small cities ≤63.40 and 63.41+ miles from the nearest large city with 50,000 or more people (table 11.5). Therefore, spatial associations of health outcomes and indicators may be equally prevalent in small cities regardless of their distance from the nearest large cities, and spatial interventions and planning policies and guidelines could affect both subsamples to similar extents but in different ways. They could affect people reporting general health conditions, people with disabilities under 65, overweight, rapes, robberies, and assaults more than the other indicators in small cities ≤63.40 miles from the nearest large city. In contrast, they could affect death rate, diabetes, people with little interest in doing things, murders, and people over 65 living alone more than the other health outcomes and indicators in small cities 63.41+ miles from the nearest large city.

Additionally, health outcomes and indicators show 92 (9.09%) and 127 (12.55%) statistically significant associations with spatial factors for cities with ≤14.90 and 14.91+ minutes of commute time (table 11.5), indicating that spatial associations of health outcomes and indicators are more frequent in cities with more commute time. Based on these findings, it can be suggested that spatial interventions and planning policies and guidelines could be relatively more effective in cities with 14.91+ minutes of commute time than in cities with ≤14.90 minutes of commute time to make an impact on health. More specifically, they could affect death rate, adult diabetes, and murders more than the other indicators in cities with ≤14.90 minutes of commute time. In contrast, they could affect people reporting general health conditions, people under 65 with disabilities, suicides, overweight, people with little interest in doing things, rapes, robberies, and assaults more than the other indicators in cities with 14.91+ minutes of commute time.

TABLE 11.5.
Ranking of significant correlations between spatial factors
and health outcomes and indicators

		Significant correlations for health outcomes and indicators	Rank
Rurality factors		n (%)	
Population	≤9,999	98 (9.68)	7
	10,000 +	146 (14.43)	2
Population density (per square mile)	≤1,834.50	97 (9.58)	8
	1,834.51+	193 (19.07)	1
Population change due to daytime travel (as percentage of total population)	≤6.25	139 (13.74)	3
	6.26+	97 (9.58)	8
Distance to nearest city (in miles)	≤63.40	122 (12.06)	5
	63.41+	119 (11.76)	6
Commute time (in minutes)	≤14.90	92 (9.09)	10
	14.91+	127 (12.55)	4

In conclusion, it may be suggested that spatial associations with health outcomes and indicators may occur more frequently in small cities with more population, higher densities, less daytime population change, and more commute time. Among the subsamples of small cities defined based on the dimensions of rurality, small cities with higher densities (1,834.51+ persons per square mile) show the greatest number of spatial associations with health outcomes and indicators (193 associations), followed by small cities with 10,000+ population (146 associations), and small cities with ≤6.25% population change due to daytime travel (139 associations). The frequency of associations found in the remaining subsample of cities varies between 92 and 127. Therefore, spatial interventions and planning policies and guidelines to improve population health could be most effective if used sensibly in small cities with 1,834.51+ persons per square mile. Spatial interventions and planning policies and guidelines to improve population health could also be effective if used sensibly in the other subsamples of cities defined based on rurality for a particular outcome or a set of outcomes that are sensitive to spatial factors.

NOTES

1. James, "All Rural Places Are Not Created Equal."
2. Gonzalez et al., "Does Increased Emergency Medical Services Prehospital Time Affect Patient Mortality?"

3. Ricketts, "The Changing Nature of Rural Health Care."
4. National Center for Health Statistics, *Urban Rural Health Chart Book.*
5. Hart et al., "Rural Health Care Providers."
6. Liese et al., "Food Store Types, Availability, and Cost of Foods."
7. Hendrickson, Smith, and Eikenberry, "Fruit and Vegetable Access."
8. Smith and Morton, "Rural Food Deserts."
9. All Things Considered, "Why Is the Risk of Youth Suicide Higher in Rural Areas?"
10. Saunderson, Haynes, and Langford, "Urban-Rural Variations in Suicides."
11. Singh and Siahpush, "Increasing Rural-Urban Gradients."
12. Caldwell, Jorm, and Dear, "Suicide and Mental Health."
13. Levin and Leyland, "Urban/Rural Inequalities in Suicide."
14. Bethea et al., "The Relationship between Rural Status, Individual Characteristics, and Self-Rated Health."
15. Maas et al., "Green Space, Urbanity, and Health."
16. Human and Wasem, "Rural Mental Health in America."
17. Skinner and Slifkin, "Rural/Urban Differences in Barriers to and Burden of Care."
18. Befort, Nazir, and Perri, "Prevalence of Obesity among Adults."
19. Bennett, Olatosi, and Probst, *Health Disparities.*
20. Jones, "Rural Populations Have Higher Rates of Chronic Disease."
21. Kuczmarski et al., "Increasing Prevalence of Overweight."
22. Flegal et al., "Overweight and Obesity in the United States."
23. Mokdad et al., "The Spread of the Obesity Epidemic."
24. Mokdad et al., "The Continuing Epidemics of Obesity and Diabetes."
25. Must et al., "The Disease Burden Associated with Overweight."
26. Blair et al., "Influences of Cardiorespiratory Fitness and Other Precursors."
27. Patterson et al., "A Comprehensive Examination of Health Conditions."
28. Ogden et al., "Prevalence of Childhood and Adult."
29. Flegal et al., "Prevalence and Trends in Obesity."
30. Jekanowski, Binkley, and Eales, "Convenience, Accessibility, and the Demand for Fast Food."
31. Prentice and Jebb, "Fast Foods, Energy Density and Obesity."
32. Garcia, Sunil, and Hinojosa, "The Fast Food and Obesity Link."
33. United States Department of Agriculture, "Rural Economy and Population."
34. Yousefian et al., "Active Living for Rural Youth."
35. Hansen et al., "Built Environments and Active Living."
36. Lutfiyya et al., "Is Rural Residency a Risk Factor."
37. Jackson et al., "A National Study of Obesity Prevalence."
38. Patterson et al., "Obesity and Physical Inactivity."
39. Davis et al., "Obesity and Related Health Behaviors."
40. Trivedi et al., "Obesity and Obesity-Related Behaviors."
41. Liu et al., "Diet, Physical Activity, and Sedentary Behaviors."
42. Durazo et al., *The Health Status and Unique Health Challenges.*
43. Kenney, Wang, and Iannotti, "Residency and Racial/Ethnic Differences."
44. Meit et al., *The 2014 Update of the Rural-Urban Chartbook.*
45. Krishna, Gillespie, and McBride, "Diabetes Burden and Access to Preventive Care."
46. Weaver et al., "Rural-Urban Disparities in Health Status."
47. Hallet et al., "Rural-Urban Disparities in Incidence."
48. Shultis et al., "Striking Rural-Urban Disparities."
49. Singh and Siahpush, "Widening Rural-Urban Disparities in All-Cause Mortality."
50. Singh and Siahpush, "Widening Rural-Urban Disparities in Life Expectancy."

51. Wallace et al., "Racial, Socioeconomic, and Rural-Urban Disparities."
52. Zhang and Smith, "Indoor Air Pollution."
53. Wang, Wen, and Xu, "Population-Adjusted Street Connectivity."
54. Xu and Wang, "Built Environment and Obesity by Urbanicity."
55. Boehmer et al., "What Constitutes an Obesogenic Environment?"
56. Doescher et al., "The Built Environment and Utilitarian Walking."
57. Veenhoven, "Greater Happiness for a Greater Number."
58. Jackson, Dannenberg, and Frumkin, "Health and the Built Environment."
59. Lenardson et al., *Access to Mental Health Services*, 1–15.
60. Rural Information Hub, "Substance Abuse in Rural Areas."
61. Agerbo, Torrey, and Mortensen, "Household Crowding in Early Adulthood."
62. Marcelis et al., "Urbanization and Psychosis."
63. Marcelis, Takei, and van Os, "Urbanization and Risk for Schizophrenia."
64. Eaton, Mortensen, and Frydenberg, "Obstetric Factors."
65. Haukka et al., "Regional Variation in the Incidence of Schizophrenia."
66. Pedersen and Mortensen, "Family History, Place and Season of Birth."
67. van Os, Pedersen, and Mortensen, "Confirmation of Synergy between Urbanicity and Familial Liability."
68. Spauwen et al., "Does Urbanicity Shift the Population Expression of Psychosis?"
69. Schelin et al., "Regional Differences in Schizophrenia Incidence."
70. McGrath et al. "A Systematic Review of the Incidence of Schizophrenia."
71. Saha et al., "A Systematic Review of the Prevalence of Schizophrenia."
72. Penkalla and Kohler, "Urbanicity and Mental Health."
73. Davis, Cook, and Cohen, "A Community Resilience Approach."
74. Kawachi and Kennedy, "Socioeconomic Determinants of Health."
75. Kawachi et al., "Social Capital, Income Inequality, and Mortality."
76. Foster and Giles-Corti, "The Built Environment, Neighborhood Crime."
77. Mason, Kearns, and Livingston, " 'Safe Going.' "
78. Stafford, Chandola, and Marmot, "Association between Fear of Crime and Mental Health."
79. Carver, Timperio, and Crawford, "Playing It Safe."
80. Lorenc et al., "Crime, Fear of Crime, Environment."
81. Hale, "Fear of Crime."
82. Lovasi et al., "Built Environments and Obesity."
83. Day, "Strangers in the Night."
84. Weisheit and Donnermeyer, "Change and Continuity in Crime."
85. Weisheit, Falcone, and Wells, *Crime and Policing*.
86. Weisheit and Wells, "Deadly Violence in the Heartland."
87. Weisheit and Wells, "Rural Crime and Justice."
88. Osgood and Chambers, "Social Disorganization Outside the Metropolis."
89. Blumstein, Rivara, and Rosenfeld, "The Rise and Decline of Homicide."
90. Grogger, "An Economic Model of Recent Trends in Violence."
91. Freudenburg and Jones, "Criminal Behavior and Rapid Community Growth."
92. Lee and Ousey, "Size Matters."
93. Jobes, "Residential Stability and Crime."
94. Agnew, "A General Strain Theory of Community Differences," 124.
95. Wells and Weisheit, "Patterns of Rural and Urban Crime."
96. Halpern, *Mental Health and the Planned Environment*.
97. Holt-Lunstad et al., "Loneliness and Social Isolation."
98. Allen, *Older People and Wellbeing*.

99. Murayama, Fujiwara, and Kawachi, "Social Capital and Health."
100. University of Rochester Medical Center, "Older Adults and the Importance of Social Interaction."
101. Bassuk, Glass, and Berkman, "Social Disengagement and Incident Cognitive Decline."
102. Halpern, *Social Capital.*
103. Bennett, "Low Level Social Engagement."
104. Institute of Medicine, *Rebuilding the Unity of Health and the Environment.*
105. Thompson and Kent, "Connecting and Strengthening Communities."

PART SIX

PROBLEMS AND PROSPECTS OF SPATIAL PLANNING AND DESIGN FOR POPULATION HEALTH IN SMALL-TOWN AMERICA

Built Environment and Population Health in Small Cities of Kansas

Study Limitations, Findings, and Implications

The purpose of this book is to study the associations between the spatial factors of the built environment and population health in isolated small towns and cities of rural America and the effects of rurality on these associations. Its aim is to help explain how built environments contribute to population health in these cities—a topic that raises significant concerns but has remained poorly studied in the United States.

For its purpose, the book uses the definition of health provided by the World Health Organization (WHO) in 1948. According to this definition, health is more than a disease-free state of an individual that includes the physical, mental, and social health and well-being of the individual. Aligning with this definition, the book uses a socio-ecological framework of population health. The framework explains the physical, mental, and social health of a population in relation to multiple spatial scales and organizational levels of its context defined by natural, built, and social environments, as described in chapter 1.

The definition of a small town or city was provided in chapter 2. Based on this definition, a sample of Kansas cities with population between 5,000 and 49,999 were selected for this study. Out of the 52 Kansas cities that fall within this population range, 36 isolated small cities were included. Nearly 560,000 people live in these cities altogether, which is about 20% of the state's population. This is also roughly the same percentage of population living in rural areas of the country. Despite their uniqueness, these small Kansas cities face some of the same problems that small towns and cities in the United States face generally (chapters 3, 4, and 5). It is hoped that the studies of this book therefore would not only identify spatial correlates of population health in small Kansas cities but also inform other similar studies elsewhere in the United States.

Guided by the socio-ecological framework described in chapter 1, the studies presented here use an area-level study design involving aggregate data to describe and understand the effects of the built environment on population health in the sample of small Kansas cities and to facilitate a systematic comparison of these cities, taking into account their rurality defined based on local and regional differences (chapter 6).

Using data collected from numerous sources, first, the book provided a description of the spatial factors, lifestyle behaviors, and the physical, mental, and social health of the sample cities (chapter 7). Correlational analyses were used to show how spatial factors are associated with lifestyle and physical, mental, and social health in these small cities (chapters 8 and 10) and in different subsamples of the sample defined based on various factors of rurality, which include population size and density, population changes due to daytime travel, distance from the nearest large city, and commute time (chapters 9 and 11).

In this chapter, the limitations of the studies of the book are discussed, focusing on issues related to the socio-ecological model of population health, the definition of small towns and cities, the factors and indicators used in these studies, the sample of small cities included in the studies, and the analysis of data. Following this, the findings of the studies and their implications for spatial design and planning in small Kansas cities are discussed from a population health perspective. Finally, this chapter discusses spatial design and planning strategies and policies for improving lifestyle and health in small towns and cities, taking into account the studies' findings.

Study Limitations
Limitations Regarding the Socio-Ecological Model of Population Health

As presented in chapter 1, a socio-ecological model of population health requires us to consider health at different levels of human organizations and at different spatial scales of the natural, built, and social environments or contexts. The levels of human organizations include individuals, groups, and communities. The spatial scales include micro, meso, and macro levels of the environments. Experts have explicitly recommended that spatial design and policy interventions related to population health should consider the interconnected levels of influence, extending from individuals to groups to communities and from micro to meso to macro scales of different environments.

It was noted in chapter 1 that the scope of a population health study depends on how it proposes to explore the interactions between human organizational levels and environments' spatial scales. Concerning this, the studies of this book considered "community" or the "city" as a unit of analysis focusing on their meso- and macro-scale spatial factors. These studies did not consider natural environments, except parks and green spaces, or social environments, except some elements of social health, demography, and rurality. The book therefore deals with a segment of the ecological model, not the whole model.

Regarding this limitation, it should be noted that the usefulness of an ecological model lies in the fact that laying out the domains and processes of population health comprehensively helps us see the gaps in the literature. Therefore, the next steps of the research presented are already evident. Any future studies should consider population health in relation to natural and social environments and in relation to the micro scale of the built environment of small towns and cities. In addition, a more complex statistical model that can simulate the complex interactions across various organizational levels and spatial scales of an ecological model of population health should be considered in future studies. In this regard, one should note that as statistical models get complicated, it becomes difficult to draw simple actionable conclusions based on these models. Qualitative studies, which can be used to replace such complex statistical models, generally work well for in-depth understanding of a handful of cases, and the results of these studies cannot easily be transferred to other cases.

Limitations Regarding the Definition of Small Towns and Cities

In this book, a small town or city is defined as *an incorporated town or a civil township that falls in the category of urban clusters (UCs) with US Census Bureau population between 2,500 and 49,999 and that is formed under the general laws of a US state or under a charter adopted by the local voters* (chapter 2). This definition of small towns and cities as territories with a certain number of people, however, does not sufficiently represent the complexities of small towns and cities as sociological units. As noted in chapter 2, in addition to having a well-defined territory with a certain number of people, a small town or city also has its peculiar social networks, institutional framework, cultural values, belief systems, myths, rituals, and celebrations. Many places may not have these sociological qualities even though they have the required number of people to be considered a small town or city. In contrast, other areas may have these qualities without having the required number of people. Put simply, a population-based definition of small towns and cities may exclude many communities that deserve to be included in a study on population health. This is important because a sociological definition takes into account the unique qualities of a community and shows what works and what does not work in the community. It is difficult, however, to see how complex sociological qualities can be operationalized for a large number of cities without in-depth qualitative studies. The studies presented here have therefore used a simple population-based definition of small cities, which was further enhanced by several scale- and place-specific attributes defining rurality in the comparative correlational analyses. As a result, it was possible to include a larger sample of cities without losing all specificity.

Limitations Regarding Spatial Factors, Lifestyle, and Health Indicators

In these studies, spatial factors included city size and density, availability of key destinations and facilities, land use type and mix, and street properties of small cities. Lifestyle behaviors included work-related travel behaviors, food shopping and eating behaviors, and physical and sedentary activities. Health indicators were related to mortality and morbidity and physical, mental, and social health. These categories represent different dimensions of a broad definition of health provided by the WHO. The selection of these spatial factors, lifestyle behaviors, and health indicators was based on the evidence presented in the literature. The selected indicators are not exhaustive but rather representative of their categories. Though many more spatial factors, lifestyle behaviors, and health indicators could have been included, it is noteworthy that the studies of this book report numerous spatial associations of lifestyle and health indicators, validating the importance of spatial factors for population health in small Kansas cities.

Limitations Regarding the Sample of Small Cities in Kansas

Small cities in Kansas may not be representative of all small towns and cities in the United States. As noted in chapters 2 and 3, there are significant variations among small towns and cities around the country in terms of geographic, socioeconomic, and demographic factors; cultural, political, and religious preferences and attitudes; and health care issues. We need to learn more about the effects of these variations on spatial associations of lifestyle and health to formulate appropriate strategies and policies aimed at eliminating health disparities in the United States. Future studies should include a larger sample of different types of small cities from different US regions to explore variations in spatial associations of lifestyle and health in small cities. Finding reliable data for such national studies will always be a significant challenge.

Limitations Regarding Data Analysis

Associations and causal relations are not the same thing. In the exploratory studies of this book, the goal was to uncover spatial associations, not causal relations. Consistent with the goal, the studies of this book have found numerous associations between spatial factors and health outcomes and indicators and between spatial factors and lifestyle. Theories explaining these associations were not offered, however. Based on the studies, we know that these associations vary based on factors of rurality, but we still do not know if these associations also vary based on socioeconomic, demographic, cultural, political, religious, and health care factors. As shown in figure 1.3, there are many pathways for spatial factors to influence lifestyle and health, most of which were not explored here. Future studies therefore must include robust statistical models to establish causal relationships between built environments and population health in small-town America.

Study Findings and Their Implications
Urban-Rural Health Disparities

The literature on population health in US small towns and cities is limited. This literature was reviewed throughout the book to provide some understanding of population health issues in these towns and cities. The review showed that regardless of how the authors of the published studies have defined urban and rural areas, urban-rural disparities exist for every dimension of population health, including lifestyle and physical, mental, and social health. Nevertheless, most comparative studies between urban and rural areas along population health dimensions have remained somewhat contrived because these areas vary in scale, structure, organization, and complexity.

More specifically, the literature reported many differences in lifestyle behaviors in urban and rural areas. For example, rural and urban areas exhibit different patterns of physical activity (PA) in different PA domains, including leisure-time PA, occupational PA, household PA, and transportation PA. Among these, transportation PA is noteworthy because there is a general lack of public transportation options in rural areas as low population density renders most public transportation infrastructure cost ineffective. Clearly, the focus to promote PA in rural areas and small towns and cities should be different from urban areas.

The literature also reported many differences in physical health in urban and rural areas. Most importantly, a higher prevalence of overweight and obesity even after adjustment for individual-level factors would suggest that rural areas might be "obesogenic" in ways that urban areas might not be. Existing studies on rural-urban health disparities, however, do not distinguish between rural and urban America in terms of obesogenic features. Since small-town America is considered an integral part of rural America in the existing literature, the unique obesogenic attributes of small-town America also remain undetermined.

Additionally, the literature reported that rural-urban health disparities generally are widespread because a general lack of accessibility, availability, and acceptability of health-related resources create more challenges in rural areas than in urban areas. Rural residents often travel long distances to receive health care services. Food deserts are found more frequently in rural areas than urban. Frequent self-reliance for health care often affects the acceptability of any physical and mental health care more in rural areas than urban. Doubts about the quality of clinical care for physical and mental health are also generally high among rural population.

One complicating factor in all this is rural residents' self-perception of social health [1–4]. Rural residents generally believe that they have better social integration and support than do urban residents. On the one hand, this perception makes rural residents self-reliant and resilient. On the other hand, this also makes them resistant to science-based health care and positive lifestyle changes. Torn apart by these often-contradictory tendencies, it is no wonder that rural residents provide poorer overall self-ratings for individual health than do urban residents. Suicide rates are generally higher for both males and females living in rural areas than their urban counterparts. Rural men may show twice the suicide rate of urban men when controlling for such variations as divorce rate and ethnicity. Rural children have more behavioral and mental health problems than urban children. Social isolation and loneliness are more prevalent among rural than urban elderly. Considered a part of rural America, small-town America probably suffers similar problems, but these problems also remain undetermined.

In general, higher crime rates indicate poorer social health. Research has consistently found that there are large differences in crime rates between rural and urban areas and that crime in rural and urban areas may be influenced by different factors or influenced differently by the same factors. To give an example, while economic prosperity reduces crime in urban areas, it does just the opposite in rural areas. Given the differences in crime between urban and rural areas, it is necessary to know where and how small-town America finds itself on this issue.

Though many problems of urban rural health disparities raised in the literature remain beyond the scope of this book, the literature makes it clear that population health in small-town America is a heavily understudied area. Since the built environment is an important dimension of a socio-ecological model of population health, the purpose of this book is to show how the built environment might be associated with population health in small-town America. Since the studies exploring these associations have already been presented in the last few chapters, here a summary of the study findings is presented, along with a discussion of the implications of these findings for spatial design and planning for population health in small cities and towns.

Spatial Factors, Lifestyle, and Health in Small Cities of Kansas: Findings and Implications

The descriptive analysis of the spatial data of the built environment of small Kansas cities was presented in chapter 7. The data include city size and density, availability of key destinations and facilities, land use type and mix, and street properties. The study shows that there are some extreme values for almost every spatial factor in one or more cities. Therefore, there is a need to consider small cities with extreme values separately from the other cities without extreme values when suggesting spatial strategies for improving the built environment of these cities. For some small cities, the distribution of values of many spatial factors shows strong peaks (where values drop sharply from the central value), while others showed weak peaks (where values drop slowly from the central value). There is therefore also a need to consider spatial properties with high peak distributions differently than spatial properties with low peak distributions in spatial strategies aimed at improving the built environment of these cities.

The descriptive analysis also shows that the values of many lifestyle and health indicators of the sample cities were different from those of the state of Kansas, while many others were similar to those of the state. For example, food shopping behaviors were worse but eating behavior was better in small cities than statewide. Likewise, the rates of murder, robbery, assault, and auto theft were lower, whereas the rates of rape, burglary, theft, arson, and people over 65 living alone were higher in small cities than the state. Based on these findings, it may be suggested that spatial strategies should focus only on some lifestyle and health indicators in small Kansas cities to improve them to the state level. If the goal of spatial strategies is to improve population health in small cities of Kansas to a level comparable to the United States overall, however, then the focus must be on improving many more lifestyle and health indicators that are worse than the national level.

Additionally, the descriptive analysis shows that the values of many physical and sedentary activities and mental health indicators are often similar in the sample of small cities and the state. Since Kansas does not do well nationally in terms of physical and sedentary activities and mental health, spatial strategies could be used for improving them to a level comparable to the national level.

Furthermore, the descriptive analysis shows that some lifestyle and health indicators show more variability than do other behaviors and indicators in the sample cities. For example, all the indicators of mortality, morbidity, and social health, and some of the indicators of lifestyle and physical health, show high variability in these cities. Spatial strategies promoting population health in each small city therefore ought to be considered separately for health indicators with high variability.

Spatial Associations of Lifestyle in Small Cities of Kansas: Findings and Implications

As reported in chapter 8, the existing literature includes studies suggesting numerous potential and empirical associations between *city size* and lifestyle focusing primarily on commuting behaviors using cars only. The literature, however, does not suggest any associations of city size with many other work-related travel behaviors, food shopping and eating behaviors, and physical and sedentary activities for both large and small cities. The studies presented in this book are relevant and important in addressing this gap. According to the findings of these studies, city size measured using land area shows significant associations with some food shopping and eating behaviors and with some physical and sedentary activities. If managed thoughtfully, city size may provide some lifestyle benefits in small Kansas cities.

The existing literature also includes studies suggesting numerous associations between *density* and travel behaviors and between density and physical activities. Conducted in urban areas, most of the studies may not be relevant to small cities because the density of an urban area within a metropolitan region and the density of a small city in a rural area may not be comparable. More significantly, there is a lack of studies reporting associations between density and food shopping and eating behaviors in both urban areas and small cities. Despite the benefits of density in urban areas as indicated in the literature, the findings of this book's studies show very few associations of census block and housing density with lifestyle in small cities of Kansas. It is possible that, despite some variations in density, densities in small cities are generally low and therefore do not affect lifestyle.

Additionally, the literature includes studies exploring associations between the *availability of key destinations and facilities* and lifestyle. According to these studies, increased availability of and access to key destinations and facilities are often associated with better lifestyle behaviors. Most of these benefits, however, seem to be related to increased availability and accessibility of parks and green spaces. Contrarily, according to the findings of the studies presented in this book, except parks and open spaces, availability of all the other key destinations and facilities shows frequent associations with lifestyle, including physical activity, in small Kansas cities. The fact that parks and open spaces do not show frequent associations with physical activity indicates that it may be possible to improve population health in small Kansas cities if small-town residents would use parks and open spaces more frequently.

The literature reports very little on the relationships between *land use type* and lifestyle. In contrast, it reports many studies on the relationships between *land use mix (LUM)* and lifestyle. According to these studies, higher LUM is generally synonymous with the presence of diverse destinations, shorter trips lengths, and hence a more permeable and walkable neighborhood; and higher LUM generally promotes more physical activity in urban areas. Similar studies in small cities and rural areas do not exist, primarily because of their smallness and their presumed lack of complexity and urbanicity. It is, however, important to note that despite being small, small cities often are functionally diverse, and they often offer functions as diverse as urban cores but at a much smaller scale. According to the findings of the studies reported here, open spaces and residential, commercial, and institutional land uses generally do not show significant associations with lifestyle in small Kansas cities. In contrast, industrial land use and LUM show several significant associations with lifestyle. Therefore, industrial land use and LUM should be considered carefully in spatial strategies for improving lifestyle in small cities.

Finally, associations between lifestyle and *street properties* have been studied extensively in existing literature. Some of these studies have reported significant relationships between street properties and physical activities, while others have found no relationships. Studies on the relationships between street properties and physical activities in rural areas generally have used national data and therefore are not sensitive to local differences. Only a few studies have looked at the associations between street properties and lifestyle in small cities. They have either a very narrow scope or a very small sample size. It is important to note that the techniques of space syntax, which have been used successfully in studies predicting travel and other behaviors in urban areas, have not been applied to behavioral studies in rural areas and small towns and cities. For these reasons, it is very difficult to draw any general conclusions on the relationships between street properties and lifestyle in small cities based on the findings reported in the literature. Given a dearth of evidence on the associations between street properties and lifestyle in rural areas and small towns and cities, the studies presented in this book are important. They show that street network properties defined using space syntax techniques have several significant associations with work-related behaviors, food shopping and eating behaviors, and physical activity in small Kansas cities. Therefore, it may be possible to improve lifestyle behaviors in these cities using street network properties describing accessibility, movement potential, and directional choices.

Spatial Associations of Health in Small Cities of Kansas: Findings and Implications

As reported in chapter 10, according to the literature, when a large sample of cities representing different sizes is considered in a study, a health gradient exists for *city size* in both developed and developing countries. The gradient shows that as city size increases, health gets better, sometimes nonlinearly. According to the findings of the studies of this book, however, city size does not seem to be an important physical and mental health factor for population health in small Kansas cities. It is still an important social health factor, showing relationships with violent and property crime.

The literature generally indicates that *density* measured in various ways can be a significant factor affecting physical, mental, and social health. However, careful spatial strategies are necessary to ensure that density produces desired health benefits. According to the findings of this study, density does not seem to affect health in any significant way in small Kansas cities and therefore may not be a critical factor for population health.

As reported in the literature, among different *key destinations and facilities*, the availability and accessibility of parks and green spaces seem to show the most beneficial health effects. In the studies involving small Kansas cities, some predictable associations between health and different categories of key destinations and facilities were found except for parks and green spaces. It is possible that parks are not maintained properly in small cities, that small-town residents do not know the health benefits of parks and green spaces, or that they are not as deprived of open spaces and green spaces as are urban residents. Nonetheless, these are good reasons why the role of parks and green spaces must be emphasized in spatial strategies aimed at improving population health in small-town America.

The associations of *land use type* and *LUM* with health have been reported frequently in the literature. Most reported studies on land use types focus on the amount or percentage of open spaces, parks, and green spaces and show significant positive associations with health. LUM also shows beneficial effects on physical and mental health, but these effects seem to vary based on how LUM is defined. For the same study areas, LUM defined based on a higher number of land use categories appears to show better associations with health outcomes than LUM defined using a lower number of land use categories. In contrast, the effects of LUM on social health remain equivocal and vary depending on the type of use included in the mix. For example, some types of mix tend to encourage crime, while others do just the opposite.

According to the findings of the studies of this book, among different land use types, the percentage of industrial areas seems to have the most health effects, and social health seems to be most affected by land use types. Neither the percentage of open areas nor LUM seems to have notable effects on health in small Kansas cities. Regardless of these findings, if improving health through spatial strategies is a goal, then the amount of open space, parks, and green space should be considered seriously in small Kansas cities. Likewise, LUM may not be as important in small cities as it is in urban areas for physical and mental health, but it should be considered carefully to avoid any unintended social consequences in small cities given the fact that LUM shows numerous associations with social health indicators in urban areas.

Finally, many previous studies did not find significant associations between *street properties* and physical health in urban areas, while other studies found significant associations between street properties and social health. More particularly, several of these studies report significant associations between street network properties measured using space syntax techniques and crime, safety, and social equity. Confirming some of the previous findings as well as going beyond, the studies of this book report many significant associations between street network properties and indicators of mortality and morbidity and between street network properties and indicators of physical, mental, and social health. There is a subsequent need to consider street network properties describing accessibility and movement potential and choices in spatial strategies aimed at improving population health in small Kansas cities.

Rurality and Spatial Associations of Lifestyle and Health in Small Cities of Kansas: Findings and Implications

Rurality is an important way to define the character of a small city. In this book it is assumed that spatial associations of lifestyle and health might be affected by the rurality of a small town. However, it is not easy to describe rurality. Different institutions have defined it using different factors. In the studies presented here, population size and density, change in population due to daytime travel, distance from the nearest large city with 50,000+ people, and commuting time were used to define the rurality of a small town, and the study sample of cities was divided into two subsamples using the low and high values of each factor to explore if rurality affects spatial associations of lifestyle and health differently in the city subsamples.

According to the findings of the comparative correlational study reported in chapters 9 and 11, spatial associations of different lifestyle and health indicators are affected differently by rurality defined using different factors. Lifestyle and health indicators show 197 and 262 significant associations with spatial factors for cities ≤9,999 and 10,000+ people, indicating that spatial associations of lifestyle and health indicators may be more frequent for small cities with more people. Taken separately, lifestyle and health indicators also show less frequent spatial associations in cities with ≤9,999 people than in cities with 10,000+ people (99 and 116 vs. 98 and 146). In other words, these two subsamples of small cities defined based on population size are different not only in terms of spatial associations of lifestyle and health indicators taken together but also in terms of spatial associations of lifestyle and health indicators taken separately. Therefore, a categorization of small cities of Kansas based on population size may be useful for spatial interventions aimed at improving both lifestyle and health. These spatial interventions may be equally effective for lifestyle in both the subsamples (99 vs. 98) and more effective for health in cities with larger population size (116 vs. 146).

These studies also find that lifestyle and health indicators show 168 and

381 significant associations with spatial factors for cities with ≤1,834.50 and 1,834.51+ people per square mile, indicating that spatial associations of lifestyle and health indicators are more frequent in cities with higher population density. Taken separately, lifestyle and health indicators show less frequent spatial associations in cities with ≤1,834.50 people per square mile than they show in cities with 1,834.51+ people per square mile (71 and 188 vs. 97 and 193). These findings indicate that these two subsamples of cities defined based on population density are different not only in terms of spatial associations of lifestyle and health indicators taken together but also in terms of spatial associations of lifestyle and health indicators taken separately. A categorization of small Kansas cities based on population density may be useful for spatial interventions aimed at improving health as well as lifestyle. However, these spatial interventions may be more effective for lifestyle in cities with higher population densities (71 vs. 97) and equally effective for health in both subsamples (188 vs. 193).

The studies also find that lifestyle and health indicators show 271 and 159 significant associations with spatial factors for cities with ≤6.25% and 6.26%+ population change due to daytime travel, indicating that spatial associations of lifestyle and health indicators are more frequent in cities with less daytime population change. Taken separately, lifestyle and health indicators show more frequent spatial associations in cities with ≤6.25% population change than in cities with 6.26%+ population change due to daytime travel (132 and 62 vs. 139 and 97). These findings indicate that these two subsamples of cities defined based on daytime population change are different not only in terms of spatial associations of lifestyle and health indicators taken together but also in terms of spatial associations of lifestyle and health indicators taken separately. A categorization of small Kansas cities based on population change due to daytime travel may be equally useful for spatial interventions aimed at improving health as well as lifestyle. These spatial interventions may be equally effective for lifestyle in both the subsamples (132 vs. 139) and more effective for health in cities with more population change due to daytime travel (62 vs. 97).

Furthermore, these studies find that lifestyle and health indicators show 246 and 184 significant associations with spatial factors for cities ≤63.40 miles and 63.41+ miles from the nearest large city, indicating that spatial associations of lifestyle and health indicators may be more frequent for cities closer to a large city. When lifestyle and health indicators are considered separately, spatial associations of lifestyle behaviors do not occur as frequently in cities ≤63.40 miles from the nearest large city as they occur in cities 63.41+ miles from the nearest large city (124 vs. 65), but spatial associations of health indicators occur almost as frequently in cities ≤63.40 miles from the nearest large city as they occur in cities 63.41+ miles from the nearest large city (122 vs. 119). In other words, these two categories of small cities defined based on distance from the nearest large city are only different in terms of the frequency of spatial associations of lifestyle and not in terms of the frequency of spatial associations of health indicators. A categorization of small Kansas cities based on distance from the nearest large city may be more useful for spatial interventions aimed at improving lifestyle behaviors (124 vs. 65) than health (122 vs. 119).

Moreover, the studies of this book find that lifestyle and health indicators show 140 and 242 significant associations with spatial factors for cities with ≤14.90 and 14.91+ minutes of commute time, indicating that spatial associations of lifestyle and health indicators are much higher in cities with more commute time. When considered separately, lifestyle and health indicators show less frequent spatial associations in cities with ≤14.90 minutes than in cities with 14.91+ minutes of commute time (48 and 115 vs. 92 and 127). These findings indicate that these two categories of cities defined based on commute time are different not only in terms of spatial associations of lifestyle and health indicators taken together but also in terms of spatial associations of lifestyle and health indicators taken separately. According to the findings, a categorization of small Kansas cities based on commute time may be significantly more useful for spatial interventions aimed at improving lifestyle (48 vs. 92) than health (115 vs. 127).

In summary, spatial associations of lifestyle and health may occur more frequently in small cities with more population, higher density, less daytime population change, less distance from the nearest city, and more commute time. Among the subsamples of small cities defined based on the dimensions of rurality, small cities with higher densities (1,834.51+ persons per square mile) show the greatest number of spatial associations with lifestyle and health indicators (381 associations). In Kansas this subsample of small cities therefore should be targeted for the most impact on population health through spatial strategies. Since every rurality factor seems to affect spatial associations of lifestyle and of health differently, when possible, each should be considered carefully in spatial strategies aimed at improving population health in small cities.

In the next few sections of this chapter, we will consider in further detail how lifestyle and health indicators in small towns and cities might be changed or improved through spatial strategies and policies developed based on the evidence presented here and in the literature.

Spatial Design and Planning for Healthy Small Towns and Cities: Some Suggestions

As shown in figure 1.3, spatial design and planning factors affecting population health may include indoor environment and interior design at the micro scale; neighborhood design, density, diversity, and accessibility at the meso scale; and city size and density, availability and accessibility of key facilities and destinations, and street grid and network properties at the macro scale. The studies of the book, however, considered mostly macro-scale spatial factors, with the exception of neighborhood accessibility defined on street network, which is a meso-scale factor. Many spatial factors were therefore not included here. Those that were included had shown significant associations with lifestyle and health not only here but also in other studies reviewed and reported throughout the book. The evidence reported in the literature along with the evidence reported in this book are used while suggesting spatial strategies and policies to improve lifestyle behaviors and health in small cities and towns.

Spatial Design and Planning for Lifestyle
SPATIAL DESIGN AND PLANNING FOR WORK-RELATED TRAVEL BEHAVIORS

Work-related travel behaviors considered in this book include working from home, driving alone, carpooling, and walking and biking to work. According to the evidence presented here, several spatial factors show frequent significant associations with these behaviors in small towns and cities. We may therefore want to use these factors in strategies and policies for making positive changes to work-related travel behaviors in small towns and cities. According to the evidence, however, density (housing density and census block density) may not be as important a factor of work-related travel behaviors in small towns as in urban areas. In contrast, the availability and accessibility of several key destinations and facilities are important factors affecting these behaviors, though their associations vary depending on the rurality of a small town.

Surprisingly, parks and green spaces did not show frequent associations with work-related travel behaviors in small Kansas cities. We should still consider improving their availability, accessibility, and usability as important strategic choices for population health because well-managed, safe parks and green spaces always provide positive benefits to those who may be able to use them. Industrial land use and LUM seem to have several significant associations with work-related travel behaviors and should therefore be considered carefully for positive population health benefits.

Street properties seem to have numerous associations with work-related travel behaviors, including walking and biking to work; therefore, they deserve careful consideration for positive health benefits in these small towns and cities. Interestingly, both walking and biking can serve utilitarian (or transportation) and recreational purposes, and both can reduce private motor vehicle dependency. According to the literature, walking is a reliable mode of transportation with demonstrated health benefits in communities that are designed to prioritize pedestrians. Similarly, biking is a great form of exercise, emission free, and one of the most efficient forms of transportation available—particularly for trips under two miles. Bike lanes support real and perceived safety for all street users [5–7]. Therefore, updating streets with pedestrians and bikers in mind should be a priority in small towns and cities because walking and biking can easily become the preferred modes of active transportation in these cities. From a spatial strategy and policy perspective, however, it should be noted that walking and biking often, but not always, need different infrastructure. Walking is more common than biking and typically needs less skill, equipment, and infrastructure. Biking allows longer distances to be traveled in less time, thereby reducing travel time to work and increasing access to amenities [6, 8, 9].

While considering work-related travel behaviors, we may want to consult urban and transportation planning literature, which has long explored ways to reduce motor vehicle use and to encourage use of public transport and active transport modes such as walking and biking for work trips [10]. The literature presents several regional and local factors and their related policies to encourage walking, biking, and public transport use while reducing private motor vehicle use in urban areas [10, 11]. At the regional level, urban and transportation planning strategies and policies may include destination accessibility (i.e., accessibility and availability of food outlets, educational facilities, and health and community services), employment distribution, and demand for driving (e.g., the ease and cost of driving and car parking) relative to active modes of transport. At the local level, they may include local neighborhoods' structure, look, feel, and convenience (e.g., street network design, availability of walking and cycling infrastructure, residential densities, the

diversity and mix of land use, and housing types); the desirability of neighborhoods (e.g., levels of crime and traffic safety); and public transport (e.g.,
convenience, affordability, service frequency, safety, and comfort). We should
carefully consider some of these regional and local factors as we develop spatial strategies and policies to promote population health in small towns and
cities without forgetting the differences between urban areas and small towns
and cities.

SPATIAL DESIGN AND PLANNING FOR FOOD SHOPPING
AND EATING BEHAVIORS

What we eat and drink directly affects our health and well-being. Unfortunately, unhealthy foods are cheap and readily available, and sugary drinks
like soda are a major contributor to today's obesity epidemic. Research shows
major disparities in access to healthy food by income level, race, and population density [12, 13]. Therefore, low-income neighborhoods are both at higher
risk of the chronic diseases associated with unhealthy food options [14] and
less likely to have access to the fresh and healthy foods that could help reduce
those health risks.

The built environment can both optimize and present barriers to choosing healthy foods over unhealthy foods. While improving the economic well-
being of the community would give residents more options to buy healthy
food, it is critical that residents have easy access to fresh and healthy food. At
minimum, there are three design and planning considerations if a food environment must ensure access to healthy food for all. These are statutory planning for food production and processing; retail planning to ensure a diversity
of outlets and ready access to these outlets; and cultural planning to create
opportunities for healthy food practices [15]. While it may be possible to optimize these outcomes by redesigning local food systems, it is important to
acknowledge that we may lack resources and capacity to do so in small towns
and cities.

In terms of what food is available in small towns and cities, it may be important to protect food producing lands and "healthy agriculture" around
these towns and cities. From an ecological perspective, such strategic choices
have several benefits: Agricultural lands perform multiple functions beyond
food production. They provide landscape amenity, eco-cultural tourism, and
environmental protection from overdevelopment. The stewardship of land
by people with a deep knowledge of its use is integral to planning for future
food security. This occurs through safeguarding agricultural lands, as well as

providing local farmers with incomes to maintain their own futures by being able to adapt to changing environmental conditions and emerging market opportunities [15].

For healthy food production and processing in small towns and cities, the following design intervention and/or policy recommendations may be useful: (1) Provide space for growing food on-site through community gardens, edible landscaping, or a small-scale farm [16, 17]. (2) Facilitate opportunities to get locally grown produce to residents [18], for example, through farm stands, farmers' markets, or community-supported agriculture arrangements. (3) Collaborate with local community organizations that offer gardening or farming expertise [19]. (4) Design a management and maintenance plan with clearly laid-out responsibilities for day-to-day gardening activities, as well as rules, security, and strategies to prevent vandalism [20].

Along with preserving food-producing land and providing support for local farmers, a mix of retail outlets (with a range of product choices), an agreeable amenity at the shopping precinct (lighting, personal safety), and limited exposure to product marketing and advertising [21, 22] are needed to ensure accessibility and affordability of foods. Findings reported here show that the availability of supermarkets, grocery stores, convenience stores with or without gas, and full-service restaurants all seem to affect food shopping and eating behaviors in small towns and cities. Hence, it may be important for small-town design and planning professionals to consider these facilities with some care for affecting food shopping and eating behaviors.

If deemed necessary, innovative financing techniques can be used to attract supermarkets to areas that lack access to healthy food or to help corner stores to carry healthier food choices. In favor of getting a supermarket in low-income communities, it has been argued that once established, a supermarket could act as an economic anchor, raising the tax base by attracting additional economic activity to an underserved neighborhood. It can also increase the number of job opportunities. However, these changes can force low-income families out of their community, a fact that small-town design and planning professionals should consider.

While many areas need a brick-and-mortar store that sells fresh produce, it is not always feasible to bring one into low-income areas with low tax base. In such cases, small-town design and planning professionals can help find venues for farmers' markets with adequate space and transportation access and utilities. Less infrastructure-intensive options, however, come with their own set of challenges. In places with extreme weather, produce is not available throughout the year. These products are sometimes pricier than equivalent produce at supermarkets, reducing their appeal to low-income populations. It may be possible to overcome this obstacle by subsidizing SNAP/food stamp purchases at farm stands.

Access to healthy food can mean increasing the likelihood of choosing healthy food over unhealthy options by putting barriers in place. While it can be difficult to adopt a comprehensive measure to restrict fast food throughout a community, it may be possible to create healthy food zones around key locations such as schools or main streets. Small-town design and planning professionals should analyze the overall food environment rather than focusing only on full-line grocery stores if they want to change consumption behavior.

Policy recommendations for food retail outlets in small towns and cities may include: (1) Provide space to accommodate a full-service grocery store, particularly in neighborhoods where there is unmet demand for healthy foods [23, 24]. (2) Host a farmers' market on-site, particularly in neighborhoods where demand for healthy foods is not met [25, 26]. (3) Help make farmers' markets more affordable by supporting pay-as-you can policies. (4) Develop farmers' markets at highly visible and accessible places with significant existing foot traffic and with parking space for farmers' trucks [27]. (5) Facilitate the delivery of fresh produce baskets directly from farmers or farmers' markets to residents. (6) Provide healthier foods in cafeterias, vending machines, and other retail sites [28, 29]. (7) Require healthy food options in vendor contracts and encourage strategic pricing, product placement, and promotional standards that favor healthy options [30].

Finally, food consumption experience is important to ensure access to healthy food. The participatory process of designing food environments and spaces can foster social connection. In turn, socially connected individuals can become motivated to organize "alternative" food systems. Small-town design and planning professionals can play a central role in making such plans possible. Local food environments can also offer opportunities for communities to engage with food, at a time when many communities and places have lost their unique qualities. Additionally, local food environments can be major catalysts for bringing people together to build trust and reciprocity [31], to enrich social capital, and to create resilient and healthy communities [32].

Some policy recommendations for health food consumption experiences in small towns and cities may include: (1) Develop local food plans in collaboration with local participants. (2) Provide regulatory and capacity building support to local agriculture and sites of food exchange. (3) Collaborate with local community organizations celebrating healthy food eating experiences. (3) Identify easily accessible places for sharing food.

SPATIAL DESIGN AND PLANNING FOR PHYSICAL AND SEDENTARY ACTIVITIES

Like with any other lifestyle behavior, the relationship between the built environment and physical activity is complex and is influenced by geographic and sociodemographic characteristics, personal and cultural variables, safety, and time constraints [33]. The pathways for the built environment to influence these and other lifestyle behaviors were shown in figure 1.3. According to the figure and the supporting literature, spatial design and planning factors—particularly density, diversity of land use, availability of multiple local destinations, and access or distance to transport and local amenities—can provide a range of active-living options. They can influence the convenience, attractiveness, and safety of walking and biking for transport, as well as the opportunities for, and desirability of, recreational physical activity.

Though the available evidence broadly suggests that diversity, design, and destination accessibility may support walking—both transport related and recreational—in small towns as they do in urban areas, caution is advised when drawing too much from urban studies for use in rural areas due to variations in measurement of spatial factors [34, 35], variations in measurement of walking [36], and variations in approaches to control for sociodemographic and other potential confounders [37]. Still, the evidence for spatial factors affecting physical activities related to active transportation—for example, walking and biking to work—is consistent in the literature [38]. In contrast, the evidence for spatial factors affecting recreational activities is less consistent [39–41]. Therefore, professionals working to improve population health in small towns are left to wonder whether the extensive evidence linking spatial factors to walking and biking in metropolitan areas is usable for their purpose.

To the comfort of these professionals, according to the evidence presented in this book, several spatial factors show frequent significant associations with physical and sedentary activities in small towns and cities. For example, city size shows significant negative correlations with people doing moderate-intensity work activities and significant positive correlations with people walking and bicycling; increased availability of key destinations and facilities increases moderate-intensity work activities and sedentary activities but decreases biking and walking; more open area reduces walking and biking;

more industrial area increases biking and walking and reduces sedentary activities; more LUM decreases moderate-intensity recreational activities and sedentary activities; and street properties are associated with moderate-intensity work activities, walking or biking, vigorous-intensity recreational activities, and moderate-intensity recreational activities. Small-town design and planning professionals may want to use some or all of these spatial factors while developing strategies and policies for positive changes in physical and sedentary activities.

Notably, the effects of land use type and mix on physical and sedentary activities in small towns are different from those in urban areas, and their effects are limited to only certain activities. This may be because land use type lacks extent, and LUM lacks complexity in small towns and cities. Small-town design and planning professionals should therefore carefully consider interventions and policies for land use type and mix, keeping in mind that findings in urban areas may not be useful for small towns.

Improvements to sidewalks, bike lanes, parks, playgrounds, and LUM have been emphasized in the literature for increasing walking and biking and decreasing obesity rates in urban areas [42]. While some of these strategies have been successfully used in some small towns and cities, especially those with established downtowns or commercial centers, other urban strategies are not appropriate for many rural and remote regions [43–46]. In rural and remote regions, dispersed settlements, low population and development density, limited transportation options, and a lack of physical activity opportunities are barriers against physical activities. Hence, participation in physical activities is generally low, and sedentary time among rural and small-town populations is generally high, leading to overweight and obesity among these populations. Establishing suitable spatial programming and policies to improve physical activities in small towns and rural areas must be a priority for small-town design and planning professionals [43, 46, 47].

In general, small-town design and planning professionals should consider categorizing key destinations and facilities of various kinds in the form of a hierarchy that reflects the catchment population they require, the proportion of the general population who use them, and the frequency with which they do so. Facilities that fall into a similar category are best located close to one another to conveniently fulfill more than one purpose with a single trip, to minimize the traffic generated by commonplace journeys, and to maximize the proportion of trips by nonmotorized modes.

Surprisingly, parks and green spaces did not show frequent associations with walking and biking. Small-town design and planning professionals might still want to consider improving the availability, accessibility, and usability of parks and green spaces as important strategic choices for population health because well-designed and well-maintained parks and playgrounds of all sizes serve as venues for physical activity and recreation, increase access to nature, and improve health [48–57]. They also boost the value of surrounding properties [58]. Parks and playgrounds shape community identity and serve as the backdrop to social interactions among different ages and groups [59]. Those living closer to a park spend more vigorous physical activity time than those who live farther away [60].

Small-town design and planning professionals may want to consider the following policies and guidelines to improve the availability, accessibility, and usability of parks and green spaces: (1) Maximize access to high-quality parks and recreation spaces [60, 61]. (2) Create adaptable, multiuse open spaces for community gathering, play, and social activity for all ages [62]. (3) Accommodate diverse uses (e.g., dog parks, skate parks, and picnic facilities) at easily accessible locations [62]. (4) Provide safe and well-lighted routes to parks. (5) Ensure parks and play spaces are in view of busy sidewalks or streets.

Street layouts have been studied extensively in relation to physical activity. It makes sense that grid layouts with frequent intersections are easier for walking than irregular layouts with frequent dead ends and cul-de-sacs, as there are more choices in getting from one place to another and distances tend to be shorter. There is enough evidence indicating that people walk more in neighborhoods with well-connected street layouts [63–66]. There is also, however, some evidence that people living in cul-de-sacs feel safer. By reducing traffic, cul-de-sacs provide safe spaces for children to play. Therefore, an ideal scenario would be grid layouts that include some low-depth cul-de-sacs, or crescents [67].

Among other things, the presence of sidewalks is consistently shown to be associated with physical activity in all pedestrian groups [68, 69]. This is particularly so for vulnerable groups such as children, adolescents, and older adults [68, 70]. There is also some evidence that the presence of street trees promotes active transport in both adults and adolescents, creating friendly and safer routes [41]. In cities with hotter climates, street trees that provide shade are particularly important to support being physically active.

Small-town design and planning professionals may want to consider the following strategies and policies for streets that promote population health benefits: (1) Provide well-connected street systems with more movement options [66, 71]. (2) Use sidewalks and bike lanes to promote walking and biking in all communities [72]. (3) Provide well-marked crosswalks, special pavers, and curb extensions to help pedestrians and slow traffic [73]. (4) Consider providing lights on streets, trails, and public spaces to minimize dark and unsafe areas [74, 75]. (5) Plant and preserve trees along streets to improve the experience of walking and biking.

Spatial Design and Planning for Health

Interest in shaping the interactions between the built environment and health using design interventions and policies is not new in the United States. In the 1920s, the first government policy was approved to regulate these interactions by separating different land uses (such as residential and commercial) to protect residents from infectious diseases caused by commercial pollution [76]. The last few decades, however, have seen a growing interest among health experts and policymakers in the built environment for health promotion [77–79].

As noted, a growing body of literature reports studies on both direct and indirect associations between the built environment and health, but only a few of these studies focus on rural areas and small towns. The studies reported in this book are interesting from a design intervention and policy perspective. They show that the associations between the built environment and health may not be limited to only urban areas, and that they may be found frequently in small towns and cities as well. The findings reported here show that city size may be associated with death rate, diabetes, overweight, and crimes; that the availability of key destinations and facilities may be associated with death rate, general health conditions, diabetes, overweight, obesity, crimes, and social isolation; that land use types and mix are associated with death rate, general health conditions, body mass index, overweight, and crime; and that street properties are associated with death rate, general health conditions, diabetes, overweight, obesity, people who have little interest in doing things, people feeling down, depressed, or hopeless, people having thoughts that they would be better off dead, murders, rapes, robberies, assaults, burglaries, and auto thefts.

Several of the associations between spatial factors and physical health problems in small Kansas cities can be partly attributed to lifestyle. Spatial strategies and policies that help improve lifestyle behaviors can therefore be considered for improving physical health in these cities. Similarly, several associations between spatial factors and mental health problems can also be partly attributed to physical inactivity and poor physical health, but declining social integration and support and increasing social isolation and loneliness can negatively affect mental health as well.

In general, social integration may promote positive social norms while simultaneously controlling antisocial behaviors that can fuel feelings of insecurity. Conversely, social stratification, in particular income inequality, is associated with higher all-cause mortality, higher infant mortality, and higher mortality from a variety of specific causes, independent of income and poverty [8, 9, 80–83]. Social support provided mainly by family, neighbors, friends, and church groups may help people cope with loneliness and depression in small towns and rural areas, particularly among rural elders. Meaningful social activities can reduce the harmful effects of stress by enhancing the body's immune response function.

Improving social integration, support, and activities through spatial design and planning, therefore, can be an effective way to fight against social isolation and its negative effects on mental health. Spatial design and planning professionals can help enhance social integration, support, and activities by encouraging higher than usual residential and land use density, improving accessibility within and across neighborhoods, and by locating parks, community services, and recreational facilities at easily accessible places, among many things. Well-connected and integrated communities are more empowered and can nurture a sense of place. This can encourage self-policing and discourage crime and deviant behavior. There is a strong link between social connection, health, and crime.

Many low-income and minority neighborhoods experience more crimes than do their counterparts due to a lack of social integration and cohesion. A lack of social integration and cohesion often breaks down social control, which can be observed in neighborhoods with missing lighting, broken windows, trash, graffiti, and other nuisances. These environmental cues are related to crime and safety issues. If residents do not perceive their environment to be safe for walking or other recreation activities, they are discouraged from using sidewalks, parks, or other amenities. Spatial design and planning professionals may want to consider Crime Prevention through Environmental Design (CPTED) strategies to maximize territorial control and defensible space, thereby reducing criminal opportunities and the fear of crime [84]. These strategies may include installing streetlights, addressing housing vacancies, enforcing development codes, minimizing isolated routes, and maximizing LUM.

In general, then, here are some policy recommendations to improve health in small towns and cities: (1) Use zoning ordinances to create communities where people live near their work; as a result, they will have more opportunities to spend time with each other. (2) Implement strategies to reduce physical inactivity that leads to overweight and obesity. (3) Implement strategies to reduce commute time, minimizing physical inactivity and saving time for social and recreational activities. (4) Use community development projects to encourage partnerships among different community stakeholders and to enhance social cohesion. (5) Provide provisions for incorporating public spaces, such as pocket parks, community gardens, and other open spaces, in land use plans to encourage social interaction and physical activity [85–87]. (6) Design spaces for maximum visibility and universal accessibility to allow people of all ages and abilities to safely participate in social activities [88]. (7) Create programs and events to enhance social interactions and to support other social goals related to health and well-being [89]. (8) Use CPTED principles and strategies to improve safety, reduce crime, improve trust among users, and increase social integration and cohesion.

Conclusions

Despite many limitations, the studies presented in this book found numerous spatial associations of lifestyle and health in small Kansas cities. Based on these findings and those reported in the existing literature, a range of spatial strategies are suggested in this chapter that small-town design and planning professionals may want to use for health promotion. In small towns and cities, these strategies include that streets, parks, and community spaces for public use are well connected, safe, and pleasant; that land use types and mix are appropriate to help existing places thrive; that local land use regulations support better access to and availability of key destinations and facilities within walking and biking distances; that local food spaces include healthy food for all; and that rural resources are protected because many communities value them as an inherent part of rural life.

Small-town spatial design and planning professionals, however, should not impose any spatial strategies for health promotion on a community. They should always consider the unique qualities of a place. It is not surprising that some communities would pursue revitalization efforts to attract growth to existing places and would provide incentives for building compact, walkable neighborhoods, whereas others would rewrite zoning ordinances and policies to limit and control development, and others still would make the connection between creating and rebuilding small rural cities and towns on the one hand and conserving working land and farms on the other.

Different spatial design and planning strategies can offer different opportunities and can help achieve different goals for a small-town community. When existing downtowns are revitalized, multiple community goals can be met, including promoting population health. Revitalized downtowns build on investments in infrastructure that communities have made in prior years, most often on a traditional, compact, interconnected street network that historically supported a range of transportation modes. They typically provide local residents and visitors with a range of conveniences like retail, civic, and employment opportunities all within easy walking distance. They also provide local residents access to local healthy food through farmers' markets and other convivial food spaces. Adjacent neighborhoods are often strengthened by these conveniences, again allowing residents to walk to work and shopping opportunities. Small cities and towns can also promote health by restricting unhealthy food outlets in walkable areas. The reuse of existing infrastructure, the revitalization of a downtown, and the increase in convenience and opportunities for local residents to participate in daily physical activity can help promote health.

Of course, new growth cannot always be accommodated in existing towns, so small communities need to have a regulatory structure that supports the creation of compact, walkable communities where residents have easy access to shops, schools, jobs, and amenities. These communities may also need to provide transportation options other than automobiles. Consequently, they should allow residents to walk to and from places as part of their daily lives and help reduce pollution resulting from car emissions. Without proper zoning ordinances and subdivision regulations, however, implementing any spatial design and planning strategies and policies promoting population health can be difficult in many small towns and cities.

Finally, farms, rangeland, forests, and grasslands are all part of what makes up rural America. Prioritizing the conservation of these places provides a number of beneficial outcomes and opportunities to rural communities, including regionally grown produce and other agriculture products, employment, recreational activity, and a diversified economy that builds on natural assets. However, how these approaches affect small towns remains an important question to ask. Preserving rural resources for recreational activities may bring in seasonal tourists to nearby small towns and cities, threatening local residents' ways of living. Preserving agricultural lands, in contrast, may preserve local residents' ways of life at the cost of more recent social innovations that promote population health.

As small-town design and planning professionals consider their options for health promotion, they should take note that unequal distribution of resources among different socioeconomic, sociodemographic, and sociocultural groups may underlie most health and social inequities. To reduce such inequities, they may need to identify areas where residents do not have equal access and stratify those areas further by socioeconomic, sociodemographic, and sociocultural characteristics. This type of analysis could help planners identify the disadvantaged areas that lack access, which could further help them prioritize their investment and design and planning strategies. They may want to align their work with local public officials for successful implementation. This could mean educating the local public officials on the population health benefits of different spatial design and planning strategies, approaches, and tools. It could also mean finding ways to measure the health benefits of walkable and well-connected streets, safe routes to school for children, and the availability of jobs, services, and retail opportunities in close proximity. However, it is never easy for small-town spatial design and planning professionals to meet their goals in a context that lacks a planning history, where planning offices never have enough people, and where populations are generally suspicious about their services and activities. We will discuss some of these difficulties and ways to overcome them in the next chapter.

NOTES

1. Wendel, "Social Capital and Health."
2. Folland, "Does 'Community Social Capital' Contribute to Population Health?"
3. Hofferth and Iceland, "Social Capital in Rural and Urban Communities."
4. Putnam, *Bowling Alone.*
5. Goodman et al., "New Walking and Cycling Routes."
6. Pucher, Dill, and Handy, "Infrastructure, Programs, and Policies."
7. New York City Department of Transportation, *Measuring the Street.*
8. Lynch et al., "Income Inequality and Mortality in Metropolitan Areas."
9. Lynch et al., "Income Inequality and Mortality."
10. Ewing and Cervero, "Travel and the Built Environment."
11. Giles-Corti et al., "City Planning and Population Health."
12. Hilmers, Hilmers, and Dave, "Neighborhood Disparities in Access."
13. Zenk et al., "Fruit and Vegetable Access Differs."
14. Seligman, Laraia, and Kushel, "Food Insecurity Is Associated with Chronic Disease."
15. Dixon and Ballantyne-Brodie, "The Role of Planning and Design."

16. Lovell, "Multifunctional Urban."
17. Castro, Samuels, and Harman, "Growing Healthy Kids."
18. Blanck et al., "Improving Fruit and Vegetable Consumption."
19. US Department of Agriculture, Natural Resources Conservation Service, *Community Garden Guide.*
20. National Policy and Legal Analysis Network to Prevent Childhood Obesity and ChangeLab Solutions, *Ground Rules.*
21. White, "Food Access and Obesity."
22. Macdonald, Ellaway, and Macintyre, "The Food Retail Environment and Area Deprivation."
23. Morland, Diez-Roux, and Wing, "Supermarkets, Other Food Stores, and Obesity."
24. Larson, Story, and Nelson, "Neighborhood Environments."
25. Larsen and Gilliland, "A Farmers' Market in a Food Desert."
26. Pitts et al., "Farmers' Market Use."
27. GrowNYC. "Green Market."
28. Kocken et al., "Promoting the Purchase of Low-Calorie Foods."
29. French, "Pricing Effects on Food Choices."
30. Liberato, Bailie, and Brimblecombe, "Nutrition Interventions."
31. Ballantyne-Brodie, Fassi, and Simone, *Coltivando.*
32. Dowler et al., " 'Doing Food Differently.' "
33. Committee on Physical Activity Health, Transportation and Land Use, Transportation Research Board, Institute of Medicine of the National Academies, *Does the Built Environment Influence Physical Activity?*
34. Brownson et al., "Measuring the Built Environment for Physical Activity."
35. Butler et al., "Identifying GIS Measures."
36. Sallis and Saelens, "Assessment of Physical Activity by Self-Report."
37. McCormack and Shiell, "In Search of Causality."
38. Doescher et al., "The Built Environment and Utilitarian Walking."
39. Van Holle et al., "Relationship between the Physical Environment and Different Domains of Physical Activity."
40. Hajna et al., "Associations between Neighbourhood Walkability and Daily Steps."
41. Sugiyama et al., "Destination and Route Attributes."
42. Ferdinand et al., "The Relationship between Built Environments and Physical Activity."
43. Yousefian et al., "Active Living for Rural Youth."
44. Boehmer et al., "What Constitutes an Obesogenic Environment in Rural Communities?"
45. Hennessy et al., "Active Living for Rural Children."
46. Umstattd et al., "Development of the Rural Active Living Perceived Environmental Support Scale."
47. Yousefian et al., "Development of the Rural Active Living Assessment Tools."
48. Sugiyama et al., "Associations of Neighbourhood Greenness."
49. Sugiyama and Thompson, "Associations between Characteristics of Neighbourhood Open Space."
50. Coutts et al., "County-Level Effects of Green Space Access."
51. De Vries et al., "Natural Environments—Healthy Environments?"
52. Giles-Corti et al., "The Influence of Urban Design and Planning on Physical Activity."
53. Croucher, Myers, and Bretherton, *The Links between Greenspace and Health.*
54. Pretty et al., "Green Exercise in the UK Countryside."
55. White et al., "Would You Be Happier Living in a Greener Urban Area?"

56. Hartig et al., "Tracking Restoration."
57. Kuo, "How Might Contact with Nature Promote Human Health?"
58. Crompton, "The Impact of Parks on Property Values."
59. Tinsley, Tinsley, and Croskeys, "Park Usage, Social Milieu, and Psychosocial Benefits."
60. Han, Cohen, and McKenzie, "Quantifying the Contribution of Neighborhood Parks."
61. Sturm and Cohen, "Proximity to Urban Parks and Mental Health."
62. Kaczynski, Potwarka, and Saelens, "Association of Park Size, Distance, and Features."
63. Leyden, "Social Capital and the Built Environment."
64. Sarkar, Gallacher, and Webster, "Urban Built Environment Configuration."
65. Sarkar, Webster, and Gallacher, *Healthy Cities.*
66. Berrigan, Pickle, and Dill, "Associations between Street Connectivity and Active Transportation."
67. Burton, "Mental Well-Being and the Influence of Place."
68. Kerr et al., "Active Commuting to School."
69. Titze et al., "Associations between Intrapersonal and Neighborhood Environmental Characteristics."
70. Burton et al., "The Relative Contributions of Psychological, Social, and Environmental Variables."
71. Sun, Oreskovic, and Lin, "How Do Changes to the Built Environment Influence Walking Behaviors?"
72. Kelly et al., "The Built Environment Predicts Observed Physical Activity."
73. Yannis, Kondyli, and Georgopoulou, "Investigation of the Impact of Low Cost Traffic Engineering Measures."
74. Sullivan and Flannagan, "Determining the Potential Safety Benefit of Improved Lighting."
75. Addy et al., "Associations of Perceived Social and Physical Environmental Supports."
76. US Supreme Court, *Village of Euclid, Ohio v. Ambler Reality Co.*
77. Ewing et al., "Relationship between Urban Sprawl and Physical Activity."
78. Saelens et al., "Neighborhood-Based Differences in Physical Activity."
79. Saelens, Sallis, and Frank, "Environmental Correlates of Walking and Cycling."
80. Kennedy, Kawachi, and Prothrow-Stith, "Income Distribution and Mortality."
81. Kaplan et al., "Income and Mortality in the United States."
82. Kaplan et al., "Inequality in Income and Mortality."
83. Kawachi et al., "Social Capital, Income Inequality, and Mortality."
84. Cozens, "Crime and Community Safety."
85. Ejlskov et al., "Individual Social Capital and Survival."
86. Fullilove, "Promoting Social Cohesion to Improve Health."
87. Mohnen et al., "Neighborhood Social Capital and Individual Health."
88. New York City Departments of Design and Construction, Health and Mental Hygiene, Transportation, and City Planning, *Active Design Guidelines.*
89. Centers for Disease Control and Prevention, *Strategies to Prevent Obesity and Other Chronic Diseases.*

CHAPTER THIRTEEN

Health Promotion in Small-Town America

Traditional and Participatory Approaches
and Some General Principles

Small-town America is experiencing many changes, including changes in population health. Poor lifestyle behaviors and poor physical, mental, and social health are common in small towns and cities across the country. Variability exists, but population health is going in the right direction in few of these places. In declining small towns and cities, population health is worsening because of failing economy, aging and decreasing population, and rising poverty. In some boomtowns with economic prosperity, population health is worsening due to social instability caused by newcomers—both young and old. In other boomtowns, it is worsening due to a lack of physical and institutional infrastructure needed to support an orderly growth. There is no one-size-fits-all design and planning approach to solving population health problems in small-town America.

As noted, the existing literature exploring the relationships between the built environment and population health in rural and small-town America is limited. In contrast, the literature exploring these relationships in urban areas is huge. Most of it provides unambiguous evidence supporting that the built environment can affect population and public health—a fact that has been intuitively known since the dawn of human civilization. Therefore, it is not surprising that the World Health Organization (WHO) European Healthy Cities Network, Phase V (2009–2013) identifies "healthy environment and design" as one of its three themes, stating that "a healthy city offers a physical and built environment that supports health, recreation and well-being, safety, social interaction, easy mobility, a sense of pride and cultural identity and that is accessible to the needs of all its citizens" [1, p. 5]. The other two themes of a healthy city are "caring and supportive environments" and "healthy living." Concerning caring and supportive environments, the network mentions that "a healthy city should be above all a city for all its citizens, inclusive, supportive, sensitive and responsive to their diverse needs and expectations" [1, p. 4]. Concerning healthy living, the network notes that "a healthy city provides conditions and opportunities that support healthy lifestyles" [1, p. 4]. Even though these themes were developed in relation to European cities, they appear equally pertinent to small American towns and cities.

Despite the importance given to healthy environment and design by the WHO and the importance of physical and built environments in the socio-ecology of health, one cannot assure positive changes in population health based only on strategies and policies aimed at changing spatial associations of lifestyle and health. For example, well-designed neighborhoods may not encourage walking if there are safety concerns. Easily accessible grocery stores may increase the frequency of trips to the store but may not increase the amount of spending on healthy foods if people are living in poverty.

Put simply, the sectoral view of traditional spatial design, planning, and research paradigms is rarely sufficient for population health promotion. This is not to say that these traditional paradigms are not required for health promotion. In fact, these paradigms must be considered essential for health promotion. If we do not build our cities with population health in mind, other promotional activities may not be enough to fix population health problems. For example, if we have sidewalks in a neighborhood but people are not walking, then we can put in place processes to change people's behaviors. If the neighborhood does not have sidewalks or if people are not able to get to places where they can walk, however, then other efforts to improve walking may not work.

In essence, small cities and towns require an intersectoral approach to health promotion, which is a collaborative approach among multiple governmental sectors and agencies, nongovernmental organizations, and relevant stakeholders and groups, with a common goal in addressing health issues. Consider the example of food environment described in the previous chapter. To make quality fresh and healthy food easily accessible and available to people in small cities, small-town designers and planners may ask a city to place supermarkets or conventional grocery stores at easily accessible locations to sell healthy and fresh food. The city would need more than a few easily accessible stores to improve food quality, availability, and accessibility, however. It would need statutory planning for food production and processing to ensure that these stores have access to fresh vegetables and foods at a reasonable cost; financial planning to pay for any infrastructure needed for the stores; retail planning to ensure a diversity of stores carrying enough good quality, healthy foods of different kinds; and cultural planning to create opportunities for healthy food practices. Upon further consideration, small-town designers and planners may question the necessity of supermarkets for health promotion in the city. They may instead find farmers' market to be a better solution for the problems related to the city's food environment. Establishing farmers' markets in the city may, however, require them to partner with local communities, which requires a shift from a traditional planning paradigm to a paradigm of intersectoral planning through community participation.

Taking an intersectoral approach to health promotion, the WHO has included four overarching action elements in its Healthy Cities projects. These include (1) action to address the determinants of health, equity in health, and the principles of health for all; (2) action to integrate and promote public health priorities; (3) action to put health on the social and political agenda of cities; and (4) action to promote good governance and integrated planning for health [1, p. 1]. Clearly, these actions involve more than what the traditional approaches to health services and planning can offer. They involve health services, planning and design, political and community activism, and much more. This chapter therefore considers the participatory design and planning approach alongside the traditional design and planning approach. It is hoped that together these two approaches will cover most of the action elements of health promotion included in the WHO's Healthy Cities projects.

The first part of this chapter discusses the traditional design and planning approach, where professionals guide the process of design and planning using institutionalized tools and techniques. The discussion covers various contextual complexities and constraints that professionals may face on a day-to-day basis as they consider spatial design and planning strategies and policies for health promotion in small-town America. These complexities and constraints may present serious challenges against any effective implementation of healthy spatial design and planning strategies and policies. This part of the chapter ends with a set of general principles for health promotion through spatial design and planning.

In contrast to the traditional spatial design and planning approach, there is no predefined approach to participatory design and planning for health promotion. It depends on people, place, politics, and purpose. Participatory design and planning strategies for improving physical activities in an urban community may not be useful for improving the same in a rural community; strategies and policies for improving physical activities may not be useful for improving access to healthy food in a community. Likewise, different communities may find similar approaches useful for promoting population health, but they may not have access to similar resources or may not have similar political environments to implement the strategies. The second part of the chapter, therefore, discusses some of these characteristics of the participatory design and planning approach, including its limitations, advantages, and status in small-town and rural communities. Based on the discussions, this part ends with a set of general principles for health promotion through participatory design and planning.

Traditional Spatial Design and Planning for Health Promotion in Small-Town America

Though spatial design and planning professionals have many opportunities to impact population health in small-town America, they also face many challenges. Their challenges include a lack of appreciation and support for spatial design and planning services; a lack of appropriately defined spatial design and planning provisions and approaches; and a lack of implementation tools and capacity. Along with these problems, small-town design and planning professionals must address many other areas of concern that urban design and planning professionals do not generally consider. For example, in big cities, natural resources have become so rare that they are rarely a basic concern for urban design and planning professionals, and small-town design and planning professionals rarely consider public transportation as an important issue like urban designers and planners do because a lack of demand generally makes public transportation ineffective in these places. This does not imply, however, that natural resources are not important for urban areas. Neither does this imply that small towns do not need public transportation. It simply means that spatial design and planning professionals must carefully consider these and other concerns to ensure that people receive the benefits of these amenities when and where they are appropriate and available.

Contexts

The work of small-town design and planning professionals is different from that of urban design and planning professionals. The nature and scale of their problems, the solutions for their problems, and the available resources to get their job done are generally different. Most importantly, small-town residents often have different attitudes toward land, institutions, and traditions, which receive too little attention in the spatial design and planning literature. In urban or suburban areas, very few people question the work of spatial design and planning professionals. They simply assume that the work of these professionals is important. But in many small towns and cities, the opposite is true. Small-town residents often question the importance of spatial design and planning professionals and do not automatically assume that the activities of these professionals are worthwhile. Small towns and cities often have no planning history, no planning bureaucracy, and no tradition and culture of planning. The burden of proof is on the professionals engaged in spatial design and planning activities to show that their products and services are important not only for economic prosperity but also for protecting the health, safety, and well-being of a population. Every spatial design and planning process, service, or product must be justified in small towns and cities [2].

It is not easy to justify spatial design and planning activities in terms of economy, health, safety, and well-being in small towns and cities. The language of the professionals engaged in these activities is often an obstacle for ordinary residents. Different planning processes, provisions, and tools leave them confused. Yet the processes of spatial design and planning in rural and small-town communities can work only when people are able to see that these processes and their outcomes are serving their own best interests—protecting their property rights, protecting their governmental services, protecting them from tax increases, and above all, giving them more control over their own lives. Small-town design and planning professionals therefore must be politically astute. They must be responsive to the needs of the people they serve. They must innovate, improvise, and rely on common sense. They must be able to do their jobs in a professional void with minimal resources. Such individuals will be spending virtually all their time working with local people. Put simply, individuals engaged in spatial design and planning activities in small towns and cities should have the ability to work with people, something that is not given much attention in urban-oriented traditional spatial design and planning education.

This, then, is the context of small-town design and planning professionals. In this context, the questions of population health would be raised rarely, if at all. These professionals would proactively bring any population health issues to the table for discussions and actions. They must muster public support, find spatial design and planning solutions for these issues on their own or with minimal support from others, and find resources for implementing these solutions. In all this, small-town design and planning professionals must be patient because any return on investment for spatial design and planning strategies and policies in terms of population health will take time.

Legal and Other Planning Provisions

While it is a fact that many US states have no law mandating local planning, each state does have the enabling legislation, which permits local units (counties, cities, and townships) to adopt plans and land use regulations for health, safety, and well-being. Yet due to a lack of resources, many small towns and cities may not adopt any plans or land use regulations at all [2]. In small towns and cities, a lack of appreciation for spatial design and planning is often accompanied by a lack of legal spatial design and planning provisions.

Regional councils are active in many states, however, providing coverage on spatial design and planning issues. Some are involved in grant assistance only, while others are involved in both grants and local technical assistance. Many have prepared local plans and land use regulations. Others have prepared model plans and regulations. These councils often have an excellent grasp of local issues and a good relationship with local elected officials. They are extremely important sources of information and assistance to county or small-town design and planning professionals.

In most states, the critical spatial design and planning work occurs at the county level because most small cities and townships in rural areas cannot support continuous design and planning activities. While county budgets are thin, they are generally larger than city and township budgets. Thus, professionals, if they are not working for a regional council, would most likely be working for a county in rural areas. Counties generally establish planning commissions for comprehensive plans. They also require a zoning ordinance to be in conformance with a comprehensive plan. In several cases, land use and subdivision regulations also exist, but these generally do not cover issues, restrictions, and regulations important for small towns and cities [2].

Counties in many states, however, have special district provisions supporting design and planning work that may help small towns and cities. They provide a variety of public services, including those related to soil conservation, water management, sanitary improvement, parks and recreation, streets, lighting, libraries, and so on, which could all potentially affect population health. Many states have an extraterritoriality jurisdiction act and an interlocal cooperation act. In an extraterritoriality act, cities with zoning ordinances are allowed to exercise zoning authority over areas outside of their city limits. Depending on the size of the city, this can run from one to several miles. An inter-local cooperation act permits cities, counties, and special districts to jointly perform a variety of services. This law would permit, for example, several counties to jointly do planning work. But in practice, the law has meant that a single county might join with several of its towns and villages to establish one planning commission and one zoning administrator for the county area [2], supporting, among other things, small-town design and planning services and activities in communities that otherwise cannot afford them.

Small-town design and planning professionals should know all the legal provisions and technical assistance available to do their job well, since no one else may know these things. Knowing these provisions may help them navigate the complex terrain of designing and planning for population health in these places, where such activities are rarely an economic priority. They may need technical support from a regional council in the process of planning, negotiations, and implementations. They may also need help from a regional council to write a grant for funding a local improvement project. Additionally, they may need to make use of an inter-local cooperation act for cities, counties, and special districts to jointly provide a variety of services, such as public transportation, to influence population health, particularly among deprived populations.

Approaches

There is no textbook approach for spatial design and planning professionals to follow in small towns and cities when planning for future development. Any approach they consider can become uncertain when they have population health priorities along with other traditional goals. Some communities would want a traditional master plan, with every opportunity carefully considered; others would be more satisfied with a "policy plan"—a relatively short statement of community goals and objectives against which any future development proposals can be measured [3]. It is important, however, that spatial design and planning professionals do not impose any standard approach on a community that does not want or need it.

Found under a variety of names—the general plan, development plan, or comprehensive plan—the master plan is characterized by a more thorough consideration of all major functions of the planning area than the policy plan and by its presentation of a "best" physical arrangement for future development. Many small communities may not prefer a master plan due to its rigidity. For the same reason, other small communities may still prefer a more traditional master plan. In contrast, general principles rather than specific proposals are the heart of a policy plan. The delineation of goals and objectives is considered a sufficient guide to future development activities in a policy plan. Although a policy plan has the advantage of flexibility, without careful follow-up it may become so general that it ends up as nothing [3].

Issues that must be considered in preparing any plan may vary depending on the needs of a small town or city. Some small towns and cities experiencing a surge of development will face a demand for roads, schools, housing, health care facilities, fire, and police, which the tax base may not be able to support for a few years. If these problems are recognized in advance of development, potential negative health, safety, and welfare impacts may be mitigated by using a plan.

Some small towns and cities with declining employment and consequent population loss may need economic development programs, which concentrate on non-farm employment. The pros and cons of recreational developments or second homes to attract tourism or the possibility of seeking out new institutions, such as a community college or a new manufacturing or processing plant, to locate in the area can be a part of an overall planning program. Small towns and cities with declining employment and population loss may also observe a rise in elderly or low-income population. Special services may be required for these population groups. The possibility of regional cooperation between adjacent municipalities or counties and the pooling of financial resources and services may be sought as a matter of planning.

Under development pressures, some small towns and cities struggle to preserve their character and ways of living. In some cases, this goal may be seen to conflict with the goal of attracting new economic development programs. Careful design of implementation tools, such as special zoning districts, performance controls, phased capital improvements programs, or special tax structures, may make it possible for a community to accommodate both goals while promoting population health.

Whether the community chooses to prepare a master plan, a policy plan, or a combination of both may depend on available resources, as well as on the preferences of people involved in the process. Most likely, a plan prepared for small towns and cities should have degrees of flexibility and comprehensiveness. It would be naive to assume that a simple list of design and planning goals and objectives will magically emerge. In the end, what is finally agreed on as the most pressing problems or most desirable goals and objectives may only represent a compromise among a group of individuals with diverse backgrounds and interests. It is for this reason that goals, plans, and implementation tools must be continually examined and reevaluated [3]. Small-town design and planning professionals, however, should try to make certain that the community commits itself explicitly to the population health goals of its planning framework before considering implementation techniques if these goals are important.

Implementation Techniques

Once the community's policies and plans have been decided, small-town design and planning professionals must consider implementation tools to use. The most common tools are land use regulations, capital improvement programs, and special funding programs. Still, many of these may not be available in small towns and cities. With only a one- or two-person staff, if any, a small town may have a hard time implementing any plan without seeking county or outside help.

Where and when available, land use regulations may take several forms. Though zoning and subdivision ordinances and building codes are more common, permitting procedures, public review processes, and other flexible procedures are also used [4]. The town may need legal assistance if it is preparing new ordinances. Again, the available planning resources in the county or city government office would be important to consider in this regard.

The capital improvement program (CIP) can be significant in implementing a community plan. CIP is a schedule of major nonrecurring public expenditures for physical facilities, usually prepared for a six-year period along with an estimate of costs and sources of revenues [3, 4]. CIP is increasingly used by cities and counties as an extension of city plans and as a fiscal tool. The impact of CIP must be carefully considered in terms of population health consequences. A decision to spend public funds to extend sewer and water lines or to develop or improve roads, for example, almost inevitably will lead to increased development activities in areas adjacent to these services and facilities. Likewise, the location of key capital facilities should be carefully considered to ensure that development occurs not only where and when the community wants it but also where and when the community gets the most health benefits. Too often, haphazard provision of facilities encourages development in a pattern that may be expensive and harmful for the community. Water lines that were intended to assist the farmer, for example, may result instead in breaking up farms for subdivisions without any regard for agricultural resources or environmental health.

Finally, new sources of funds may have to be sought to help implement any spatial design and planning programs promoting health and well-being. Small-town design and planning professionals will therefore have to be acquainted with the tax structure and the possibilities of local tax adjustment, the legality and acceptability of local development fees, and the intricacies of applying for outside grants. None of these activities by local governments can stand alone, and any wide use of planning and land use controls will depend heavily on local leadership and resources. People will have to take the time to learn about the tools available to manage their community's resources. In this regard, the two most widely used planning and land use control tools are zoning and subdivision regulations. The relevance of these tools to small-town design and planning is questionable, however.

IS THERE A NEED FOR ZONING IN SMALL TOWNS AND CITIES?

A zoning ordinance is generally made up of two parts: (1) a map showing the location and boundaries of each zoning district, and (2) an accompanying text that specifies the zoning requirements. The basic aim of zoning is to segregate incompatible uses. This is both the strength and weakness of zoning. By designating specific areas for different uses, zoning provides one of the easiest forms of regulations to administer. Zoning specifies what residents can or cannot do with their land. Likewise, it gives the best protection to current land uses. However, for small communities with large amounts of undeveloped land, which is often the case for small cities and towns, zoning may block off too many options if not done with care. To avoid the problem, a small town may want to draw zoning districts for some of its land and leave the rest in a more general category. As the community grows and land use patterns become better established, the ordinance can be amended to reflect the state of current land use patterns and trends.

In addition to zoning districts, zoning ordinances also include dimensional requirements and other standards, such as the height of buildings in feet and/or stories; the minimum size of front, side, and rear yards; minimum lot width; minimum lot size; and requirements for water and sewer. These requirements could have significant population health impacts. For example, in areas without public sewer systems, the minimum lot size may be set as whatever is required to obtain approval for a septic tank. In contrast, in areas with sewers, the minimum lot size can be used to set the overall eventual pattern and density of development, with significant effects on public facility and service costs. In agricultural areas, it can be used to discourage development.

Originally, the intent of zoning requirements was only to ensure adequate light, air, and protection from fire hazards. Today, zoning requirements have been expanded to include such purposes as preserving interesting street faces, preventing buildings from blocking sight lines at intersections, and keeping potentially noxious uses at significant distances from adjoining property. An opportunity exists for small-town design and planning professionals to use zoning ordinances for population health benefits.

Zoning can be useful in small towns and cities because people do not have to worry about incompatible land uses. When zoning is in place, small-town residents do not have to worry whether a fast food restaurant might be built next door or a mobile home parked on a lot across the street. The difficulty for spatial design and planning professionals in sparsely populated areas, however, is that most people will be indifferent to zoning, and everyone will probably have misconceptions about it [5]. For most, zoning may not solve any perceived problems. Unless the town or rural area is experiencing development pressures, land use is probably not a major problem. In small towns and cities, the amount of development is small anyway, and most people develop their land in the same way as their neighbors have. Sometimes low density helps, and distance serves as a buffer. Conflicts are few and generally can be handled ad hoc. Zoning may seem somewhat overkill in such a context. Using bits and pieces from traditional land use controls to tackle specific problems is common. Many places have a floodplain ordinance or a wetland ordinance or a mobile home ordinance without having established formal zoning. When necessary, these ordinances can be instrumental in convincing the local population that land use controls have their place in small towns and cities. It is typical for a small town or rural area to begin with a junk car ordinance, move on to a mobile home ordinance, and end up with a comprehensive plan and zoning ordinance [5].

As in other cities, in small towns and cities the basic reason for land controls through zoning ordinances must be to protect individual and community interests related to economy, health, safety, and welfare. In a town, the land may be changing ownership. The risks are different if land transfers are internal to the current population or to outsiders—corporate farmers, second-home buyers, or others—who may not use the land in ways the community is used to. There may also be risks of quick, dramatic change with significant population health consequences. Having a poultry farm or a meat processing plant next to a town may provide employment opportunities, but it may also put population health at risk. If natural resources, such as gas or coal, become available for extraction, a quiet town may suddenly become a boomtown. It is easier for people to complain about their current problems than to figure out what they want for their community in the next five, ten, or twenty years. Small-town design and planning professionals can give advice about the future: what the probabilities are of things going wrong in terms of health, economy, and environment because of an economic development decision, and what can be done now to reduce these probabilities. If the risks of future changes are substantial, it may be important to convince the local government and residents that zoning is necessary, even if disliked.

In many cases where comprehensive zoning ordinances are absent, spatial design and planning professionals will need to develop land use control systems that are more compatible with the needs of a small town or city. Most of these systems fall under the rubric of "development permit systems." Different from traditional zoning, these systems lack land use districts defining residential, commercial, industrial, and other uses. Instead, development permit systems set up standards by which each development is reviewed, and acceptance or denial of a development is based on whether the proposed project meets these standards. In practice, the systems operate like a hybrid of subdivision and zoning. The standards generally include considerations for streets, sanitation, water, storm drainage, and utilities, much like subdivision ordinances, and for compatibility with surrounding uses, much like zoning [5].

IS THERE A NEED FOR SUBDIVISION REGULATIONS IN SMALL TOWNS AND CITIES?

Subdivision regulations specify responsibilities, requirements, and standards for subdivisions. In principle, any division of land into two or more separate parcels, no matter how large, might be considered a subdivision. In practice, not all divisions are subject to subdivision regulations. Those divisions that do not significantly affect the overall plan of the area, or do not require public improvements or the creation of new roads, are often exempt from regulations [6]. Concerning population health, subdivision regulations assure that necessary public facilities are provided, that the quality of the improvements is adequate, that the public is protected against hazards resulting from natural and manmade forces, and that the layout is safe and serviceable as per a community's expectations.

Requirements and Standards for Improvement. Improvement requirements and standards are central issues in subdivision regulations. This is true for small towns and cities, as it is for urban areas. Subdivision improvements can be divided into "basic" and "optional" ones [6]. The basic ones involving streets, sanitation, water, storm drainage, utilities, survey monuments, and reservations are generally required of subdivision developers. Optional ones, including parks, sidewalks, and streetlights, may be necessary or desired in some communities but not others. For example, sidewalks and streetlights may be necessary for safety in a high-density subdivision but not in a low-density one. Optional design requirements cannot be fully specified in subdivision regulations since subdivisions vary. Yet at the discretion of the planning board, these requirements often provide more opportunity for negotiation with subdivision developers. In the absence of a planning board, small-town design and planning professionals generally work with the city government to determine basic and optional requirements for subdivision improvement.

Streets improved to adequate width and standards for expected functions and loads are essential for population health, safety, and welfare and should be required at the expense of the developer. Streets should generally be dedicated to the locality. Width of streets, right-of-way, and paving and curving requirements in various situations should all be specified in regulations. Lengths of blocks, numbers of lots per block, shapes and proportions of lots, and related matters may be included in subdivision regulations as optional requirements to ensure that lots are suitable for building purposes and that they minimize streets and utilities. Sidewalks and bikeways are generally discussed as optional improvements as well since they may not be necessary in low-density rural communities. When included, they should be considered in relation to vehicular traffic and should connect appropriate destinations. Standards for these requirements should be established by the locality in response to local needs and conditions if population health is a concern, and they should not be simply adopted from elsewhere, such as model subdivision regulations or state highway standards.

Both sewer and water systems are often handled by reference to applicable county and state health requirements; and those requirements are generally controlling unless the subdivision standards require more. All such provisions should require approval of health authorities and local consulting engineers, and standards in subdivision regulations should include which types, locations, and densities of subdivisions might be required to have public or community systems rather than individual facilities.

Subdivision regulations related to stormwater management are meant to prevent flooding of lots within the subdivision, to avoid water load in down-hill or downstream areas by keeping both stormwater on-site and runoff to what they were before development, and to prevent water pollution resulting from runoff from the subdivision. All drainage and related grading plans should be certified by an engineer, subject to review by the local engineer and soil conservation service.

It is increasingly prevalent to require electric lines, telephone cables, and cable TV to be installed underground in a subdivision for safety, aesthetic, and maintenance advantages, as well as reduction in service interruptions due to storms. This requirement will generally not apply below a certain density for cost reasons, but cost questions need to be explored locally with the utility company to determine a cutoff point. For technical and safety reasons, power lines above a certain level of voltage cannot be buried.

As a matter of standard, public or semipublic parks and open spaces are required in subdivisions above a minimal density. Reasonable requirements for lot size and fees can be stipulated in case developers are not willing to provide parks and open spaces within a subdivision. In small towns and low-density areas, however, it may be more advantageous to provide larger community parks for recreational and health benefits, which are not treated by dedication requirements, but can be reserved and purchased later. In small boomtowns, it is important to provide open spaces within newly developing areas since open space will become rare as more development occurs.

An Assessment of Subdivision Regulations for Small Towns and Cities. In small towns and cities, subdivision regulations are often more important than zoning [6]. Zoning determines the uses to which parcels can be put, as well as the size of parcels and hence density. In many small towns and cities, however, there is little public concern as to whether parcels are used for recreation, housing, or commerce. As noted previously, many may not even have zoning provisions. Instead, the concern is that subdivisions include adequate roads and fire access, utilities, and sanitary conditions to ensure health, safety, and welfare. The community is concerned that any lots sold should be able to be built on and that steep slopes and floodplains should be protected from development because of hazards that may result.

Regardless of due care, some subdivisions will create public problems, for example, in providing fire protection, school bus service, road maintenance, and sewer and water or other sanitation in small towns and cities. Some will create a hazard due to mistreatment of the natural environment such as flood-plains, slopes, wetlands, and water recharge areas. Others will affect land ownership patterns in such a way that future use of the land, according to reasonable community plans, is threatened. Divisions of land that are not likely to create such problems are often exempt from subdivision regulations. For other land divisions, subdivision review provides the city or the town an opportunity to negotiate with the developer of a subdivision. Even though it is desirable that local standards and policies are clear, subdivision review is a design process providing room for differences of opinion and negotiations, which can be used for population health benefits.

Other Areas of Concerns

Besides contexts, provisions, approaches, and implementation techniques, there are many other areas of spatial design and planning concerns in small towns and cities. Concerns most relevant to population health are natural resources, public transportation, and community services.

NATURAL RESOURCES

Natural resources are an important part of spatial design and planning in rural areas and in small towns and cities. Yet they are frequently overlooked by professionals trained to deal with urban situations where natural resources have long since disappeared. Subdivision regulations in small towns and cities often include design requirements for natural resources. The significance of natural resources is rarely limited to subdivisions, however. Spatial design and planning based on natural resources is motivated not only by the desire to conserve and protect desirable natural features (although this is an important point) but also to determine the optimum location of development and save the community from problems related to environment, health, and safety in the future [7]. Once the natural characteristics of the land are mapped and classified, a clear pattern of development that constrains or permits future growth often becomes apparent. Natural resources that have the most important effects on health as well as future development are topography, soil, and water.

Topography. Topography can determine land use by elevation and slope. Historically, development progressed through lowlands, into valleys, and around hills and mountains. Although this general pattern remains true, today there are far fewer restrictions on developing steep slopes and other areas once considered inaccessible or undesirable. For this reason, the shape of the terrain must be known if land use is to be properly planned. Care must also be exercised when tampering with the harmony of slope, soil, vegetation, drainage patterns, and geological foundation because such tampering may harm human health, safety, and welfare. The removal of vegetation during site development increases runoff that would ordinarily be retained and transpired by trees and other vegetation. The detrimental effects of site disturbance are increased by the addition of impervious surfaces, such as paving and buildings, further reducing groundwater percolation, thus adding to the amount of runoff, destruction of water quality, and potential for flooding, creating population health problems. Disturbance of sites can destroy a community's aesthetic resources and reduce the psychological benefits of natural beauty. A range of hills frequently marks a community's boundary and provides an attractive scenic setting for homes and buildings. Degradation of hillsides, because of erosion and loss of vegetation, deprives a community of its attractive and distinct setting and decreases real estate values. In essence, site development can have a far-reaching impact on a region's population health by affecting land, water, economic, and scenic resources of the region.

Water and Related Resources. Water and related resources are found as lakes, rivers, estuaries, streams, and creeks; flood lands and wetlands; aquifers; and so on. They contribute to a region's total water resource and affect general environmental and population health and well-being. In regions where agriculture is a major land use, water availability and quality are as important as soil. Surface waters are generally valuable as a source of water supply, food, and recreation. They are also important for waste dispersion, transportation, and power generation. Therefore, the planning of development within a region must expand beyond the watercourses themselves and look to the whole concept of the watershed system. The desired degree of control should vary for the type of area where development would affect water resources.

Flood lands are the land area adjacent to a body of water, which is covered by excess water during periods of flooding. Flood lands may be divided into zones based on the frequency of inundation, often categorized as channels, floodways, and floodplains. It is especially important to make these distinctions for land use and development controls because building on flood lands endangers human life and property. Filling, damming, or leveling floodplains decreases storage capacity and increases flood velocity and downstream flood potential. Agriculture is often an ideal use in floodplains as the soils are very fertile, there is usually substantial groundwater, and the effect on flat land is minimal.

Wetlands are tracts of low-lying lands that are saturated with moisture and usually overgrown with vegetation. Wetlands absorb excess runoff and thus reduce flooding potential. They provide important wildlife habitats and often have scenic beauty. Wetlands generally possess recreational, educational, scientific, or agricultural value. Protecting these wetlands may help save human lives and the environment.

Subsurface waters in the form of aquifers—water-bearing layers of sand, gravel, or porous rock—are as important and delicate as surface waters. As a major source of water supply for human use, their quality must be maintained and the removal of water from them must not exceed the rate of replenishment. Because aquifers serve as a reservoir, a filter, and part of the hydrological cycle, they are important regional resources and are particularly sensitive in terms of development. It is best to avoid development over deep aquifers to minimize harmful effects on population and environmental health.

Soil. Soil composition directly affects building and highway construction, septic systems, water availability, and agriculture; therefore, it is relevant to both population and environmental health. Since everything that touches soil is affected by it, it is essential that accurate soil data be used in land use planning. A soil suitability study should be used to assess (1) the engineering property of soils in order to determine the appropriate pattern of residential, commercial, industrial, agricultural, and recreational use; (2) the suitability of soils for sewage dispersion, drainage systems, and water storage; (3) the soil and plant relationship so that prime agricultural areas can be identified; and (4) the location of important mineral deposits [7].

Vegetation and Wildlife (Biotic Resources). Too often, if vegetation and wildlife are considered at all in land use planning, it is only in terms of parks and other open spaces for recreation [4, 7]. Little thought is given to the ecologically delicate relationship among plants, animals, and humans. Since uncontrolled development and the subsequent loss of groundcover can often have serious consequences, it is important that spatial designers and planners should have at least a working acquaintance with ecology and should gather as much information as possible about areas in their region sensitive to development.

Development should be watched in woodlands especially since they play an important role in the protection of watersheds. Aside from aesthetic pleasures, trees, shrubs, and other vegetation also prevent erosion by binding the soil together with their roots. In addition, as water percolates downward, plant life aids in its cleansing.

Unique vegetation habitats should be preserved for the benefits of a community. Virgin forest, unbroken prairie, and other features support complex animal communities that are intrinsically important. The tolerance of these areas to intensive nearby development varies but must be taken into consideration in any event for the long-term benefits of a community.

PUBLIC TRANSPORTATION

Transportation Trends in Small-Town America. Transportation problems of small towns and cities in rural areas are not restricted to people living in poverty or with disabilities or people over the age of 65 [8–11]. With increasing poverty, out-of-town job opportunities, and automobile-operating expenses, more and more rural and small-town residents are facing serious transportation problems. If current trends continue, transportation problems will worsen, and many small-town and rural residents will become transportation disadvantaged, regardless of mobility being essential for small-town and rural residents. Many such residents are dependent on non-farm activities for their income and often must commute to distant employment centers. Besides commuting, they may need mobility for shopping, education, health care, recreation, and all other matters related to everyday life that are rarely available locally [8, 12, 13].

A need for flexible and affordable transportation options has been present in small towns and rural areas for several decades now. Recent deregulations have heightened the need. Unable to take advantage of economies of scale, regional rail and bus systems have abandoned many remote areas [10, 14]. Transportation infrastructure has improved during the last few decades, but the problems of deteriorated road surfaces, narrow and unsound bridges, unprotected railroad crossings, inadequate lane widths, and a lack of emergency medical care transportation still remain [8, 15]. In general, small towns and cities in rural areas have many transportation problems—each with potentials to, directly or indirectly, affect population health. Some are more pressing than are others. Some can be solved locally, while others would require external support. But most of these problems cannot be solved by spatial design and planning professionals working independently.

Small-Town Transportation Characteristics. In general, there is a primacy of personal automobile use in small towns and rural areas. Most trips in these areas are made by automobile, and public transit typically does not exist or is constrained to limited routes, schedules, and old equipment [8, 14]. Even though a very high percentage of families in rural areas and small towns have access to an automobile, many households still may not own an automobile [8]. Still other households may indicate automobile ownership when they own inoperable automobiles. Some, who indicate having a means of transportation, may need to obtain rides from friends or relatives at a high cost. Even in a household with a functioning vehicle, some family members may remain stranded when others in the household use the vehicle [11, 12].

From a population health perspective, a lack of transportation raises serious problems [11]. A very large percent of households with a head 65 or older do not have a vehicle in nonmetropolitan areas. Small-town and rural residents make more and longer auto trips than urban residents. People in unincorporated areas and incorporated small towns (between 5,000 and 24,999 people) often make the most trips per day of all Americans. Many small-town residents in rural areas must own cars at the expense of other basic needs. There is little carpooling in these areas. Overt efforts to increase carpooling have not been very successful. The aversion to carpooling seems to be greater in towns under 25,000 in population, perhaps because to serve the same number of people drivers take more trips in these places than they do in urban areas; and the destinations are widely scattered. It is a myth that small-town people help one another with rides [15].

In general, the private automobile is likely to remain the dominant transportation mode in small towns and rural areas for the same reasons it will remain so in larger urban areas: it is the most convenient and fastest mode. It becomes the least expensive mode if the value of one's time is considered as a cost when comparing alternative ways to travel. It has been argued that public transit in small towns and rural areas could be both fruitless and wasteful because people will continue to rely on cars [16]. Even in the face of higher energy costs, it will be more economical to operate cars in small towns and rural areas. The only people opting for public transit when it is available will be those with physical and income limitations. It may be true that the number people without cars increases as urban areas get bigger, but bigger urban areas also have public transit systems that most nonmetropolitan areas do not have.

Public Transit in Small Towns. Public transit does not exist in many small towns and cities. Where it does, it carries a much smaller percentage of total trips than public transit services in larger cities [14]. It may be limited in frequency and coverage, may not serve outlying areas, and may not provide evening or weekend service. Taxi service may not exist, and persons without phones may have difficulty sharing rides in these small towns and cities. In recent years, the rise in the numbers of mobile phone users and the availability of ride-hailing services have affected transportation in many cities but probably not in economically deprived small cities and towns [17].

It may not be convenient for car users in small towns and rural areas to give up their cars in favor of public transit. Nonetheless, there remains a need for public transit. Unfortunately, very few small towns have public transit systems because of low demand and high operating costs. Intercity bus service is more common, particularly in small cities that are fortunate enough to be located along intercity bus routes. Buses have been able to provide the service for lower rates than other modes because they use the existing road network and obtain a low cost-per-seat mile by adapting to the demand characteristics of small towns and rural areas. But by being able to respond quickly to demand, particularly decreasing demand, bus systems have been able to cut back and eliminate service in areas with low demand. Although some cities have taken over failing private bus systems, the smaller the city, the less likely the ability to do so. Rail and air passenger services to small towns in rural areas are almost nonexistent [14]. Yet many people, particularly those over 65, in these areas need to get from one town to another to obtain specialized services like health care that they cannot obtain in their own town.

Alternatives for Public Transit. If both a need and demand for public transportation exist, the question arises as to what type of system should be provided. The answer depends, of course, on the population to be served, the population density, the distribution of trip-generating activities, financing, and other related factors. The fixed-route system—the type of system found in larger cities—is used when potential riders are located along major routes and the demand and density are such that buses can pass fixed pickup points at regular intervals. This system works well in high-density areas and when people are traveling to many activity centers. It does not work well for physically handicapped persons or in areas where distances make it difficult for persons to walk to pickup points.

Many communities have adopted paratransit—the use of bus-like vehicles, often run by nontraditional transit operators, and usually providing demand-responsive service—as an alternative. A demand-responsive system is routed in response to the requests of users. Typically involving minibuses or vans, door-to-door service is provided to persons who call for a ride. Usually, the calls are received in advance at a central location and routes are established so that passengers are picked up as others are being taken to their destinations.

Demand-responsive systems have the advantage of greater flexibility in destinations, door-to-door service, elimination of the need to transfer, and ability to more easily serve physically handicapped persons. Demand-responsive systems can be less reliable, however, since travel times can be affected by such things as the demand on the system, variation in routing, and delays in waiting for passengers.

Whenever possible, spatial design and planning for small-town and rural transit service ideally should take place as part of a comprehensive planning process since transportation needs are closely related to other factors, including population density, land use patterns, and economic activities. A focus on transit, however, should not imply that small towns in rural areas have no other transportation problems. On the contrary, many towns could benefit from several other things, including a redesign of the major street system, construction of railroad grade separations, improved signalization and channelization, resurfacing, and bridge replacement. These needs should be identified through the general planning process, and assistance should be obtained from relevant agencies.

PUBLIC SERVICES

Relative to urban residents, small-town and rural residents have less access to health care services because of geographic isolation and transportation barriers [18]. Environmental conditions, such as inadequate waste treatment and chemicals from field runoff, significantly affect the health of small-town and rural residents [19]. Access to education needs attention in small towns and cities. No matter how testing or evaluation is done, the academic performance is worse for rural and small-town children than urban children. Fewer school-aged children are enrolled in school in rural areas and small towns than urban areas. Rural and small-town adults generally have less schooling than urban adults [20]. Overall, public services in small towns in rural areas are fragmented, uncoordinated, and fraught with problems [21]. They are affected by the absence of population concentrations that permit specialization [22].

The demand for public services generally increases as small towns and cities grow. The demand comes in part from new residents who bring with them expectations of higher service levels. They move to small towns for their amenities, but they eventually begin to desire some of the urban services they had used in larger urban areas where they lived previously. The increased demand also comes from long-term residents with better access to information.

The complexity and variability of public service needs in small-town America make small-town design and planning difficult.

Small-town design and planning professionals may therefore become involved in the development of a wide variety of public services, though the actual delivery of these services may be done by another organization. These professionals may be involved in estimating the demand, determining the cost, locating funding sources, and undertaking construction activities related to these services. Although the development of some physical facilities and services such as roads, water, and sewer have been generally agreed on, this is not the case with services such as health care, education, law enforcement, and recreation. For these types of services, opinions may vary considerably as to what constitutes an adequate level of service and whether existing services are enough for the community. In these and many other cases, design and planning professionals will need to work with communities. The second part of this chapter describes these processes.

General Principles for Health Promotion through Traditional Design and Planning

In small towns and cities of rural America, where the need for sensible spatial design and planning strategies and policies for health promotion is great, nothing seems to work in favor of spatial design and planning professionals. Often, they would work in an intellectual and a professional vacuum and would lack the most basic political, economic, and social resources to do their job well. Lonely, they would pursue their goals to promote and protect the health, safety, and well-being of a population. All too frequently, they will need to overlook long-term population health benefits in favor of more immediate technical, economic, social, and political priorities. The result of their failures can be seen in the impoverished built environments of many small towns and cities around the country, where convenience, equity, effectiveness, and aesthetics are absent, in addition to health, safety, and well-being. It is not easy for small-town design and planning professionals to overcome this predicament. In this regard, it may be helpful for them to consider the following general principles.

TAKE A SOCIO-ECOLOGICAL VIEW OF HEALTHY PLACEMAKING

Human experiences shaping health are complex. For example, one's racial experience cannot be separated from one's experiences of economic and food deprivation, homelessness, and loneliness when these social stressors are present. The combined experiences of these stressors often produce numerous negative health effects. These effects vary from one to another and commonly include overweight, obesity, diabetes, hypertension, cardiovascular disease, stroke, asthma, and other immune-related illnesses.

Pathways from complex human experiences to health outcomes, described in chapter 1, would indicate that spatial design and planning professionals must pay attention to harmful environmental, social, and economic stressors because these professionals often help co-produce these stressors through their institutionalized responses to the problems of health, race, poverty, mobility, housing, or food. The far-reaching effects of their spatial design and planning activities, however, are not easy to isolate and recognize in everyday practices. Nor is it easy to avoid any unintended effects of these activities because of the complex decision-making and implementation processes involved.

A socio-ecological framework can be useful in this regard. This framework, also described in chapter 1, identifies population health as a product of human interactions with various coexisting factors of the physical, social, and natural environments. These interactions occur at different spatial scales of buildings, neighborhoods, and cities and at different organizational levels of individuals, groups, and communities. Sometimes, the extent and significance of some of these interactions in terms of spatial scales and organizational levels remains difficult to determine. For example, population health in a small city observing fast growth may be affected not only by internal factors but also by external factors that cannot be precisely known.

Put simply, human interactions with various coexisting factors of the physical, social, and natural environments are not static and homogeneous. Rather, they are dynamic and heterogeneous, creating ever-changing experiences that shape population health. In response to these interactions, spatial design and planning professionals can never be too general in their approaches to protect and promote the health, safety, and welfare of the population they serve. They must remain focused on the qualities of a place and the compositions of a society along with many other internal and external factors as they consider population health.

AVOID ONE-SIZE-FITS-ALL APPROACHES

According to the socio-ecological model of population health, significant place- and population-based variabilities may exist in spatial associations of health, safety, and well-being. We have seen that in this book's studies, where spatial associations of lifestyle and health in small Kansas cities were differently affected by different factors of rurality. According to the findings of these studies, there are no one-size-fits-all spatial design and planning strategies, policies, and programs for promoting population health, even in these small cities. These strategies, policies, and programs may need to be tailored to the needs of a place and a population. For example, effective programs for older adults in one place may not be as effective for older adults in another place. Similarly, effective programs for older adults may not be as effective for younger adults living in the same place. For effective spatial strategies, policies, and programs promoting population health, it is necessary to know what issues of life and place are truly driving population health disparities and what can be done to address those issues for the greatest impact on rurality-based health disparities in small-town America.

According to the findings of the studies presented in this book, important place-based (spatial) factors driving population health disparities among small Kansas cities may include street network properties for their pervasive associations with lifestyle and physical, mental, and social health indicators. Important spatial factors also include industrial land use, for it shows frequent associations with several lifestyle and physical, mental, and social health indicators. Industrial land use is even more important than open spaces in these small cities in terms of how frequently they are associated with lifestyle and physical, mental, and social health indicators. Other important factors related to population health in small cities may include the availability of key destinations and functions. Density and land use mix, however, are not as important in small towns and cities as they are in urban areas.

TAKE INTO ACCOUNT THE QUALITY OF EVIDENCE

For effective spatial design and planning that protects and promotes population health, research-based evidence is needed on design and planning issues (how to build healthy communities), policy issues (how to engage policymakers and to put incentives in place to encourage needed environmental and behavioral changes), and behavioral issues (how to motivate people to change lifestyle behaviors). It is, however, necessary to acknowledge that the very meaning of evidence is highly problematic. It has been argued, repeatedly and cogently, that evidence is socially constructed and negotiated and is contested within and across professions [23, 24].

Like every other field of study, while a complete agreement on the nature of evidence and its use in spatial design and planning may remain contested in population health, population health presents many opportunities for collaboration among design and planning professionals, policymakers, and researchers. They could work together in framing population health problems and hence in determining methodologies that could be used to produce evidence. The quality of evidence rests on the methodology that produces the evidence. Concerning this, the following well-established hierarchy of evidence [25, 26] may help increase specificity, reduce bias in decision-making, and improve effectiveness in spatial design and planning processes:

1. Systematic reviews and meta-analysis
2. Randomized controlled trials with definitive results
3. Randomized controlled trials with nondefinitive results
4. Cohort studies
5. Case-controlled studies
6. Cross-sectional surveys
7. Case reports

In this hierarchy, the most robust methodological approaches are systematic reviews. Meta-analysis is a subset of systematic reviews that systematically combines pertinent qualitative and quantitative study data from several selected studies to develop a single conclusion with greater statistical power. The conclusions of a meta-analysis are statistically stronger than the conclusions of an analysis of any single study due to increased numbers of subjects, greater diversity among subjects, or accumulated effects and results.

Randomized controlled trials (RCTs) provide the next best quality of evidence. They use a study design that randomly assigns participants into an experimental group or a control group. As the study is conducted, the only expected difference between the control and experimental groups in an RCT is the outcome variable being studied. Though expensive in terms of time and money, good randomization helps eliminate population bias. It is also easier to mask or blind the participants in these studies. In an RCT, the populations of participants are clearly identified, but often participants may not be representative of their populations.

In a cohort study design, one or more samples (called cohorts) are followed prospectively, and subsequent status evaluations with respect to a disease or outcome to determine which initial participants exposure characteristics (risk factors) are associated with it. As the study is conducted, outcome from participants in each cohort is measured and relationships with specific characteristics determined. This study design helps limit the influence of confounding variables since the participants in one or more cohorts can be matched. It is also easier and cheaper than an RCT.

A case control study compares cases that show outcomes of interest with controls that do not show outcomes of interest and looks back retrospectively to compare how frequently the exposure to a risk factor is present in each case to determine the relationship between the risk factor and the outcome. Case control studies are observational because no intervention is attempted and no attempt is made to alter the course of the outcome. The goal is to retrospectively determine the exposure to the risk factor of interest from each of the two study groups: cases and controls. These studies are designed to estimate odds.

The weakest among the evidence are those provided by cross-sectional studies and case reports. Cross-sectional studies use a convenient or randomized sample of participants from a population for a study, whereas a case report describes and interprets an individual case, often written in the form of a detailed story. Case studies can help identify new trends or disease and adverse or beneficial effects of a treatment, and they can be an easy way of sharing lessons learned.

USE EVIDENCE-BASED METRICS

Metrics help measure, assess, and evaluate performance using evidence-based criteria. Appropriate metrics can help integrate population health–related goals and policies with spatial design and planning processes. They can play a key part in determining how to prioritize spatial design and planning interventions and track health outcomes and impacts. Spatial design and planning professionals can share data as well as analysis done based on shared metrics to develop strategic partnerships with stakeholders from other sectors, including public health and health care. Metrics can be useful in community engagement and to develop new cross-sector partnerships and collaborations. Data collected using shared metrics to assess current conditions can spark discussions at neighborhood associations, city and county boards, and public meetings. Such discussions could potentially increase public awareness about current issues and garner support for spatial solutions to population health problems.

Regarding metrics, however, it is important to note that political, social, cultural, economic, and environmental conditions are different in each community, and so are its population health issues and challenges. Due to these differences, population health priorities change, making some metrics less appropriate than others. There is no reason to abandon all the metrics when only some of them are less useful, however. Others can still be used to analyze conditions, help prioritize a community's goals and objectives, and support the implementation of appropriate spatial policies and programs. Concerning this, a participatory approach to health promotion may be helpful.

Participatory Design and Planning for Health Promotion in Small-Town America
Participatory Design and Planning and Levels of Participation

In the difficult population health context of small cities and towns, design and planning through community participation (or participatory design and planning) may be a more sustainable approach to health promotion than traditional spatial design and planning. A WHO publication provides the following working definition of community participation:

> A process by which people are enabled to become actively and genuinely involved in defining the issues of concern to them, in making decisions about factors that affect their lives, in formulating and implementing policies, in planning, developing and delivering services and in taking action to achieve change [27, p. 10].

A participatory process of design and planning assumes that community participation works best when people take action to improve their situations; when people are allowed to build on their knowledge and skills; when they develop skills to monitor their own progress; when they can see if their activities are having an impact; and when resources are used effectively and efficiently by the people for their own good [28]. When communities are given the opportunity to work out their own problems, they will find solutions that will have a more lasting effect.

The revised Health for All policy for the WHO European Region [29] therefore suggests that the active participation of communities is essential for environmentally, economically, and socially sustainable development, urging local authorities to undertake a consultative and consensus-building process with citizens and local organizations and to help formulate their own sustainable development strategy. It also suggests that a participatory health development process, one that reaches out "to empower individuals, local communities and private and voluntary organizations in different settings for health, e.g., homes, workplaces, schools and cities," is essential for health promotion [29, p. 68].

The nature and level of community participation can vary, however, and communities are not always empowered, nor do they have the capacity, to do the things they should do or would like to do. Recognizing this, Arnstein provides a ladder of participation with eight rungs. At the bottom of the ladder is *non-participation*, which includes manipulation and therapy. The next level up is *tokenism*, which includes informing, consultation, and placation. The topmost level of the ladder is *citizen power*, which includes partnership, delegated power, and citizen control [30]. In contrast, Davidson identifies four types of community participation in a wheel of participation: providing information, consulting with the public, enabling participation through representation, and empowering individuals and communities [31]. Others describe participation as an umbrella term, suggesting an ongoing, active relationship with shared power and ownership, understood in different ways by different people [32].

Limitations and Advantages of Participatory Design and Planning for Health Promotion in Small Cities and Towns

Depending on the level and nature of community participation, the participatory design and planning approach can have many limitations and advantages for health promotion in small cities and towns. Among the limitations, it should be noted that broad support for participatory design and planning may generally be absent in small cities and towns. Even in cases where it may enjoy some support from a local government, it may generally lack a stable institutional framework supported by human, financial, and physical resources. Without people in appropriate roles, a budget to plan with, and physical resources for its day-to-day activities, participatory design and planning may lack the capacity, stability, and continuity of traditional spatial design and planning activities performed by a local government. It takes time and effort to acquire resources for participatory or community-engaged activities. As these resources are being acquired, the problem that needs to be solved may change due to forces beyond the control of a community.

It should also be noted that, due to a lack of resources, participatory design and planning activities must have a narrow focus in small cities and towns. For example, food deserts, crime, and physical activity may be interrelated, but small communities may not always have the resources necessary to deal with all of them at the same time. The broader the scope of community-led participatory design and planning activities, the more these activities depend on various outside (governmental and nongovernmental) supports. This eventually makes community-led activities bureaucratic and inflexible. Ironically, these are among the problems that community-led participatory design and planning activities want to eliminate.

One very important limitation of community participation that needs mention here is that some community organizations, due to their religious, cultural, or political affiliations, may do just the opposite of what needs to be done concerning health promotion in small-town communities. For example, they may discourage mental health patients from seeking medical help, hold unfavorable views about immigrants, or discourage people from taking medical treatments that could potentially save lives. Community beliefs are among the hardest things to change concerning population health.

Finally, it should be mentioned that community-led participatory design and planning activities pose many difficulties for evaluation. First, various actors and groups, sometimes with opposing interests, may be involved in these activities, disallowing a common set of metrics and outcomes of interest for these activities. Second, participatory activities are generally developmental, and their outcomes are unpredictable. Third, participants, goals and objectives, and resources change frequently. Fourth, process is integral in community-led participatory design and planning activities; therefore, process needs evaluation as much as any outcomes of the process. However, it is difficult to evaluate a process, which changes constantly [28].

Despite limitations, community participation in design and planning activities is widely accepted to have many important benefits [33]. These benefits include increasing democracy, mobilizing local resources and energy, developing more holistic and integrated approaches, achieving better decisions and more effective services, ensuring the ownership and sustainability of programs, and actively empowering people [27]. Skills learned through participation can be extended to other aspects of people's lives, including their political awareness, and can be expressed in the wider community. The experience of participation can lead to a general increase in confidence [34]. It has been suggested that the changes that have taken place in people themselves are probably more important than the physical improvements effected within a community in the process of community participation [35].

There is little rigorous evidence of the effectiveness of community-led participatory design and planning activities for health promotion, however. Still, it is generally accepted that community organizations may be able to serve many different purposes for health promotion, including providing essential leadership in population health–related activities, creating the preconditions for healthier living and participatory governance, and facilitating intersectoral actions for health promotion. In times of economic downturns, they may be able to play a key role as advocates and guardians of the health needs of the people who are most vulnerable and socially disadvantaged.

Among other advantages, local communities and community organizations can help tackle unusual problems that lie beyond the scope of traditional spatial design and planning bodies. For example, they can help launch campaigns at the grassroots level when citizens lack interest for a farmers' market that could improve access to healthy foods; when citizens are physically inactive despite having access to physical activity resources; when citizens prefer unhealthy foods despite having access to healthy foods; or when they want to reduce crime through eyes on the street because neighborhood design or law enforcement has failed.

Local communities and community organizations can respond to a problem more quickly than can traditional spatial design and planning bodies and local government experts. They can easily mobilize local resources and energy. When neighborhood crime is no longer a problem, they may be able to modify their mission to curb social isolation among elderly; when getting people to a farmers' market is no longer a problem, they can provide help at neighborhood gardens that grow fresh produce for these markets; or when resident participation in physical activities is no longer a problem, they can focus on the maintenance and safety of streets and sidewalks. In essence, local communities and community organizations are nimble. As the solution of a problem is found or as the resources for an existing program run out, they can regroup for another more urgent health problem for which resources have become available.

Projects and programs developed by local communities and community organizations are generally more sustainable. They empower communities and are owned by communities. They are also more relevant because local communities and community organizations know their health needs and their strengths and weaknesses better than outside experts. Therefore, it is easy to garner community support for projects and programs conceived and developed by local communities and community organizations. Even on matters that fall squarely on the shoulders of local government and outside experts, any steps taken by these experts without consulting local communities and community organizations may not be prudent.

Status of Community Participation in Small Towns and Rural Areas

Nationally and internationally, social, political, and economic changes in rural environments continue to contribute to a "circle of decline" in many small cities and towns with significant negative health impacts. Considering this decline, many have highlighted the significance of community participation for the health of rural and small-town communities [36–39]. This assumes that community participation will somehow build resilient, self-determining communities capable of dealing with complex population health problems. What happens in the practice of community participation for health promotion in rural and small-town communities, however, is less clear.

In this regard, the successful experiences of Healthy Cities projects sponsored by the WHO can be used as the basis for meaningful multisectoral local government partnerships with rural and small-town communities to ensure acceptable, appropriate, and effective responses to health inequities in small cities and towns [40]. As exemplified by the Healthy Cities projects discussed in chapter 1, local governments through community partnerships can provide shared advantages in terms of survival, resilience, sustainability, and fiscal responsibility [41]. Community partnerships can help rebuild or harness community capacity, which is integral to developing locally responsive health services [37]. They can help draw together local resources and can take advantage of the innate, adaptive, inventive, and innovative nature of local communities [42]. They can also lead to empowered communities capable of developing local solutions [43]. The underpinning proposition in all this is that by giving decision-making powers to community members, health care will be locally responsive, costs will be contained, and health outcomes will improve [36, 44].

The World Health Organization identified the centrality of communities in health planning and decision making in 1978 [45]. Soon after, it launched the Healthy Cities programs. Almost four decades after the Healthy Cities programs were launched, nationally and internationally, rural and small-town communities continue to remain disempowered and distanced from urban centers of power [46, 47]. A lack of knowledge is consistently identified on how to build effective community partnerships that empower small-town communities and encourage citizen control and responsibility in local decision-making [37]. This lack is more noticeable in the participatory design and planning processes because these processes do not have any ideal predefined set of steps, approaches, or implementation tools for local communities and community organizations to use for health promotion. The following general principles may be useful in guiding successful community participatory processes.

General Principles for Health Promotion through Participatory Design and Planning

The literature has generally indicated that community projects and programs need to have many characteristics to be successful. Some of these characteristics include strong political support, effective leadership, high visibility within a community, a strong strategic orientation supported by adequate and appropriate resources, broad community ownership and strong community participation, intersectoral collaboration, and political and managerial accountability [48]. At this time, an elaborate description of these characteristics seems less important because they will likely vary from one community to another, from one problem to another. Instead, a few general principles are provided for successful health promotion through participatory design and planning projects and programs in small cities and towns.

THINK BEYOND "HEALTH PLANNING" AND "TRADITIONAL PLANNING"

"Health planning" commonly deals with health care services. The emphasis is on serving people who are ill with acute or chronic conditions while sidelining socio-ecological factors that make them ill. In contrast, according to the definition provided by the WHO, discussed in chapter 1, health is not a concern for only health care professionals. Rather, it is a concern for all agencies with abilities to change the social, economic, and environmental determinants of health. Population health embraces this expanded view of health for promotion and considers the lifestyle behaviors and the physical, mental, and social health and well-being of a population in relation to its socio-ecological context. It promotes policies and action for health promotion at the local and regional levels, with an emphasis on the social and ecological determinants of health.

Clearly, several areas of population health are beyond the scope of traditional spatial design and planning. Narrowly focused tools and techniques of traditional design and planning, such as the bureaucratic process of land use control, capital improvements programs, and special funding development programs, are rarely enough to deal with health promotion in a comprehensive manner. Small-town communities should also consider participatory design and planning as another important approach for health promotion.

There is a need to be cognizant of the complexity and changing nature of the population health of rural and small-town communities prior to embarking on community participation initiatives. To assume that communities will welcome participation opportunities and will engage as "well-behaved" citizens is at best naive. Almost two decades ago, Oakley made the following comments about rural people, which are still a timely reminder of rural complexities:

> Participation . . . cannot merely be proclaimed or wished upon rural people. . . . It must begin by recognizing the powerful, multi-dimensional and, in many instances, anti-participatory forces which dominate the lives of rural people. Centuries of domination and subservience will not disappear overnight just because we have "discovered" the concept of participation [49].

EMPHASIZE PROCESS OVER PROJECT

Process is central in different activities and initiatives of health promotion. A city, whether small or big, must be engaged in an ongoing process of health promotion at multiple spatial and organizational levels to improve health and well-being. Most often, health promotion requires a process or a set of processes that engages communities. Yet communities remain a neutral participant, not an engaged agent, in traditional design and planning processes.

To be successful, the process of community participation requires long-term commitment, which pays off in several ways. Over time, the process becomes more visible on the political agenda of a community, and the practical understanding of policies that promote health is broadened. Along with this comes the successful accumulation of practical knowledge about the organizational structures and management strategies needed to put community ideas into practice. With long-term engagement, it is also possible to learn what predicts success in health promotion at the local level.

This emphasis on the long-term in community participatory processes can, however, be a problem. People, accustomed to seeing concrete outcomes, may want status information and short-term results. Such expectations can be unrealistic in community participatory processes. It is important to acknowledge that the process of making a city healthier does not produce quick and easily measurable results [50].

The implications for research concerning community-engaged processes of health promotion are obvious. Research needs to inform what works and what does not in such processes. Some of that research should provide answers about how to measure short-term changes and impacts to meet political demand [51]. The research should also provide information on the long-term development and implementation of processes for health promotion considering that many unknowns can potentially derail the processes.

CONSIDER COMMUNITY PARTICIPATION TO PROMOTE "HEALTH IN ALL POLICIES"

A healthy environment is not merely a product of spatial design and planning activities. It is also determined by policies and actions beyond these activities. Health and well-being are increasingly becoming shared values across societal sectors. Indeed, there is solid evidence showing that actions beyond spatial design and planning can significantly influence the environmental risk factors of major diseases and the determinants of health. "Health in all policies" addresses policies influencing transportation, housing and urban development, and the environment, as well as education, agriculture, fiscal policies, tax policies, economic policies, and more.

Strategies to develop healthy public policies covering all aspects of a society are fundamental to the processes of health promotion. In this regard, local governments can help by establishing health-promoting policies and providing mechanisms and structures allowing intersectoral collaboration. In many small cities and towns, intersectoral collaboration is not an issue because local governments do not have many sectors. People may already be working with one another in these small governments. Their issues may be finding the extra time and resources to develop and implement health promotion policies in partnership with local communities.

Leveraging their own limited resources, local governments can help establish mechanisms that allow community organizations to work collaboratively with various sectors or units of these governments to formulate health-promoting policies. When collaboration is difficult, local governments should at least provide these community organizations with appropriate resources for the work they need or want to do. When internal resources are scarce, local governments should help these community organizations connect with external resources. The last thing local governments need to do is to discourage these community organizations because that will be an opportunity missed for health promotion.

Even though it is not always easy for communities and local governments to work together on policies regarding health promotion, experience has shown that a broad concept of health can provide a useful strategic umbrella beneath which they can work collaboratively toward a common goal [51]. There is, however, a lack of evidence showing that widespread policy changes are possible through citizen inputs, particularly in rural areas, and that such changes can promote locally appropriate and diversified health care delivery models [52]. There is also a lack of evidence demonstrating that short-term efforts through community participation can result in cost-effective policy solutions for health improvement objectives of small towns and cities, such as reducing the burden of chronic disease and health spending [43, 53, 54]. Additionally, there is a lack of research on models to assess the possible impacts of various policy options as well as mechanisms to assess the actual impacts of policies once implemented. Therefore, a need for more research focusing on how community participation may help promote health policies for all in small towns and rural areas exists in the United States and elsewhere.

RECOGNIZE THE NEED FOR NEW KINDS OF RESEARCH

Whatever its purpose may be, community participation requires new and creative approaches to interdisciplinary research. While there is work in many fields that is of great potential relevance to health promotion through community participation, these links are not self-evident. Before interdisciplinary research can develop, questions need to be formulated in a way that attracts the interests of different disciplines. For example, it will be necessary to know which groups come to be represented in a project through the process of community participation, whose interests prevail, and how far the results of these processes are successfully translated into policies to promote equity. It will also be necessary to know how one measures what works and what does not work in a participatory process, how progress is measured in such a process, and how programs can be justified in terms of improved health and effective use of limited resources.

Differences in research paradigm, methodological approach, or political position need to be considered when researching community participation. Applied research can tell us which approaches are effective and worth implementing more widely, and policy analysis can bring out the rationale and implications of strategic decisions. Research can provide useful topics for local campaigns, and it can play an important strategic role in showing how local government policies need to be changed if actions at the community level are to have any impact. Above all, traditional research approaches are unlikely to prove satisfactory in health promotion through community participation. Realignments within research and between researchers and local community leaders and organizations may therefore be called for. New partnerships may be needed to build a coherent research response. Research practices need to become more open and participative; and researchers should be made accountable to local people when they do research in communities.

EMPOWER COMMUNITIES

The promotion of health in a community clearly requires a high level of participation that promotes active and genuine involvement and empowerment rather than the more passive processes of providing information and consultation. People must be empowered individually and through their local communities to take control of their health. Empowering individuals and communities and allowing them to define their own needs increases self-confidence, self-esteem, knowledge, and skills. The process of community participation is considered as important and health promoting as any outcomes. When communities are empowered, equal opportunities are promoted and anti-discriminatory practices developed simultaneously [55].

High-level participation is not always possible, however. Different political, social, economic, and organizational contexts may create different conditions, offering different opportunities and constraints for community participation [55]. It has been noted that empowerment cannot be bestowed by others but that those who have power (e.g., health practitioners) and those who want it (e.g., clients) must cooperate to create the conditions necessary to make empowerment possible [56]. This can be done by building capacity and enabling social action to address the underlying social, structural, and economic conditions that impact health.

There are at least two implications for research on community empowerment in US small cities and towns. The first is the need to understand what makes for successful community empowerment and what works against it. The second is that research itself should be sensitive to the issue of community empowerment. Action or participatory research strategies should be utilized so that the community is fully involved in defining the research problem, developing the research model, conducting the research, and analyzing and interpreting the results.

PROMOTE HEALTH EQUALITY

In praising the virtues of community participation, it is naive to think that grassroots work and some local or state government responsiveness will dramatically improve health equality. The major challenge in rural small-town communities is unequal positions of power, stemming from differences in social class, knowledge and expertise, and other educational and occupational advantages [57]. Reducing inequalities requires a redistribution of resources and power and political change, which is beyond the capacity of these communities.

Dealing with health inequality is particularly difficult in small-town communities because they frequently lack power and resources to deal with the fundamental economic and social determinants underlying such problems as unemployment, malnutrition, and inferior education associated with poverty. In areas where they lack power and resources, communities can and must advocate to state and national governments (preferably in conjunction with other communities) policy changes that will address the basic determinants of health, reduce health inequalities, and improve the health and well-being of their citizens. A participatory approach to health promotion can help exert an influence on the local government and create a momentum for change.

It has been argued that strong governance is a necessary preparatory step for meaningful community participation promoting health equality [58]. There are a few examples of governance structures that have partnered community members, health care, and other service stakeholders to bring together lay and expert knowledge and community resources [59, 60], but the paucity of evidence-based governance processes provides a major challenge for local implementation. Even in situations where governance mechanisms are established, government regulations may conflict with ways small-town communities have traditionally governed themselves. This can delegitimize the communities' own forms of self-organization [61].

There are other issues or challenges when dealing with inequalities in health through community participation. One challenge is simply whether adequate data exist at the city level to document and describe inequalities in health within the city for strategic decision-making. Another challenge is identifying cost-effective, socially responsible strategies for participatory processes to address inequality in access to basic determinants of health while acknowledging a city's limited power and jurisdiction [51].

Yet another challenge is related to the questions of who participates, who does not, and whether it matters. These are challenging questions to answer for rural communities. In participatory activities, community members are generally assumed to share a vested interest in making their community a good place to live. For small-town communities in rural areas, this can mean appointing "local champions" or the "usual suspects" to attend structured meetings and provide opinions or feedback [59, 60]. However, by only including those who are available, participation may become compromised. Sometimes, participation may exclude others with diverse perspectives by including only those who self-elect. As a result, participation of the disadvantaged and marginalized remains elusive [62].

Although there are some examples of inclusion involving disadvantaged or marginalized people and subcultures [63], there is limited evidence to suggest that participatory approaches alone, without specific strategies to target marginalized groups, result in an inclusive model of community participation [43, 62]. Since it is impossible to adequately represent those who are not directly participating, "translation agents"—those who are comfortable in the circles of both the powerful and the powerless and who are able to facilitate transactions among groups—are important [64]. "Participation fatigue" can also develop among those who are pulled into many activities [65–67]. This can pose a barrier to participation in small-town communities. Community members who have been involved in participation processes have reported negative physical and psychological health consequences, including exhaustion and stress [68].

Still another challenge is related to the need to acknowledge that different forms of community knowledge exist. Local community knowledge is grounded in context, which challenges those external to rural communities to accept local knowledge as a legitimate form of understanding [69]. Sometimes, longstanding community members can dismiss the views of others who are not considered "real locals" as they do not have familial roots within the community. Sometimes, residents may have lived in the community for extensive time periods, yet they are not viewed as having legitimate claims to knowledge about the community until they have lived there for decades [32]. Sometimes, dialogue is made complicated by "the persisting assumption that experts are still holding the only real 'knowledge'" [69, p. 34].

Finally, concerning inequality, it should be noted that one group (often endogenous and usually the more powerful) may try to "engage" the other group by using its own spaces and processes in community participation. This may include having workshops or meetings that are presented in a format and language that makes sense to one group but can alienate the other [70, 71]. Critics argue that these "invited spaces" are "still structured and owned by those who provide them" as compared to spaces that people create for themselves [66]. Finding ways to encourage people to create their own spaces and to give them ownership of these spaces, therefore, may be the essential first step to promote health equality.

NOTES

1. WHO European Healthy Cities Network, *Phase V.*
2. Toner, "Getting to Know the People and the Place."
3. Getzels, "Policies and Plans."
4. Getzels and Thurow, *Rural and Small Town Planning.*
5. Thurow, "Zoning and Development Permit Systems."
6. Friedman, "Rural and Small Town Subdivision Regulations."
7. Turnbull, "Using Natural Resources as a Planning Guide."
8. Economic Research Service, *Rural Transportation at a Glance.*
9. Shoup and Homa, *Principles for Improving Transportation Options.*
10. Kidder, *The Challenges of Rural Transportation.*
11. Litman and Hughes-Cromwick, *Public Transportation's Impact on Rural and Small Towns.*
12. Patton, "Rural Public Transportation."
13. Casavant et al., *Study of Rural Transportation Issues,* 116–127.
14. Stommes and Brown, "Transportation in Rural America."
15. Coates and Weiss, *Revitalization of Small Communities.*
16. Rupprecht, "Private Motor Vehicles."
17. Henning-Smith et al., *Rural Transportation.*
18. Meit et al., *The 2014 Update of the Rural-Urban Chartbook.*
19. W. K. Kellogg Foundation, *Perceptions of Rural America.*
20. Zajacova and Lawrence, "The Relationship between Education and Health."
21. Rogers and Whiting, *Aspects of Planning.*
22. Schreiner, "A Planning Framework for Rural Public Sector Analysis."
23. Rashid, "The Question of Knowledge in Evidence-Based Design."
24. Chan and Chan, "Medicine for the Millennium."
25. Evans, "Hierarchy of Evidence."
26. Barton, "Which Clinical Studies Provide the Best Evidence?"
27. WHO Regional Office for Europe, *Community Participation in Local Health and Sustainable Development.*
28. Smithies and Adams, "Walking the Tightrope," 59.
29. WHO Regional Office for Europe, *Health 21.*
30. Arnstein, "Eight Rungs on a Ladder of Citizen Participation."
31. Davidson, "Spinning the Wheel of Empowerment."
32. Kenny et al., "Community Participation in Rural Health: A Scoping Review."
33. Zakus and Lysack, "Revisiting Community Participation."
34. Liffman, *Power For the Poor.*
35. Anyanwu, "The Technique of Participatory Research."
36. Corrigan et al., *Quality through Collaboration.*
37. Kulig and Williams, *Health in Rural Canada.*
38. World Health Organization, *Rural Poverty and Health Systems.*
39. Commonwealth of Australia, *National Strategic Framework.*
40. Kenny et al., "Community Participation for Rural Health: A Review of Challenges."

41. Alford, *Engaging Public Sector Clients*.
42. Farmer and Kilpatrick, "Are Rural Health Professionals Also Social Entrepreneurs?"
43. Needham, "Realizing the Potential of Co-Production."
44. MacKinney, Mueller, and McBride, "The March to Accountable Care Organizations."
45. World Health Organization, *Primary Health Care*.
46. Nimegeer et al., "Addressing the Problem of Rural Community Engagement."
47. Farmer et al., "Territorial Tensions."
48. Tsouros, "Healthy Cities Means Community Action."
49. Oakley, *Projects with People*, 4.
50. Hancock and Duhl, "WHO Healthy Cities Paper 1."
51. Hancock, "The Healthy City from Concept to Application."
52. Montoya and Kent, "Dialogical Action."
53. Mitton et al., "Public Participation in Health Care Priority Setting."
54. Head, "Community Engagement."
55. Heritage and Dooris, "Community Participation and Empowerment."
56. Laverack, "Improving Health Outcomes through Community Empowerment."
57. Organization for Economic Co-operation and Development, *Strategies to Improve Rural Service Delivery*.
58. Kilpatrick, "Multi-Level Rural Community Engagement."
59. Huttlinger, "Research and Collaboration."
60. Johns, Kilpatrick, and Whelan, "Our Health in Our Hands."
61. Eversole and Martin, *Participation and Governance in Regional Development*.
62. Taylor, Wilkinson, and Cheers, "Is It Consumer or Community Participation?"
63. Kidd, Kenny, and Endacott, "Consumer Advocate and Clinician Perceptions."
64. Eversole, "Empowering Institutions."
65. Attree et al., "The Experience of Community Engagement."
66. Cornwall, A., "Unpacking 'Participation.'"
67. Scerri and James, "Communities of Citizens and 'Indicators' of Sustainability."
68. Ziersch and Baum, "Involvement in Civil Society Groups."
69. Eversole, "Community Agency and Community Engagement."
70. Crawford et al., "Systematic Review of Involving Patients."
71. Glasziou et al., "Taking Healthcare Interventions from Trial to Practice."

Ablah, E., F. Dong, A. P. Cupertino, K. Konda, J. A. Johnston, and T. Collins. "Prevalence of Diabetes and Pre-Diabetes in Kansas." *Ethnicity and Disease* 23, no. 4 (Autumn 2013): 415–20.

Acevedo-Garcia, Dolores, Kimberly A. Lochner, Theresa L. Osypuk, and Sukanya V. Subramanian. "Future Directions in Residential Segregation and Health Research: A Multilevel Approach." *American Journal of Public Health* 93, no. 2 (2003): 215–21.

Addy, Cheryl L., Dawn K. Wilson, Karen A. Kirtland, Barbara E. Ainsworth, Patricia Sharpe, and Dexter Kimsey. "Associations of Perceived Social and Physical Environmental Supports with Physical Activity and Walking Behavior." *American Journal of Public Health* 94, no. 3 (2004): 440–43.

Adler, Nancy E., and Joan M. Ostrove. "Socioeconomic Status and Health: What We Know and What We Don't." *Annals of the New York Academy of Sciences* 896, no. 1 (1999): 3–15.

Agerbo, Esben, E. Fuller Torrey, and Preben Bo Mortensen. "Household Crowding in Early Adulthood and Schizophrenia Are Unrelated in Denmark: A Nested Case-Control Study." *Schizophrenia Research* 47, no. 2–3 (2001): 243–46.

Agnew, Robert. "A General Strain Theory of Community Differences in Crime Rates." *Journal of Research in Crime and Delinquency* 36, no. 2 (1999): 123–55.

Ahmad, Aqeel, Anuradha Ghosh, Coby Schal, and Ludek Zurek. "Insects in Confined Swine Operations Carry a Large Antibiotic Resistant and Potentially Virulent Enterococcal Community." *BMC Microbiology* 11, no. 1 (2011): 1–13.

Alberti, L. B. *On the Art of Building in Ten Books.* Cambridge, MA: MIT Press, 1988. http://books.google.com/books?id=OFGTd1gQBXEC.

Albrecht, Don E. "The Industrial Transformation of Farm Communities: Implications for Family Structure and Socioeconomic Conditions." *Rural Sociology* 63, no. 1 (1998): 51–64.

Albrecht, Don E., and Carol Mulford Albrecht. "Metro/Nonmetro Residence, Nonmarital Conception, and Conception Outcomes." *Rural Sociology* 69, no. 3 (2004): 430–52.

Alexander, Leslie M., Jo Inchley, Joanna Todd, Dorothy Currie, Ashley R. Cooper, and Candace Currie. "The Broader Impact of Walking to School among Adolescents: Seven Day Accelerometry Based Study." *BMJ: British Medical Journal* 331, no. 7524 (2005): 1061–62.

Alford, John. *Engaging Public Sector Clients: From Service-Delivery to Co-Production.* London: Palgrave Macmillan, 2009.

Allen, Jessica. *Older People and Wellbeing.* London: Institute for Public Policy Research, 2008.

Allen, Matilda, and Jessica Allen. "Health Inequalities and the Role of the Physical and Social Environment." In *The Routledge Handbook of Planning for Health and Well-Being: Shap-*

ing a Sustainable and Healthy Future, edited by Hugh Barton, Susan Thompson, Sarah Burgess, and Marcus Grant, 89–107. New York: Routledge, 2015.

All Things Considered. "Why Is the Risk of Youth Suicide Higher in Rural Areas?" NPR, March 15, 2015, https://www.npr.org/2015/03/15/393192543/why-is-the-risk-of-youth -suicide-higher-in-rural-areas.

Ameli, S. Hassan, Shima Hamidi, Andrea Garfinkel-Castro, and Reid Ewing. "Do Better Urban Design Qualities Lead to More Walking in Salt Lake City, Utah?" *Journal of Urban Design* 20, no. 3 (2015): 393–410.

American Diabetes Association. "Economic Costs of Diabetes in the U.S. in 2017." *Diabetes Care* (2018): dci180007. https://doi.org/10.2337/dci18-0007.

American Hospital Association. *Rural Report 2020: Challenges Facing Rural Communities and the Roadmap to Ensure Local Access to High-Quality, Affordable Care.* Chicago: American Hospital Association, 2019. https://www.aha.org/guidesreports/2019-02-04-rural-report -2019.

Andersen, Lars Bo, Peter Schnohr, Marianne Schroll, and Hans Ole Hein. "All-Cause Mortality Associated with Physical Activity during Leisure Time, Work, Sports, and Cycling to Work." *Archives of Internal Medicine* 160, no. 11 (2000): 1621–28. https://doi.org/10.1001 /archinte.160.11.1621.

Antonovsky, Aaron. "The Salutogenic Model as a Theory to Guide Health Promotion." *Health Promotion International* 11, no. 1 (1996): 11–18.

Antonovsky, Aaron. "The Structure and Properties of the Sense of Coherence Scale." *Social Science and Medicine* 36, no. 6 (1993): 725–33. https://doi.org/https://doi.org/10.1016/0277 -9536(93)90033-Z.

Antonovsky, Aaron. *Unraveling the Mystery of Health: How People Manage Stress and Stay Well.* San Francisco: Jossey-bass, 1987.

Anyanwu, C. N. "The Technique of Participatory Research in Community Development." *Community Development Journal* 23, no. 1 (1988): 11–15.

Appleyard, D. *Livable Streets, Protected Neighborhoods.* Berkeley: University of California Press, 1980.

Aristotle. *Aristotle in Twenty-Three Volumes: Politics*, bk 2, section 1267b. Translated by H. Rackham. Cambridge, MA: Harvard University Press, 1944. Accessed July 4, 2019 from Perseus Digital Library. http://data.perseus.org/citations/urn:cts:greekLit:tlg0086.tlg035 .perseus-eng1:2.1267b.

Aristotle. *Aristotle in Twenty-Three Volumes: Politics*, bk 7, section 1330b. Translated by H. Rackham. Cambridge, MA: Harvard University Press, 1944. Accessed July 4, 2019. http://data.perseus.org/citations/urn:cts:greekLit:tlg0086.tlg035.perseus-eng1:7.1330b.

Arnstein, S. "Eight Rungs on a Ladder of Citizen Participation." *Journal of the Institute of American Planners* 35, no. 4 (1969): 216–24.

Ashida, Sato, and Catherine A. Heaney. "Differential Associations of Social Support and Social Connectedness with Structural Features of Social Networks and the Health Status of Older Adults." *Journal of Aging and Health* 20, no. 7 (2008): 872–93.

Ashton, John, ed. *Healthy Cities.* Milton Keynes: Open University Press, 1992.

Ashton, John, Paula Grey, and Keith Barnard. "Healthy Cities—WHO's New Public Health Initiative." *Health Promotion International* 1, no. 3 (1986): 319–24.

Attree, Pamela, Beverley French, Beth Milton, Susan Povall, Margaret Whitehead, and Jennie Popay. "The Experience of Community Engagement for Individuals: A Rapid Review of Evidence." *Health and Social Care in the Community* 19, no. 3 (2011): 250–60.

Auchincloss, Amy H., and Ana V. Diez-Roux. "A New Tool for Epidemiology: The Usefulness of Dynamic-Agent Models in Understanding Place Effects on Health." *American Journal of Epidemiology* 168, no. 1 (2008): 1–8.

Auchincloss, Amy H., Kari A. B. Moore, Latetia V. Moore, and Ana V. Diez-Roux. "Improving Retrospective Characterization of the Food Environment for a Large Region in the United States During a Historic Time Period." *Health and Place* 18, no. 6 (2012): 1341–47.

Babey, Susan H., Theresa A. Hastert, Hongjian Yu, and E. Richard Brown. "Physical Activity among Adolescents: When Do Parks Matter?" *American Journal of Preventive Medicine* 34, no. 4 (2008): 345–48.

Babisch, Wolfgang. "Road Traffic Noise and Cardiovascular Risk." *Noise and Health* 10, no. 38 (2008): 27.

Bader, Michael D. M., Marnie Purciel, Paulette Yousefzadeh, and Kathryn M. Neckerman. "Disparities in Neighborhood Food Environments: Implications of Measurement Strategies." *Economic Geography* 86, no. 4 (2010/10/01 2010): 409–30. https://doi.org/10.1111/j.1944-8287.2010.01084.x.

Badland, Hannah M., Mitch J. Duncan, and W. Kerry Mummery. "Travel Perceptions, Behaviors, and Environment by Degree of Urbanization." *Preventive Medicine* 47, no. 3 (2008): 265–69.

Bailey, Conner, Leif Jensen, and Elizabeth Ransom, eds. *Rural America in a Globalizing World: Problems and Prospects for the 2010s.* Morgantown: West Virginia University Press, 2014.

Ball, K., K. Lamb, N. Travaglini, and A. Ellaway. "Street Connectivity and Obesity in Glasgow, Scotland: Impact of Age, Sex and Socioeconomic Position." *Health and Place* 18 (2012): 1307–13.

Ballantyne-Brodie, E., D. Fassi, and G. Simone. *Coltivando: Making a University Convivial Garden.* Sweden: European Academy of Design, 2013.

Banyard, Victoria L. "Measurement and Correlates of Prosocial Bystander Behavior: The Case of Interpersonal Violence." *Violence and Victims* 23, no. 1 (2008): 83–97.

Baran, Perver K., Daniel A. Rodríguez, and Asad J. Khattak. "Space Syntax and Walking in a New Urbanist and Suburban Neighbourhoods." *Journal of Urban Design* 13, no. 1 (2008): 5–28.

Bar-Massada, Avi, Volker C. Radeloff, Susan I. Stewart, and Todd J. Hawbaker. "Wildfire Risk in the Wildland-Urban Interface: A Simulation Study in Northwestern Wisconsin." *Forest Ecology and Management* 258, no. 9 (2009): 1990–99.

Barros, Ana Paula Borba Gonçalves, Erika Cristine Kneib, Mariana de Paiva, and Giovanna Megumi Ishida Tedesco. "Analysis of Trip Generating Developments by Space Syntax: A Case Study of Brasília, Brazil." *Journal of Transport Literature* 8 (2014): 07–36. http://www.scielo.br/scielo.php?script=sci_arttext&pid=S2238-10312014000300002&nrm=iso.

Barros, Ana Paula Borba Gonçalves, Paulo Cesar Marques da Silva, and Frederico Rosa Borges de Holanda. "Exploratory Study of Space Syntax as a Traffic Assignment Tool." Paper presented at the Proceedings of the 6th International Space Syntax Symposium, Istanbul, Turkey, 2007.

Barton, Hugh, and Marcus Grant. "A Health Map for the Local Human Habitat." *Journal for the Royal Society for the Promotion of Health* 126, no. 6 (2006): 252–53.

Barton, Hugh, and Marcus Grant. "Urban Planning for Healthy Cities." *Journal of Urban Health* 90, no. 1 (2013): 129–41.

Barton, Hugh, Susan Thompson, Sarah Burgess, and Marcus Grant. *The Routledge Handbook of Planning for Health and Well-Being: Shaping a Sustainable and Healthy Future.* New York: Routledge, 2015.

Barton, Hugh, and Catherine Tsourou. *Healthy Urban Planning: A WHO Guide to Planning for People.* London: Spon Press, 2000.

Barton, J., and J. Pretty. "What Is the Best Dose of Nature and Green Exercise for Improving Mental Health? A Multi-Study Analysis." *Environmental Science and Technology* 44 (2010): 3947–55.

Barton, Stuart. "Which Clinical Studies Provide the Best Evidence?" *BMJ* 321, no. 7256 (2000): 255.

Bassett, David R. "Encouraging Physical Activity and Health through Active Transportation." *Kinesiology Review* 1, no. 1 (2012): 91–99.

Bassuk, Shari S., Thomas A. Glass, and Lisa F. Berkman. "Social Disengagement and Incident Cognitive Decline in Community-Dwelling Elderly Persons." *Annals of Internal Medicine* 131, no. 3 (1999): 165–73.

Batty, Michael. "The Size, Scale, and Shape of Cities." *Science* 319, no. 5864 (2008): 769–71.

Batty, Michael. "A Theory of City Size." *Science* 340, no. 6139 (2013): 1418–19.

Baum, Andrew, J. P. Garofalo, and Ann Marie Yali. "Socioeconomic Status and Chronic Stress: Does Stress Account for Ses Effects on Health?" *Annals of the New York Academy of Sciences* 896, no. 1 (1999): 131–44.

Bauman, Adrian E., Rodrigo S. Reis, James F. Sallis, Jonathan C. Wells, Ruth J. F. Loos, Brian W. Martin, and Lancet Physical Activity Series Working Group. "Correlates of Physical Activity: Why Are Some People Physically Active and Others Not?" *Lancet* 380, no. 9838 (2012): 258–71.

Beale, Calvin L. "Anatomy of Nonmetro High-Poverty Areas Common in Plight, Distinctive in Nature." *Amber Waves* 2, no. 1 (2004): 20.

Beavon, Daniel J. K., Patricia L. Brantingham, and Paul J. Brantingham. "The Influence of Street Networks on the Patterning of Property Offenses." In *Crime Prevention Studies*, edited by Ronald V. Clarke. Monsey, NY: Criminal Justice Press, 1994.

Beck, Madelyn. "Wind-Blown Pesticides an Issue in Courtrooms, Communities across U.S." Illinois Public Media, August 13, 2018. https://will.illinois.edu/news/story/wind-blown -pesticides-an-issue-in-courtrooms-communities-across-u.s.

Befort, Christie A., Niaman Nazir, and Michael G. Perri. "Prevalence of Obesity among Adults from Rural and Urban Areas of the United States: Findings from NHANES (2005–2008)." *Journal of Rural Health* 28, no. 4 (2012): 392–97. https://doi.org/https://doi.org/10.1111/j .1748-0361.2012.00411.x.

Beil, Kurt, and Douglas Hanes. "The Influence of Urban Natural and Built Environments on Physiological and Psychological Measures of Stress: A Pilot Study." *International Journal of Environmental Research and Public Health* 10, no. 4 (2013): 1250–67.

Belay, Ermias D. "Transmissible Spongiform Encephalopathies in Humans." *Annual Reviews in Microbiology* 53, no. 1 (1999): 283–314.

Belden, J. N., and R. J. Wiener. *Housing in Rural America: Building Affordable and Inclusive Communities.* Thousand Oaks, CA: SAGE Publications, 1998. https://books.google.com /books?id=oG2PAAAAIAAJ.

Belkic, Karen L., Paul A. Landsbergis, Peter L. Schnall, and Dean Baker. "Is Job Strain a Major Source of Cardiovascular Disease Risk?" *Scandinavian Journal of Work, Environment and Health* 30, no. 2 (2004): 85–128.

Bellamy, Gail R., Jane Nelson Bolin, and Larry D. Gamm. "Rural Healthy People 2010, 2020, and Beyond: The Need Goes On." *Family and Community Health* 34, no. 2 (2011): 182–88.

Bennett, Kate Mary. "Low Level Social Engagement as a Precursor of Mortality among People in Later Life." *Age and Ageing* 31, no. 3 (2002): 165–68.

Bennett, Kevin J., Bankole Olatosi, and Janice C. Probst. *Health Disparities: A Rural-Urban Chartbook.* Columbia: South Carolina Rural Health Research Center, 2008.

Berger, Michael L. *The Devil Wagon in God's Country: The Automobile and Social Change in Rural America, 1893–1929.* Hamden, CT: Archon Books, 1979.

Berke, Ethan M. "Geographic Information Systems (GIS): Recognizing the Importance of Place in Primary Care Research and Practice." *Journal of the American Board of Family Medicine* 23, no. 1 (2010): 9–12.

Berrigan, David, Linda W. Pickle, and Jennifer Dill. "Associations between Street Connectivity and Active Transportation." *International Journal of Health Geographics* 9, no. 1 (2010): 20.

Besser, Terry L., and Margaret M. Hanson. "Development of Last Resort: The Impact of New State Prisons on Small Town Economies in the United States." *Community Development* 35, no. 2 (2004): 1.

Bethea, Traci N., Russell P. Lopez, Yvette C. Cozier, Laura F. White, and Michael D. McClean. "The Relationship between Rural Status, Individual Characteristics, and Self-Rated Health in the Behavioral Risk Factor Surveillance System." *Journal of Rural Health* 28, no. 4 (2012): 327–38.

Bettencourt, Luís M. A., José Lobo, Dirk Helbing, Christian Kühnert, and Geoffrey B. West. "Growth, Innovation, Scaling, and the Pace of Life in Cities." *Proceedings of the National Academy of Sciences* 104, no. 17 (2007): 7301–06.

Bevis, C., and J. Nutter. *Changing Street Layouts to Reduce Residential Burglary.* Minneapolis, MN: Crime Prevention Center, 1978.

Beyer, Kirsten M. M., Sara Comstock, Renea Seagren, and Gerard Rushton. "Explaining Place-Based Colorectal Cancer Health Disparities: Evidence from a Rural Context." *Social Science and Medicine* 72, no. 3 (2011): 373–82.

Bickel, Amy. "Downward Flow's Ripples: Oil, Gas Downturn Hitting Counties on Many Levels." *Hutchinson News*, February 13, 2016. https://www.hutchnews.com/story/news /local/2016/02/13/downward-flow-s-ripples-oil/20971196007/.

Bickel, Amy. "Faith Still Strong in Ghost Town of Willowdale." *Hutchinson News*, July 30, 2017. https://www.hutchnews.com/news/20170730/faith-still-strong-in-ghost-town-of -willowdale/1.

Biesecker, Michael, and Gary D. Robertson. "Hurricane Florence Breaches Manure Lagoon, Coal Ash Pit in North Carolina." PBS NewsHour, September 17, 2018. https://www.pbs .org/newshour/nation/hurricane-florence-breaches-manure-lagoon-coal-ash-pit-in -north-carolina.

Billings, C. G., and P. Howard. "Damp Housing and Asthma." *Monaldi Archives for chest Disease / Archivio Monaldi per le malattie del torace* 53, no. 1 (1998): 43–49.

Black, J. L., J. Macinko, L. B. Dixon, and J. G. E. Fryer. "Neighborhoods and Obesity in New York City." *Health and Place* 16 (2010): 489–99.

Blackwell, Debra L., Jacqueline W. Lucas, and Tainya C. Clarke. "Summary Health Statistics for US Adults: National Health Interview Survey, 2012." *Vital and Health Statistics* 260 (2014).

Blair, Steven N., James B. Kampert, Harold W. Kohl, Carolyn E. Barlow, Caroline A. Macera, Ralph S. Paffenbarger, and Larry W. Gibbons. "Influences of Cardiorespiratory Fitness and Other Precursors on Cardiovascular Disease and All-Cause Mortality in Men and Women." *Journal of the American Medical Association* 276, no. 3 (1996): 205–10.

Blalock, Hubert M., and Paul H. Wilken. *Intergroup Processes: A Micro-Macro Perspective.* New York: Free Press, 1979.

Blanck, Heidi Michels, Linda Nebeling, Amy L. Yaroch, and Olivia M. Thompson. "Improving Fruit and Vegetable Consumption: Use of Farm-to-Consumer Venues among US Adults." *Preventing Chronic Disease* 8, no. 2 (2011): A49.

Block, Jason P., Richard A. Scribner, and Karen B. DeSalvo. "Fast Food, Race/Ethnicity, and Income: A Geographic Analysis." *American Journal of Preventive Medicine* 27, no. 3 (2004): 211–17.

Block, Melissa. "Despite Economic Troubles, Residents of Kansas Town Remain Proud." NPR, January 26, 2017. https://www.npr.org/2017/01/26/511851731/despite-economic-troubles -residents-of-kansas-town-remain-proud.

Bluestone, Barry, and Bennett Harrison. *The Deindustrialization of America: Plant Closings,*

Community Abandonment, and the Dismantling of Basic Industry. New York: Basic Books, 1982.

Blumstein, A., F. P. Rivara, and R. Rosenfeld. "The Rise and Decline of Homicide—and Why." In *Annual Review of Public Health*, edited by J. E. Fielding, 505–41. Palo Alto, CA: Annual Reviews, 2000.

Boehmer, Tegan K., C. M. Hoehner, A. D. Deshpande, L. K. Brennan Ramirez, and R. C. Brownson. "Perceived and Observed Neighborhood Indicators of Obesity among Urban Adults." *International Journal of Obesity* 31 (2007): 968–77.

Boehmer, Tegan K., Sarah L. Lovegreen, Debra Haire-Joshu, and Ross C. Brownson. "What Constitutes an Obesogenic Environment in Rural Communities?" *American Journal of Health Promotion* 20, no. 6 (2006): 411–21.

Boer, R., Y. Zheng, A. Overton, G. K. Ridgeway, and D. A. Cohen. "Neighborhood Design and Walking Trips in Ten U.S. Metropolitan Areas." *American Journal of Preventive Medicine* 32 (2007): 298–304.

Bolin, Jane N., Gail R. Bellamy, Alva O. Ferdinand, Ann M. Vuong, Bita A. Kash, Avery Schulze, and Janet W. Helduser. "Rural Healthy People 2020: New Decade, Same Challenges." *Journal of Rural Health* 31, no. 3 (2015): 326–33.

Bopp, Melissa, Andrew T. Kaczynski, and Gina Besenyi. "Active Commuting Influences among Adults." *Preventive Medicine* 54, no. 3–4 (2012): 237–41.

Bopp, Melissa, Andrew T. Kaczynski, and Matthew E. Campbell. "Social Ecological Influences on Work-Related Active Commuting among Adults." *American Journal of Health Behavior* 37, no. 4 (2013): 543–54.

Bowers, K., S. Johnson, and A. Hirschfield. "Closing-Off Opportunities for Crime: An Evaluation of Alley-Gating." *European Journal on Criminal Policy and Research* 10, no. 4 (2005): 285–308.

Boyer, Corrine. "Tyson Plant Fire Sends Ripples of Uncertainty through Western Kansas, Cattle Industry." High Plains Public Radio, August 22, 2019. https://www.harvestpublic media.org/post/tyson-plant-fire-sends-ripples-uncertainty-through-western-kansas -cattle-industry.

Boyer, Corrine. "Why the Cattle Industry Might Not Use a Drug That Cuts the Pollution of Manure and Pee." High Plains Public Radio, July 9, 2019. https://www.kcur.org/2019-07 -09/why-the-cattle-industry-might-not-use-a-drug-that-cuts-the-pollution-of-manure -and-pee.

Brauer, M., G. Hoek, P. Van Vliet, K. Meliefste, P. H. Fischer, A. Wijga, L. P. Koopman, et al. "Air Pollution from Traffic and the Development of Respiratory Infections and Asthmatic and Allergic Symptoms in Children." *American Journal of Respiratory and Critical Care Medicine* 166 (2002): 1092–98.

Braveman, Brent. "AOTA's Statement on Health Disparities." *American Journal of Occupational Therapy* 60, no. 6 (2006): 679.

Briggs, Ronald, and William A. Leonard IV. "Mortality and Ecological Structure: A Canonical Approach." *Social Science and Medicine (1967)* 11, no. 14–16 (1977): 757–62.

Britt, Karrey. "New Health Assessment Identifies 13 Challenges That Douglas County Residents Face." *Baldwin City (KS) Signal*, April 30, 2012. http://signal.baldwincity.com/news /2012/apr/30/new-health-assessment-identifies-13-challenges-dou/.

Britton, M., A. J. Fox, P. Goldblatt, D. R. Jones, and M. Rosato. *The Influence of Socio-Economic and Environmental Factors on Geographic Variation in Mortality.* London: Office of Population, Censuses and Surveys, 1990.

Broadway, Michael. "Meatpacking and the Transformation of Rural Communities: A Comparison of Brooks, Alberta and Garden City, Kansas." *Rural Sociology* 72, no. 4 (2007): 560–82.

Brown, Barbara B., Ken R. Smith, Heidi Hanson, Jessie X. Fan, Lori Kowaleski-Jones, and Cathleen D. Zick. "Neighborhood Design for Walking and Biking: Physical Activity and Body Mass Index." *American Journal of Preventive Medicine* 44, no. 3 (2013): 231–38.

Brown, Barbara B., Ikuho Yamada, Ken R. Smith, Cathleen D. Zick, Lori Kowaleski-Jones, and Jessie X. Fan. "Mixed Land Use and Walkability: Variations in Land Use Measures and Relationships with BMI, Overweight, and Obesity." *Health and Place* 15, no. 4 (2009): 1130–41.

Brown, Caroline, Glen Bramley, and David Watkins. *Urban Green Nation: Building the Evidence Base*. London: Chartered Association of Building Engineers, 2010.

Brown, David L., John B. Cromartie, and Laszlo J. Kulcsar. "Micropolitan Areas and the Measurement of American Urbanization." *Population Research and Policy Review* 23, no. 4 (2004): 399–418.

Brown, David L., Glenn V. Fuguitt, Tun B. Heaton, and Saba Waseem. "Continuities in Size of Place Preferences in the United States, 1972–1992." *Rural Sociology* 62, no. 4 (1997): 408–28.

Brown, David L., and Nina Glasgow. *Rural Retirement Migration*. Vol. 21. N.p.: Springer Science and Business Media, 2008.

Brown, David L., and L. E. Swanson. *Challenges for Rural America in the Twenty-First Century*. University Park: Pennsylvania State University Press, 2010. https://books.google.com /books?id=pgfsiynCAXYC.

Brown, Susan L., and Anastasia R. Snyder. "Residential Differences in Cohabitors' Union Transitions." *Rural Sociology* 71, no. 2 (2006): 311–34.

Brownson, Ross C., Laura Hagood, Sarah L. Lovegreen, Betty Britton, Nicole M. Caito, Michael B. Elliott, Jennifer Emery, et al. "A Multilevel Ecological Approach to Promoting Walking in Rural Communities." *Preventive Medicine* 41, no. 5–6 (2005): 837–42.

Brownson, Ross C., C. M. Hoehner, K. Day, A. Forsyth, and J. F. Sallis. "Measuring the Built Environment for Physical Activity: State of the Science." *American Journal of Preventive Medicine* 36 (2009): S99–123.e12.

Brownson, Ross C., Robyn A. Housemann, David R. Brown, Jeannette Jackson-Thompson, Abby C. King, Bernard R. Malone, and James F. Sallis. "Promoting Physical Activity in Rural Communities: Walking Trail Access, Use, and Effects." *American Journal of Preventive Medicine* 18, no. 3 (2000): 235–41.

Buck, Andrew J., Simon Hakim, and Uriel Spiegel. "Endogenous Crime Victimization, Taxes and Property Values." *Social Science Quarterly* 74, no. 2 (1993): 334–48.

Bureau of Epidemiology and Public Health Informatics. *Kansas: Annual Summary of Vital Statistics, 2019*. Topeka: Kansas Department of Health and Environment, 2020. http:// www.kdheks.gov/bephi/.

Bureau of Health Promotion. "Diabetes Control and Prevention—Numbers to Know." Kansas Department of Health and Environment, 2021. Accessed September 18, 2021. https://www .kdheks.gov/diabetes/numbers_to_know.htm.

Burgoine, T., S. Alvanides, and A. A. Lake. "Assessing the Obesogenic Environment of North East England." *Health and Place* 17 (2011): 738–47.

Burr, M. L., A. S. St Leger, and J. W. G. Yarnell. "Wheezing, Dampness, and Coal Fires." *Journal of Public Health* 3, no. 3 (1981): 205–9.

Burton, Libby. "Mental Well-Being and the Influence of Place." In *The Routledge Handbook of Planning for Health and Well-Being: Shaping a Sustainable and Healthy Future*, edited by Hugh Barton, Susan Thompson, Sarah Burgess, and Marcus Grant, 150–61. New York: Routledge, 2015.

Burton, Libby M., R. Garrett-Peters, and J. M. Eason. "Mortality, Identity, and Mental Health in Rural Ghettos." In *Communities, Neighborhoods, and Health: Expanding the Boundaries of Place*, edited by L. M. Burton, S. P. Kemp, M. Leung, S. A. Matthews, and D. T. Takeuchi, 91–110. New York: Springer, 2011.

Burton, Nicola W., Gavin Turrell, Brian Oldenburg, and James F. Sallis. "The Relative Contributions of Psychological, Social, and Environmental Variables to Explain Participation in Walking, Moderate-, and Vigorous-Intensity Leisure-Time Physical Activity." *Journal of Physical Activity and Health* 2, no. 2 (2005): 181–96.

Butler, Colin. *Climate Change and Global Health.* Oxfordshire, UK: CABI, 2016.

Butler, Eboneé N., Anita M. H. Ambs, Jill Reedy, and Heather R. Bowles. "Identifying GIS Measures of the Physical Activity Built Environment through a Review of the Literature." *Journal of Physical Activity and Health* 8, no. s1 (2011): S91–S97.

Caldwell, Tanya M., Anthony F. Jorm, and Keith B. G. Dear. "Suicide and Mental Health in Rural, Remote and Metropolitan Areas in Australia." *Medical Journal of Australia* 181 (2004): S10–S14.

Calhoun, John B. "Population Density and Social Pathology." *Scientific American* 206, no. 2 (1962): 139–49.

Campoli, J. *Made for Walking.* Cambridge, MA: Lincoln Institute of Land Policy, 2012.

Carlson, Susan A., Janet E. Fulton, Michael Pratt, Zhou Yang, and E. Kathleen Adams. "Inadequate Physical Activity and Health Care Expenditures in the United States." *Progress in Cardiovascular Diseases* 57, no. 4 (2015): 315–23.

Carr, P., and M. Kefalas. *Hollowing Out the Middle: The Rural Brain Drain and What It Means for America.* Boston: Beacon Press, 2009.

Carrion-Flores, Carmen, and Elena G. Irwin. "Determinants of Residential Land-Use Conversion and Sprawl at the Rural-Urban Fringe." *American Journal of Agricultural Economics* 86, no. 4 (2004): 889–904.

Carver, Alison, Anna Timperio, and David Crawford. "Playing It Safe: The Influence of Neighborhood Safety on Children's Physical Activity—a Review." *Health and Place* 14, no. 2 (2008): 217–27.

Carver, Alison, Anna Timperio, Kylie Hesketh, and David Crawford. "Are Safety-Related Features of the Road Environment Associated with Smaller Declines in Physical Activity among Youth?" *Journal of Urban Health* 87, no. 1 (2010): 29–43.

Casavant, Ken, Marina R. Denicoff, Eric Jessup, April Taylor, Daniel Nibarger, David Sears, Hayk Khachatryan, et al. *Study of Rural Transportation Issues (No. 147544).* Washington, DC: Department of Agriculture, Agricultural Marketing Service, Transportation and Marketing Program, 2010.

Casperson, C. J., K. E. Powell, and G. M. Christenson. "Physical Activity, Exercise, and Physical Fitness." *Public Health Reports* 100 (1985): 125–31.

Caspi, Caitlin E., Glorian Sorensen, S. V. Subramanian, and Ichiro Kawachi. "The Local Food Environment and Diet: A Systematic Review." *Health and Place* 18, no. 5 (2012): 1172–87.

Castro, Dina C., Margaret Samuels, and Ann E. Harman. "Growing Healthy Kids: A Community Garden–Based Obesity Prevention Program." *American Journal of Preventive Medicine* 44, no. 3 (2013): S193–S99.

Cauthon, P. "Health Improvement Initiative Launched to Identify State's Priorities." KHI News Service, August 29, 2012. https://www.khi.org/news/article/health-improvement-initiative -launched-identify-st.

Cavill, Nick, Sonja Kahlmeier, Harry Rutter, Francesca Racioppi, and Pekka Oja. "Economic Analyses of Transport Infrastructure and Policies Including Health Effects Related to Cycling and Walking: A Systematic Review." *Transport Policy* 15, no. 5 (2008): 291–304.

Cecil G. Sheps Center for Health Services Research. "Rural Hospital Closures." Accessed September 19, 2021. https://www.shepscenter.unc.edu/programs-projects/rural-health /rural-hospital-closures/.

Center on the Developing Child at Harvard University. *The Foundations of Lifelong Health Are Built in Early Childhood.* Cambridge, MA: Center on the Developing Child at Harvard University, 2010.

Centers for Disease Control and Prevention. "Behavioral Risk Factor Surveillance System." US Department of Health and Human Services, August 30, 2021. https://www.cdc.gov/brfss/index.html.

Centers for Disease Control and Prevention. "CDC Health Disparities and Inequalities Report-United States, 2011." In *Morbidity and Mortality Weekly Report (MMWR), Vol. 60 (Supplement).* Atlanta, GA: Department of Health and Human Services, 2011. http.//www.cdc.gov/mmwr/pdf/other/su6001.pdf.

Centers for Disease Control and Prevention. "Healthy Weight, Nutrition, and Physical Activity: About Adult BMI." Division of Nutrition, Physical Activity, and Obesity, National Center for Chronic Disease Prevention and Health Promotion, updated August 27, 2021, https://www.cdc.gov/healthyweight/assessing/bmi/adult_bmi/index.html#.

Centers for Disease Control and Prevention. *National Diabetes Statistics Report.* Atlanta, GA: Department of Health and Human Services, 2020. https://www.cdc.gov/diabetes/pdfs/data/statistics/national-diabetes-statistics-report.pdf.

Centers for Disease Control and Prevention. "Only 1 in 10 Adults Get Enough Fruits or Vegetables." February 16, 2021. https://www.cdc.gov/nccdphp/dnpao/division-information/media-tools/adults-fruits-vegetables.html.

Centers for Disease Control and Prevention. "Physical Activity." Updated January 14, 2020. https://www.cdc.gov/physicalactivity/data/index.html?CDC_AA_refVal=https%3A%2F%2Fwww.cdc.gov%2Fphysicalactivity%2Fdata%2Ffacts.htm.

Centers for Disease Control and Prevention. "Places: Local Data for Better Health." US Department of Health and Human Services, December 8, 2020. https://www.cdc.gov/places/.

Centers for Disease Control and Prevention. *Strategies to Prevent Obesity and Other Chronic Diseases: The CDC Guide to Strategies to Increase Physical Activity in the Community.* Atlanta, GA: Department of Health and Human Services, 2011.

Centers for Disease Control and Prevention. "Suicide Increasing among American Workers." CDC Newsroom news release, November 15, 2018. https://www.cdc.gov/media/releases/2018/p1115-Suicide-american-workers.html.

Cerin, Ester, and Eva Leslie. "How Socio-Economic Status Contributes to Participation in Leisure-Time Physical Activity." *Social Science and Medicine* 66, no. 12 (2008): 2596–609.

Cerin, Ester, Eva Leslie, and Neville Owen. "Explaining Socio-Economic Status Differences in Walking for Transport: An Ecological Analysis of Individual, Social and Environmental Factors." *Social Science and Medicine* 68, no. 6 (2009): 1013–20.

Cerin, Ester, Duncan J. Macfarlane, Hin-Hei Ko, and Kwok-Cheung A. Chan. "Measuring Perceived Neighborhood Walkability in Hong Kong." *Cities* 24, no. 3 (2007): 209–17.

Cervero, Robert. "Land-Use Mixing and Suburban Mobility." *Transportation Quarterly* 42 (1988): 429–46.

Cervero, Robert. "Linking Urban Transport and Land Use in Developing Countries." *Journal of Transport and Land Use* 6, no. 1 (2013): 7–24.

Cervero, Robert. "Mixed Land-Uses and Commuting: Evidence from the American Housing Survey." *Transportation Research Part A: Policy and Practice* 30 (1996): 361–77.

Cervero, Robert, and K. Kockelman. "Travel Demand and the 3Ds: Density, Diversity, and Design." *Transportation Research Part D: Transport and Environment* 2 (1997): 199–219.

Chan, Jonathan J., and Julienne E. Chan. "Medicine for the Millennium: The Challenge of Postmodernism." *Medical Journal of Australia* 172, no. 7 (2000): 332–34.

Charreire, Hélène, Romain Casey, Paul Salze, Chantal Simon, Basile Chaix, Arnaud Banos, Dominique Badariotti, Christiane Weber, and Jean-Michel Oppert. "Measuring the Food

Environment Using Geographical Information Systems: A Methodological Review." *Public Health Nutrition* 13, no. 11 (2010): 1773–85.

Chavez, Sergio. "Community, Ethnicity, and Class in a Changing Rural California Town." *Rural Sociology* 70, no. 3 (2005): 314–35.

Chee-Sanford, Joanne C., Roderick I. Mackie, Satoshi Koike, Ivan G. Krapac, Yu-Feng Lin, Anthony C. Yannarell, Scott Maxwell, and Rustam I. Aminov. "Fate and Transport of Antibiotic Residues and Antibiotic Resistance Genes Following Land Application of Manure Waste." *Journal of Environmental Quality* 38, no. 3 (2009): 1086–108.

Chen, Juan, Deborah S. Davis, Kaming Wu, and Haijing Dai. "Life Satisfaction in Urbanizing China: The Effect of City Size and Pathways to Urban Residency." *Cities* 49 (December 2015): 88–97. https://doi.org/https://doi.org/10.1016/j.cities.2015.07.011.

Chetty, Raj, Michael Stepner, Sarah Abraham, Shelby Lin, Benjamin Scuderi, Nicholas Turner, Augustin Bergeron, and David Cutler. "The Association between Income and Life Expectancy in the United States, 2001–2014." *Journal of the American Medical Association* 315, no. 16 (2016): 1750–66. https://doi.org/10.1001/jama.2016.4226.

Cheung, Monit, Patrick Leung, and Peter Viet Nguyen. "City Size Matters: Vietnamese Immigrants Having Depressive Symptoms." *Social Work in Mental Health* 15, no. 4 (July 2017): 457–68. https://doi.org/10.1080/15332985.2016.1231156.

Chiaradia, Alain, Edouard Moreau, and Noah Raford. "Configurational Exploration of Public Transport Movement Networks: A Case Study, the London Underground." Paper presented at the Proceedings of the 5th International Space Syntax Symposium. Delft, 2005.

Chillón, Palma, Kelly R. Evenson, Amber Vaughn, and Dianne S. Ward. "A Systematic Review of Interventions for Promoting Active Transportation to School." *International Journal of Behavioral Nutrition and Physical Activity* 8, no. 1 (2011): 10.

Chilson, Morgan. "'A Huge Blow': SKF to Close Seneca Factory, Eliminating 170 Jobs." *Topeka Capital-Journal*, October 24, 2017. https://www.cjonline.com/news/business/2017-10-24/huge-blow-skf-close-seneca-factory-eliminating-170-jobs.

Cho, W. K., and S. Ogunwole. "Black Workers in Southern Rural Labor Markets." In *Research in Rural Sociology and Development*, edited by W. W. Falk and T. A. Lyson, 189–206. Greenwich, CT: JAI, 1989.

Christenson, Bruce A., and Nan E. Johnson. "Educational Inequality in Adult Mortality: An Assessment with Death Certificate Data from Michigan." *Demography* 32, no. 2 (1995): 215–29.

Christian, W. Jay. "Using Geospatial Technologies to Explore Activity-Based Retail Food Environments." *Spatial and Spatio-Temporal Epidemiology* 3, no. 4 (2012): 287–95.

Clark, Charlotte, and Stephen A. Stansfeld. "The Effect of Transportation Noise on Health and Cognitive Development: A Review of Recent Evidence." *International Journal of Comparative Psychology* 20, no. 2 (2007).

Clark, Jill K., Ronald McChesney, Darla K. Munroe, and Elena G. Irwin. "Spatial Characteristics of Exurban Settlement Pattern in the United States." *Landscape and Urban Planning* 90, no. 3–4 (2009): 178–88.

Clark, P., N. Mapes, J. Burt, and S. Preston. *Greening Dementia: A Literature Review of the Benefits and Barriers Facing Individuals Living with Dementia in Accessing the Natural Environment and Local Greenspace.* Worcester: Natural England, 2013.

Clean Air Partnership. *Bike Lanes, On-Street Parking and Business: Year 2 Report—a Study of Bloor Street in Toronto's Bloor West Village.* Toronto: Clean Air Partnership, 2010. https://www.cleanairpartnership.org/wp-content/uploads/2016/08/BikeLanes_Parking_Business_BloorWestVillageNewCover.pdf.

Clem, Marcus. "Fargo Factory to Shut Down." *Atchison Globe*, May 2, 2019. https://www

.atchisonglobenow.com/news/local_news/fargo-factory-to-shut-down/article_5e8cfa3a
-6ce2-11e9-8098-d795d7578df8.html.

Cloke, Paul. "Conceptualizing Rurality." In *Handbook of Rural Studies*, edited by P. Cloke,
T. Marsden, and P. H. Mooney, 18–28. London: Sage, 2006.

Coates, Vary, and Ernest Weiss. *Revitalization of Small Communities: Transportation Options.
Second Year Report.* Vol. 1. Washington, DC: Department of Transportation, 1975.

Cohen, Deborah A., J. Scott Ashwood, Molly M. Scott, Adrian Overton, Kelly R. Evenson,
Lisa K. Staten, Dwayne Porter, Thomas L. McKenzie, and Diane Catellier. "Public Parks
and Physical Activity among Adolescent Girls." *Pediatrics* 118, no. 5 (2006): e1381–e89.

Cohen, Deborah A., Scott Ashwood, Molly Scott, Adrian Overton, Kelly R. Evenson,
Carolyn C. Voorhees, Ariane Bedimo-Rung, and Thomas L. McKenzie. "Proximity
to School and Physical Activity among Middle School Girls: The Trial of Activity for
Adolescent Girls Study." *Journal of Physical Activity and Health* 3, no. s1 (2006): S129–S38.

Cohen, Deborah A., C. Mason, A. Bedimo, R. Scribner, V. Basolo, and T. A. Farley. "Neighborhood Physical Conditions and Health." *American Journal of Public Health* 93 (2003):
467–71.

Cohen, Steven A., Sarah K. Cook, Lauren Kelley, Julia D. Foutz, and Trisha A. Sando. "A
Closer Look at Rural-Urban Health Disparities: Associations between Obesity and
Rurality Vary by Geospatial and Sociodemographic Factors." *Journal of Rural Health* 33,
no. 2 (2017): 167–79.

Colclough, Glenna. "Uneven Development and Racial Composition in the Deep South." *Rural
Sociology* 53, no. 1 (1988): 73–86.

Coleman-Jensen, Alisha, Matthew P. Rabbitt, Christian A. Gregory, and Anita Singh. *Household Food Security in the United States in 2016, Err-237.* Washington, DC: Department of
Agriculture, Economic Research Service, 2017.

Collins, Peter, Yahya Al-Nakeeb, Alan Nevill, and Mark Lyons. "The Impact of the Built Environment on Young People's Physical Activity Patterns: A Suburban-Rural Comparison
Using GPS." *International Journal of Environmental Research and Public Health* 9, no. 9
(2012): 3030–50.

Committee on Capitalizing on Social Science and Behavioral Research to Improve the Public's
Health, Division of Health Promotion Disease Prevention, and Institute of Medicine.
"Promoting Health: Intervention Strategies from Social and Behavioral Research." *Amer-
ican Journal of Health Promotion* 15, no. 3 (2001): 149–66.

Committee on the Medical Effects of Air Pollutants. *The Mortality Effects of Long-Term Exposure to Particulate Air Pollution in the UK.* London: HMSO, 2010.

Committee on Physical Activity Health, Transportation and Land Use, Transportation Research Board, Institute of Medicine of the National Academies. *Does the Built Environment
Influence Physical Activity? Examining the Evidence.* Washington, DC: National Academy
of Sciences, 2005.

Commonwealth Fund Commission on Elderly People Living Alone. *Old, Alone, and Poor: A
Plan for Reducing Poverty among Elderly People Living Alone.* New York: Commonwealth
Fund, 1987.

Commonwealth of Australia. *National Strategic Framework for Rural and Remote Health.*
Canberra: Commonwealth of Australia, 2012.

Connor, Robert A., John E. Kralewski, and Steven D. Hillson. "Measuring Geographic Access
to Health Care in Rural Areas." *Medical Care Review* 51, no. 3 (1994): 337–77.

Cooper, Ashley R., Lars Bo Andersen, Niels Wedderkopp, Angie S. Page, and Karsten Fro-
berg. "Physical Activity Levels of Children Who Walk, Cycle, or Are Driven to School."
American Journal of Preventive Medicine 29, no. 3 (2005): 179–84.

Corburn, Jason. *Toward the Healthy City: People, Places, and the Politics of Urban Planning.* Cambridge, MA: MIT Press, 2009.

Corburn, Jason. "Urban Inequities, Population Health and Spatial Planning." Chap. 3 in *The Routledge Handbook of Planning for Health and Well-Being: Shaping a Sustainable and Healthy Future,* edited by Hugh Barton, Susan Thompson, Sarah Burgess, and Marcus Grant, 37–47. New York: Routledge, 2015.

Cornwall, Andrea. "Unpacking 'Participation': Models, Meanings and Practices." *Community Development Journal* 43, no. 3 (2008): 269–83.

Cornwell, Erin York. "Social Resources and Disordered Living Conditions: Evidence from a National Sample of Community-Residing Older Adults." *Research on Aging* 36, no. 4 (2014): 399–430.

Corrigan, J. M., P. Aspden, L. P. Snyder, J. Wolcott, G. Wunderlich, and B. Russell. *Quality through Collaboration: The Future of Rural Health.* Washington, DC: Institute of Medicine, National Academies Press, 2004.

Costello, Anthony, Mustafa Abbas, Adriana Allen, Sarah Ball, Sarah Bell, Richard Bellamy, Sharon Friel, et al. "Managing the Health Effects of Climate Change: Lancet and University College London Institute for Global Health Commission." *Lancet* 373, no. 9676 (2009): 1693–733.

Courtin, Emilie, and Martin Knapp. "Social Isolation, Loneliness and Health in Old Age: A Scoping Review." *Health and Social Care in the Community* 25, no. 3 (2017): 799–812.

Coutts, Christopher, Timothy Chapin, Mark Horner, and Crystal Taylor. "County-Level Effects of Green Space Access on Physical Activity." *Journal of Physical Activity and Health* 10, no. 2 (2013): 232–40.

Coveney, John, and Lisel A. O'Dwyer. "Effects of Mobility and Location on Food Access." *Health and Place* 15, no. 1 (2009): 45–55.

Cozens, P. "Crime and Community Safety: Challenging the Design Consensus." In *The Routledge Handbook of Planning for Health and Well-Being: Shaping a Sustainable and Healthy Future,* edited by Hugh Barton, Susan Thompson, Sarah Burgess, and Marcus Grant, 87–107. New York: Routledge, 2015.

Cozens, P., and T. Love. "Permeability as a Process for Controlling Crime: A View from Western Australia." *Built Environment* 35, no. 3 (2009): 346–65.

Crawford, Mike J., Deborah Rutter, Catherine Manley, Timothy Weaver, Kamaldeep Bhui, Naomi Fulop, and Peter Tyrer. "Systematic Review of Involving Patients in the Planning and Development of Health Care." *BMJ* 325, no. 7375 (2002): 1263.

Crimmins, Eileen, Jung Ki Kim, and Sarinnapha Vasunilashorn. "Biodemography: New Approaches to Understanding Trends and Differences in Population Health and Mortality." *Demography* 47, no. 1 (2010): S41–S64.

Cromartie, John, and Shawn Bucholtz. "Defining the 'Rural' in Rural America." *Amber Waves* 6, no. 3 (2008).

Crompton, John L. "The Impact of Parks on Property Values: A Review of the Empirical Evidence." *Journal of Leisure Research* 33, no. 1 (2001): 1–31.

Crosby, R. A., M. L. Wendel, R. C. Vanderpool, and B. R. Casey. *Rural Populations and Health: Determinants, Disparities, and Solutions.* San Francisco: Wiley, 2012. https://books.google.com/books?id=6owvQM1FAEgC.

Croucher, K., L. Myers, and J. Bretherton. *The Links between Greenspace and Health: A Critical Literature Review.* Stirling: Greenspace Scotland, 2007.

Crowley, Martha, and Daniel T. Lichter. "Social Disorganization in New Latino Destinations?" *Rural Sociology* 74, no. 4 (2009): 573–604.

Cubit Planning. "Kansas Cities by Population." 2020, accessed August 3, 2020, https://www.kansas-demographics.com/cities_by_population.

Cummins, Steven, Sarah Curtis, Ana V. Diez-Roux, and Sally Macintyre. "Understanding and Representing 'Place' in Health Research: A Relational Approach." *Social Science and Medicine* 65, no. 9 (2007): 1825–38.

Cummins, Steven, and Sally Macintyre. "Food Environments and Obesity—Neighborhood or Nation?" *International Journal of Epidemiology* 35, no. 1 (2006): 100–104.

Cummins, Steven C. J., Laura McKay, and Sally MacIntyre. "McDonald's Restaurants and Neighborhood Deprivation in Scotland and England." *American Journal of Preventive Medicine* 29, no. 4 (2005): 308–10.

Curric, Janct, Stefano DellaVigna, Enrico Moretti, and Vikram Pathania. "The Effect of Fast-Food Restaurants on Obesity and Weight Gain." *American Economic Journal: Economic Policy* 2, no. 3 (2010): 32–63.

Curry, Susan J., Edward H. Wagner, Paula Diehr, Allen Cheadle, Thomas Koepsell, Bruce Psaty, and Colleen McBride. "Assessment of Community-Level Influences on Individuals' Attitudes about Cigarette Smoking, Alcohol Use, and Consumption of Dietary Fat." *American Journal of Preventive Medicine* 9, no. 2 (1993): 78–84.

Cutler, David M., and Adriana Lleras-Muney. "Education and Health: Evaluating Theories and Evidence." In *Making Americans Healthier: Social and Economic Policy as Health Policy*, edited by R. F. Schoeni, J. S. House, G. A. Kaplan, and H. Pollack, 29–60. New York: Russell Sage Foundation, 2008.

Cutler, David M., and Adriana Lleras-Muney. "Understanding Differences in Health Behaviors by Education." *Journal of Health Economics* 29, no. 1 (2010): 1–28.

Cutler, Stephen J., and Raymond T. Coward. "Residence Differences in the Health Status of Elders." *Journal of Rural Health* 4, no. 3 (1988): 11–26.

Cutumisu, N., and J. C. Spence. "Exploring Associations between Urban Environments and Children's Physical Activity: Making the Case for Space Syntax." *Journal of Science and Medicine in Sport* 12 (2009): 537–8.

Dahlgren, Göran, and Margaret Whitehead. *Policies and Strategies to Promote Social Equity in Health.* Stockholm: Institute for Future Studies, 1991.

Dáil, P. W. *Hard Living in America's Heartland: Rural Poverty in the 21st Century Midwest.* Jefferson, NC: McFarland, 2015. https://books.google.com/books?id=ozFzBgAAQBAJ.

Dalbey, M. "Implementing Smart Growth Strategies in Rural America: Development Patterns That Support Public Health Goals." *Journal of Public Health Management and Practice*, no. 14 (2008): 238–43.

Daniel, Terry C. "Measuring the Quality of the Natural Environment: A Psychophysical Approach." *American Psychologist* 45, no. 5 (1990): 633.

Dannenberg, Andrew L., Howard Frumkin, and Richard J. Jackson, eds. *Making Healthy Places.* Washington, DC: Island Press, 2011.

Danzinger, Sheldon. "Explaining Urban Crime Rates." *Criminology* 14 (1976): 291–96.

"Data USA." Accessed September 26, 2021. https://datausa.io/.

Davidson, O. G. *Broken Heartland: The Rise of America's Rural Ghetto.* Iowa City: University of Iowa Press, 1996.

Davidson, Scott. "Spinning the Wheel of Empowerment." *Planning* 1262, no. 3 (1998): 14–15.

Davies, John K., and Michael Kelly, eds. *Healthy Cities: Research and Practice.* New York: Routledge, 1993.

Davis, Adrian, and John Parkin. "Active Travel: Its Fall and Rise." In *The Routledge Handbook of Planning for Health and Well-Being: Shaping a Sustainable and Healthy Future*, edited by Hugh Barton, Susan Thompson, Sarah Burgess, and Marcus Grant, 108–20. New York: Routledge, 2015.

Davis, Ann McGrath, Kevin J. Bennett, Christie Befort, and Nikki Nollen. "Obesity and Related Health Behaviors among Urban and Rural Children in the United States: Data from the National Health and Nutrition Examination Survey 2003–2004 and 2005–2006." *Journal of Pediatric Psychology* 36, no. 6 (2011): 669–76.

Davis, Rachel, Danice Cook, and Larry Cohen. "A Community Resilience Approach to Reducing Ethnic and Racial Disparities in Health." *American Journal of Public Health* 95, no. 12 (2005): 2168–73.

Davison, Elizabeth, and William Smith. "Exploring Accessibility Versus Opportunity Crime Factors." *Sociation Today: The Journal of The North Carolina Sociological Association* 1, no. 1 (2003).

Day, Kristen. "Strangers in the Night: Women's Fear of Sexual Assault on Urban College Campuses." *Journal of Architectural and Planning Research* (1999): 289–312.

de Leeuw, Evelyne. "Evaluating Who Healthy Cities in Europe: Issues and Perspectives." *Journal of Urban Health* 90, no. 1 (2013): 14–22.

de Leeuw, Evelyne, and Jean Simos. "Healthy Cities Move to Maturity." In *Healthy Cities: The Theory, Policy, and Practice of Value-Based Urban Planning*, edited by Evelyne de Leeuw and Jean Simos, 75–86. New York: Springer, 2017.

Dempsey, Nicola, Caroline Brown, and Glen Bramley. "The Key to Sustainable Urban Development in UK Cities? The Influence of Density on Social Sustainability." *Progress in Planning* 77, no. 3 (2012): 89–141.

Dengel, Donald R., Mary O. Hearst, Joe H. Harmon, Ann Forsyth, and Leslie A. Lytle. "Does the Built Environment Relate to the Metabolic Syndrome in Adolescents?" *Health and Place* 15, no. 4 (2009): 946–51.

Deshpande, Anjali D., Elizabeth A. Baker, Sarah L. Lovegreen, and Ross C. Brownson. "Environmental Correlates of Physical Activity among Individuals with Diabetes in the Rural Midwest." *Diabetes Care* 28, no. 5 (2005): 1012–18.

De Vries, Sjerp, Robert A. Verheij, Peter P. Groenewegen, and Peter Spreeuwenberg. "Natural Environments—Healthy Environments? An Exploratory Analysis of the Relationship between Greenspace and Health." *Environment and Planning A* 35, no. 10 (2003): 1717–31.

Dibner, J. J., and J. D. Richards. "Antibiotic Growth Promoters in Agriculture: History and Mode of Action." *Poultry Science* 84, no. 4 (2005): 634–43.

Diehr, P., T. Koepsell, A. Cheadle, B. M. Psaty, E. Wagner, and S. Curry. "Do Communities Differ in Health Behaviors?" *Journal of Clinical Epidemiology* 46 (1993): 1141–49.

Diepenbrock, George. "Political Climate Spurs Kansas Immigrants to Fear Interactions in Daily Life, Study Finds." University of Kansas, April 16, 2018. https://news.ku.edu/2018 /04/11/political-climate-spurs-kansas-immigrants-fear-interactions-daily-life-study -finds.

Diez-Roux, A. V. "Investigating Neighborhood and Area Effects on Health." *American Journal of Public Health* 91, no. 11 (2001): 1783–89.

Diez-Roux, A. V. "On the Distinction—or Lack of Distinction—between Population Health and Public Health." *American Journal of Public Health* 106, no. 4 (2016): 619.

Diez-Roux, A. V., K. R. Evenson, A. P. McGinn, D. G. Brown, L. Moore, S. Brines, and D. R. Jacobs Jr. "Availability of Recreational Resources and Physical Activity in Adults." *American Journal of Public Health* 97 (2007): 493–99.

Diez-Roux, A. V., F. J. Nieto, C. Muntaner, H. A. Tyroler, G. W. Comstock, E. Shahar, L. S. Cooper, R. L. Watson, and M. Szklo. "Neighborhood Environments and Coronary Heart Disease: A Multilevel Analysis." *American Journal of Epidemiology* 146 (1997): 48–63.

Dimitri, Carolyn, Anne Effland, and Neilson C. Conklin. *The 20th Century Transformation of US Agriculture and Farm Policy*. Washington, DC: Department of Agriculture, Economic Research Service, 2005.

Dixon, Jane, and Emily Ballantyne-Brodie. "The Role of Planning and Design in Advancing a Bio-Nutrition-Sensitive Food System." In *The Routledge Handbook of Planning for Health and Well-Being: Shaping a Sustainable and Healthy Future*, edited by Hugh Barton, Susan Thompson, Sarah Burgess, and Marcus Grant, 178–94. New York: Routledge, 2015.

Dockery, Douglas W., C. Arden Pope, Xiping Xu, John D. Spengler, James H. Ware, Martha E. Fay, Benjamin G. Ferris Jr., and Frank E. Speizer. "An Association between Air Pollution and Mortality in Six US Cities." *New England Journal of Medicine* 329, no. 24 (1993): 1753–59.

Doescher, Mark P., Chanam Lee, Ethan M. Berke, Anna M. Adachi-Mejia, Chun-kuen Lee, Orion Stewart, Davis G. Patterson, et al. "The Built Environment and Utilitarian Walking in Small US Towns." *Preventive Medicine* 69 (2014): 80 86.

Domina, T. "What Clean Break? Education and Nonmetropolitan Migration Patterns, 1989–2004." *Rural Sociology* 71, no. 3 (2006): 373–98.

Douglass, Harlan Paul. *The Little Town: Especially in Its Rural Relationships*. New York: Macmillan, 1919.

Dowd, Rebecca. "Fracking Divides Small Town of Anthony, Kansas." *University Daily Kansan*, July 12, 2015. https://www.kansan.com/news/fracking-divides-small-town-of-anthony -kansas/article_f6c59722-2901-11e5-a0b8-2317e0115117.html.

Dowler, E. A., and B. M. Dobson. "Nutrition and Poverty in Europe: An Overview." *Proceedings of the Nutrition Society* 56, no. 1A (1997): 51–62.

Dowler, Elizabeth, Moya Kneafsey, Rosie Cox, and Lewis Holloway. "'Doing Food Differently': Reconnecting Biological and Social Relationships through Care for Food." *Sociological Review* 57, no. 2 (2009): 200–221.

Draper, R., L. Curtice, J. Hooper, and M. Goumans. *WHO Healthy Cities Project: Review of the First Five Years (1987–2002)*. Copenhagen: World Health Organization Regional Office for Europe, 1993.

Dreiling, Larry. "Small Town Works Together to End Population Bust." *High Plains Journal* (Dodge City, KS), updated July 19, 2018. https://www.hpj.com/ag_news/small-town-works -together-to-end-population-bust/article_6ef6cc48-5849-11e7-ba62-935f255936e4.html.

Duffey, Kiyah J., Penny Gordon-Larsen, David R. Jacobs Jr., O. Dale Williams, and Barry M. Popkin. "Differential Associations of Fast Food and Restaurant Food Consumption with 3-Y Change in Body Mass Index: The Coronary Artery Risk Development in Young Adults Study." *American Journal of Clinical Nutrition* 85, no. 1 (2007): 201–08.

Duhl, Leonard J. "The Healthy City: Its Function and Its Future." *Health Promotion International* 1, no. 1 (1986): 55–60.

Duncan, Craig, Kelvyn Jones, and Graham Moon. "Context, Composition and Heterogeneity: Using Multilevel Models in Health Research." *Social Science and Medicine* 46, no. 1 (1998): 97–117.

Duncan, Craig, Kelvyn Jones, and Graham Moon. "Do Places Matter? A Multi-Level Analysis of Regional Variations in Health-Related Behavior in Britain." *Social Science and Medicine* 37, no. 6 (1993): 725–33.

Duncan, Craig, Kelvyn Jones, and Graham Moon. "Psychiatric Morbidity: A Multilevel Approach to Regional Variations in the UK." *Journal of Epidemiology and Community Health* 49, no. 3 (1995): 290–95.

Duncan, M., and K. Mummery. "Psychosocial and Environmental Factors Associated with Physical Activity among City Dwellers in Regional Queensland." *Preventive Medicine* 40 (2005): 363–72.

Dunstan, David, Elizabeth Barr, Genevieve Healy, Jo Salmon, Jonathan Shaw, Beverley Balkau, Dianna Magliano, et al. "Television Viewing Time and Mortality: The Australian Diabetes, Obesity and Lifestyle Study (Ausdiab)." *Circulation* 121, no. 3 (2010): 384.

Dunstan, David W., Bethany Howard, Genevieve N. Healy, and Neville Owen. "Too Much Sitting—a Health Hazard." *Diabetes Research and Clinical Practice* 97, no. 3 (2012): 368–76.

Durazo, E. M., M. R. Jones, S. P. Wallace, J. Van Arsdal, M. Aydin, and C. Stewart. *The Health Status and Unique Health Challenges of Rural in California.* Los Angeles: UCLA Center for Health Policy Research, 2011.

Dutko, Paula, Michele Ver Ploeg, and Tracey L. Farrigan. *Characteristics and Influential Factors of Food Deserts.* Washington, DC: Department of Agriculture, Economic Research Service, 2012.

Dye, Thomas R. "Population Density and Social Pathology." *Urban Affairs Quarterly* 11, no. 2 (1975): 265–75.

Eames, Margaret, Yoav Ben-Shlomo, and Michael G. Marmot. "Social Deprivation and Premature Mortality: Regional Comparison across England." *British Medical Journal* 307, no. 6912 (1993): 1097–102.

Eason, John. "Mapping Prison Proliferation: Region, Rurality, Race and Disadvantage in Prison Placement." *Social Science Research* 39, no. 6 (2010): 1015–28.

Easterling, Doug, Ross Conner, and Carl E. Larson. "Creating a Healthy Civic Infrastructure: The Legacy of the Colorado Healthy Communities Initiative." *National Civic Review* 101, no. 1 (2012): 35–48.

Eaton, William W., Preben Bo Mortensen, and Morten Frydenberg. "Obstetric Factors, Urbanization and Psychosis." *Schizophrenia Research* 43, no. 2–3 (2000): 117–23.

Eberhardt, Mark Stephen, Virginia M. Freid, Sam Harper, Deborah D. Ingram, Diane M. Makuc, Elsie Pamuk, and Kate Prager. *Health, United States, 2001; with Urban and Rural Health Chartbook.* Hyattsville, MD: National Center for Health Statistics, 2001.

Economic Research Service. "Food Access Research Atlas: State-Level Estimates of Low Income and Low Access Populations." Department of Agriculture, September 30, 2019. https://www.ers.usda.gov/data-products/food-access-research-atlas/state-level-estimates-of-low-income-and-low-access-populations/.

Economic Research Service. "Rural America at a Glance." In *Economic Information Bulletin, No. 59.* Washington, DC: Department of Agriculture, 2009.

Economic Research Service. *Rural Transportation at a Glance, Agriculture Information Bulletin Number 795.* Washington, DC: Department of Agriculture, 2005.

Ejlskov, Linda, Rikke N. Mortensen, Charlotte Overgaard, Line R. B. U. Christensen, Henrik Vardinghus-Nielsen, Stella R. J. Kræmer, et al. "Individual Social Capital and Survival: A Population Study with 5-Year Follow-Up." *BMC Public Health* 14, no. 1025 (2014).

Elder, K., and J. Retrum. *Framework for Isolation in Adults over 50: AARP Foundation/Isolation Framework Project.* San Diego, CA: Research Works, 2012.

Ellaway, Anne, Michaela Benzeval, Michael Green, Alastair Leyland, and Sally Macintyre. " 'Getting Sicker Quicker': Does Living in a More Deprived Neighborhood Mean Your Health Deteriorates Faster?" *Health and Place* 18, no. 2 (2012): 132–37.

Elliott, S. J., D. C. Cole, P. Krueger, N. Voorberg, and S. Wakefield. "The Power of Perception: Health Risk Attributed to Air Pollution in an Urban Industrial Neighborhood." *Risk Analysis* 19 (1999): 621–34.

Ellis, Blake. "Oil Boom Strikes Kansas." CNN Money, May 23, 2012. https://money.cnn.com/2012/05/23/pf/america-boomtown-kansas/index.htm?iid=F_Jump.

Ellis, Blake. "Where Trailer Homes Rent for $2,000 a Month." CNN Money, June 1, 2012. https://money.cnn.com/2012/06/01/pf/kansas-housing-america-boomtown/.

Elo, Irma T., and Samuel H. Preston. "Educational Differentials in Mortality: United States, 1979–1985." *Social Science and Medicine* 42, no. 1 (1996): 47–57.

Ely, Andrea C., Christie Befort, Angela Banitt, Cheryl Gibson, and Debra Sullivan. "A Qualitative Assessment of Weight Control among Rural Kansas Women." *Journal of Nutrition Education and Behavior* 41, no. 3 (2009): 207–11.

Eng, Eugenia, Marla E. Salmon, and Fitzhugh Mullan. "Community Empowerment: The

Critical Base for Primary Health Care." *Family and Community Health: The Journal of Health Promotion and Maintenance* 15, no. 1 (1992): 1–12.

Epstein, Leonard H., Samina Raja, Samuel S. Gold, Rocco A. Paluch, Youngju Pak, and James N. Roemmich. "Reducing Sedentary Behavior: The Relationship between Park Area and the Physical Activity of Youth." *Psychological Science* 17, no. 8 (2006): 654–59.

Epstein, Paul R. "Climate Change and Human Health." *New England Journal of Medicine* 353, no. 14 (2005): 1433–36.

Erwin, Paul Campbell, Eugene C. Fitzhugh, Kathleen C. Brown, Shannon Looney, and Timothy Forde. "Health Disparities in Rural Areas: The Interaction of Race, Socioeconomic Status, and Geography." *Journal of Health Care for the Poor and Underserved* 21, no. 3 (2010): 931–45.

Evans, David. "Hierarchy of Evidence: A Framework for Ranking Evidence Evaluating Healthcare Interventions." *Journal of Clinical Nursing* 12, no. 1 (2003): 77–84.

Evans, Gary W. "The Built Environment and Mental Health." *Journal of Urban Health* 80, no. 4 (2003): 536–55.

Evans, Gary W., and Elyse Kantrowitz. "Socioeconomic Status and Health: The Potential Role of Environmental Risk Exposure." *Annual Review of Public Health* 23, no. 1 (2002): 303–31.

Evans, Gary W., and Stephen J. Lepore. "Household Crowding and Social Support: A Quasi-experimental Analysis." *Journal of Personality and Social Psychology* 65, no. 2 (1993): 308.

Evans, Gary W., Madan N. Palsane, Stephen J. Lepore, and Janea Martin. "Residential Density and Psychological Health: The Mediating Effects of Social Support." *Journal of Personality and Social Psychology* 57, no. 6 (1989): 994–99.

Evans, Isobel E. M., David J. Llewellyn, Fiona E. Matthews, Robert T. Woods, Carol Brayne, Linda Clare, and CFAS-Wales Research Team. "Living Alone and Cognitive Function in Later Life." *Archives of Gerontology and Geriatrics* 81 (2019): 222–33.

Evans, Robert G., and George L. Stoddart. "Consuming Health Care, Producing Health." *Social Science and Medicine* 33 (1990): 1347–63.

Evans, Robert G., and George L. Stoddart. "Producing Health, Consuming Health Care." In *Why Are Some People Healthy and Others Not?*, 27–64. New York: Routledge, 2017.

Evenson, Kelly R., Molly M. Scott, Deborah A. Cohen, and Carolyn C. Voorhees. "Girls' Perception of Neighborhood Factors on Physical Activity, Sedentary Behavior, and BMI." *Obesity* 15, no. 2 (2007): 430–45.

Evenson, Kelly R., Daniela Sotres-Alvarez, Amy H. Herring, Lynne Messer, Barbara A. Laraia, and Daniel A. Rodríguez. "Assessing Urban and Rural Neighborhood Characteristics Using Audit and GIS Data: Derivation and Reliability of Constructs." *International Journal of Behavioral Nutrition and Physical Activity* 6, no. 1 (2009): 44.

Evers, Adalbert, Wendy Farrant, and Alf Trojan. *Healthy Public Policy at the Local Level.* Frankfurt: Campus Verlag, 1990.

Eversole, Robyn. "Community Agency and Community Engagement: Re-Theorizing Participation in Governance." *Journal of Public Policy* 31, no. 1 (2011): 51–71.

Eversole, Robyn. "Empowering Institutions: Indigenous Lessons and Policy Perils." *Development* 53, no. 1 (2010): 77–82.

Eversole, R., and J. Martin. *Participation and Governance in Regional Development: Global Trends in an Australian Context.* Farnham, UK: Ashgate, 2005. https://books.google.com/books?id=pZTZwAEACAAJ.

Ewing, Reid, and Robert Cervero. "Travel and the Built Environment: A Meta-Analysis." *Journal of the American Planning Association* 76, no. 3 (2010): 265–94.

Ewing, Reid, Christopher V. Forinash, and William Schroeer. "Neighborhood Schools and Sidewalk Connections: What Are the Impacts on Travel Mode Choice and Vehicle Emissions?" *Transportation Research News*, no. 237 (2005): 4–10.

Ewing, Reid, Padma Haliyur, and G. William Page. "Getting around a Traditional City, a Suburban Planned Unit Development, and Everything in Between." *Transportation Research Record* 1466 (1994): 53.

Ewing, Reid, S. Handy, R. C. Brownson, O. Clemente, and E. Winston. "Identifying and Measuring Urban Design Qualities Related to Walkability." *Journal of Physical Activity and Health* 3 (2006): 223.

Ewing, Reid, T. Schmid, R. Killingsworth, A. Zlot, and S. Raudenbush. "Relationship between Urban Sprawl and Physical Activity, Obesity, and Morbidity." *American Journal of Health Promotion* 18 (2003): 47–57.

Ewing, Reid, William Schroeer, and William Greene. "School Location and Student Travel Analysis of Factors Affecting Mode Choice." *Transportation Research Record* 1895, no. 1 (2004): 55–63.

Fan, Jessie X., Ming Wen, and Lori Kowaleski-Jones. "An Ecological Analysis of Environmental Correlates of Active Commuting in Urban US." *Health and Place* 30 (2014): 242–50.

Fan, Jessie X., Ming Wen, and Lori Kowaleski-Jones. "Rural-Urban Differences in Objective and Subjective Measures of Physical Activity: Findings from the National Health and Nutrition Examination Survey (Nhanes) 2003–2006." *Preventing Chronic Disease* 11 (2014). https://doi.org/10.5888/pcd11.140189.

Fan, Jessie X., Ming Wen, and Neng Wan. "Built Environment and Active Commuting: Rural-Urban Differences in the US." *SSM-Population Health* 3 (2017): 435–41.

Farley, Thomas A., Rebecca A. Meriwether, Erin T. Baker, Liza T. Watkins, Carolyn C. Johnson, and Larry S. Webber. "Safe Play Spaces to Promote Physical Activity in Inner-City Children: Results from a Pilot Study of an Environmental Intervention." *American Journal of Public Health* 97, no. 9 (2007): 1625–31.

Farmer, Frank L., and Zola K. Moon. "An Empirical Examination of Characteristics of Mexican Migrants to Metropolitan and Nonmetropolitan Areas of the United States." *Rural Sociology* 74, no. 2 (2009): 220–40.

Farmer, Jane, and Sue Kilpatrick. "Are Rural Health Professionals Also Social Entrepreneurs?" *Social Science and Medicine* 69, no. 11 (2009): 1651–58.

Farmer, Jane, Lorna Philip, Gerry King, John Farrington, and Marsaili MacLeod. "Territorial Tensions: Misaligned Management and Community Perspectives on Health Services for Older People in Remote Rural Areas." *Health and Place* 16, no. 2 (2010): 275–83.

Farrigan, Tracey. *Rural Income, Poverty, and Welfare.* Washington, DC: Economic Research Service, USDA, 2004.

Farrigan, Tracey. "Rural Poverty and Well-Being." USDA Economic Research Service, November 29, 2022. https://www.ers.usda.gov/topics/rural-economy-population/rural-poverty-well-being/#demographics.

Federal Bureau of Investigation. "Crime in the U.S." Accessed September 19, 2021, https://ucr.fbi.gov/crime-in-the-u.s.

Feeding America. "Food Insecurity in Kansas: Before Covid-19." Map the Meal Gap, accessed September 19, 2021. https://map.feedingamerica.org/county/2019/overall/kansas.

Feldman, Jacob J., Diane M. Makuc, Joel C. Kleinman, and Joan Cornoni-Huntley. "National Trends in Educational Differentials in Mortality." *American Journal of Epidemiology* 129, no. 5 (1989): 919–33.

Felson, Marcus, and Rachel L. Boba. *Crime and Everyday Life.* Thousand Oaks, CA: Sage Publications, 2010.

Fennelly, Katherine. "Prejudice toward Immigrants in the Midwest." In *New Faces in New Places: The Changing Geography of American Immigration*, edited by Douglas S. Massey, 151–78. New York: Russell Sage Foundation, 2008.

Ferdinand, Alva O., Bisakha Sen, Saurabh Rahurkar, Sally Engler, and Nir Menachemi. "The

Relationship between Built Environments and Physical Activity: A Systematic Review." *American Journal of Public Health* 102, no. 10 (2012): e7–e13.

Ferré, Céline, Francisco H. G. Ferreira, and Peter Lanjouw. "Is There a Metropolitan Bias? The Relationship between Poverty and City Size in a Selection of Developing Countries." *World Bank Economic Review* 26, no. 3 (2012): 351–82. https://doi.org/10.1093/wber /lhs007.

Findholt, Nancy E., Yvonne L. Michael, Linda J. Jerofke, and Victoria W. Brogoitti. "Environmental Influences on Children's Physical Activity and Eating Habits in a Rural Oregon County." *American Journal of Health Promotion* 26, no. 2 (2011): e74–e85.

Fischer, Claude S. *Made in America: A Social History of American Culture and Character.* Chicago: University of Chicago Press, 2010.

Fitzpatrick, J. J., and E. Merwin. *Focus on Rural Health.* N.p.: Springer, 2008. https://books .google.com/books?id=zkj-qxuBOVYC.

Fitzpatrick, K., and M. LaGory. *Unhealthy Cities: Poverty, Race, and Place in America.* New York: Taylor and Francis, 2013. https://books.google.com/books?id=RLI0O5l2iOoC.

Flaherty, Jeremy, and Ralph B. Brown. "A Multilevel Systemic Model of Community Attachment: Assessing the Relative Importance of the Community and Individual Levels." *American Journal of Sociology* 116, no. 2 (2010): 503–42.

Flegal, Katherine M., Margaret D. Carroll, Robert J. Kuczmarski, and Clifford L. Johnson. "Overweight and Obesity in the United States: Prevalence and Trends, 1960–1994." *International Journal of Obesity* 22, no. 1 (1998): 39–47.

Flegal, Katherine M., Margaret D. Carroll, Cynthia L. Ogden, and Lester R. Curtin. "Prevalence and Trends in Obesity among US Adults, 1999–2008." *Journal of the American Medical Association* 303, no. 3 (2010): 235–41.

Flegal, Katherine M., and Barry I. Graubard. "Estimates of Excess Deaths Associated with Body Mass Index and Other Anthropometric Variables." *American Journal of Clinical Nutrition* 89, no. 4 (2009): 1213–19.

Flora, Cornelia Butler, Jan L. Flora, and Stephen P. Gasteyer. *Rural Communities: Legacy and Change.* New York: Routledge, 2018.

Flowerdew, R., D. J. Manley, and C. E. Sabel. "Neighbourhood Effects on Health: Does It Matter Where You Draw the Boundaries?" *Social Science and Medicine* 66 (2008): 1241–55.

Flynn, Beverly Collora. "Healthy Cities: Toward Worldwide Health Promotion." *Annual Review of Public Health* 17, no. 1 (1996): 299–309.

Flynn, Beverly Collora. "Healthy Cities within the American Context." Chap. 9 in *Healthy Cities: Research and Practice,* edited by John K. Davies and Michael Kelly, 112–26. New York: Routledge, 1993.

Folland, Sherman. "Does 'Community Social Capital' Contribute to Population Health?" *Social Science and Medicine* 64, no. 11 (2007): 2342–54.

Fonseca, Walter, Betty R. Kirkwood, Cesar Gomes Victora, S. R. Fuchs, J. A. Flores, and C. Misago. "Risk Factors for Childhood Pneumonia among the Urban Poor in Fortaleza, Brazil: A Case-Control Study." *Bulletin of the World Health Organization* 74, no. 2 (1996): 199.

FoodPrint. "Antibiotics in Our Food System." Updated February 14, 2020, https://foodprint .org/issues/antibiotics-in-our-food-system/.

Forsyth, A., M. Hearst, J. M. Oakes, and K. H. Schmitz. "Design and Destinations: Factors Influencing Walking and Total Physical Activity." *Urban Studies* 45 (2008): 1973–96.

Foster, Sarah, and Billie Giles-Corti. "The Built Environment, Neighborhood Crime and Constrained Physical Activity: An Exploration of Inconsistent Findings." *Preventive Medicine* 47, no. 3 (2008): 241–51.

Foster, Sarah, Billie Giles-Corti, and Matthew Knuiman. "Neighborhood Design and Fear of

Crime: A Social-Ecological Examination of the Correlates of Residents' Fear in New Suburban Housing Developments." *Health and Place* 16, no. 6 (2010): 1156–65.

Foster, Sarah, Lisa Wood, Hayley Christian, Matthew Knuiman, and Billie Giles-Corti. "Planning Safer Suburbs: Do Changes in the Built Environment Influence Residents' Perceptions of Crime Risk?" *Social Science and Medicine* 97 (2013): 87–94.

Foulkes, M., and K. A. Schafft. "The Impact of Migration on Poverty Concentrations in the United States, 1995–2000." *Rural Sociology* 75, no. 1 (2010): 90–110.

Fowler, Michael J. "Microvascular and Macrovascular Complications of Diabetes." *Clinical Diabetes* 26, no. 2 (2008): 77–82.

Fox, Anthony John, and P. O. Goldblatt. *Longitudinal Study: Socio-Demographic Mortality Differentials: A First Report on Mortality in 1971–1975 According to 1971 Census Characteristics, Based on Data Collected in OPCS Longitudinal Study.* London: HMSO, 1982.

Fox, Anthony John, D. R. Jones, and P. O. Goldblatt. "Approaches to Studying the Effect of Socio-Economic Circumstances on Geographic Differences in Mortality in England and Wales." *British Medical Bulletin* 40, no. 4 (1984): 309–14.

Fragkias, Michail, José Lobo, Deborah Strumsky, and Karen C. Seto. "Does Size Matter? Scaling of CO2 Emissions and US Urban Areas." *PLoS One* 8, no. 6 (2013): e64727.

Frank, Lawrence, M. A. Andresen, and T. L. Schmid. "Obesity Relationships with Community Design, Physical Activity, and Time Spent in Cars." *American Journal of Preventive Medicine* 27 (2004): 87–96.

Frank, Lawrence, Jacqueline Kerr, Jim Chapman, and James Sallis. "Urban Form Relationships with Walk Trip Frequency and Distance among Youth." *American Journal of Health Promotion* 21, no. 4 (2007): 305–11.

Frank, Lawrence D., and G. Pivo. "The Impacts of Mixed Use and Density on the Utilization of Three Modes of Travel: The Single Occupant Vehicle, Transit, and Walking." *Transportation Research Record* 1466 (1994): 44–52.

Frank, Lawrence D., James F. Sallis, Terry L. Conway, James E. Chapman, Brian E. Saelens, and William Bachman. "Many Pathways from Land Use to Health: Associations between Neighborhood Walkability and Active Transportation, Body Mass Index, and Air Quality." *Journal of the American Planning Association* 72, no. 1 (2006): 75–87.

Freedman, David S., Mary Horlick, and Gerald S. Berenson. "A Comparison of the Slaughter Skinfold-Thickness Equations and BMI in Predicting Body Fatness and Cardiovascular Disease Risk Factor Levels in Children." *American Journal of Clinical Nutrition* 98, no. 6 (2013): 1417–24.

Freedman, David S., Peter T. Katzmarzyk, William H. Dietz, Sathanur R. Srinivasan, and Gerald S. Berenson. "Relation of Body Mass Index and Skinfold Thicknesses to Cardiovascular Disease Risk Factors in Children: The Bogalusa Heart Study." *American Journal of Clinical Nutrition* 90, no. 1 (2009): 210–16.

French, Simone A. "Pricing Effects on Food Choices." *Journal of Nutrition* 133, no. 3 (2003): 841S–43S.

Freudenberg, Nicholas, S. Galea, and D. Vlahov. *Cities and the Health of the Public.* Nashville: Vanderbilt University Press, 2006. https://books.google.com/books?id=f-w4AQAAIAAJ.

Freudenberg, Nicholas, Susan Klitzman, and Susan Saegert. *Urban Health and Society: Interdisciplinary Approaches to Research and Practice.* San Francisco: Wiley, 2009. https://books.google.com/books?id=1ov6QpamXT8C.

Freudenburg, William R., and Robert Emmett Jones. "Criminal Behavior and Rapid Community Growth: Examining the Evidence." *Rural Sociology* 56, no. 4 (1991): 619–45.

Friedland, William H. "Agriculture and Rurality: Beginning the 'Final Separation'?" *Rural Sociology* 67, no. 3 (2002): 350–71.

Friedland, William H. "The End of Rural Society and the Future of Rural Sociology." *Rural Sociology* 47, no. 4 (1982): 589.

Friedman, Stephen B. "Rural and Small Town Subdivision Regulations." In *Rural and Small Town Planning*, edited by Judith Getzels and Charles Thurow, 97–160. Chicago: Planners Press, 1979.

Friedrich, Eva, Bill Hillier, and Alain Chiaradia. "Anti-Social Behavior and Urban Configuration Using Space Syntax to Understand Spatial Patterns of Socio-Environmental Disorder." Paper presented at the Proceedings of the 7th International Space Syntax Symposium, 2009.

Friel, Sharon, O. Walsh, and D. McCarthy. "The Irony of a Rich Country: Issues of Financial Access to and Availability of Healthy Food in the Republic of Ireland." *Journal of Epidemiology and Community Health* 60, no. 12 (2006): 1013–19.

Frontier Education Center. *Frontier: A New Definition*. Ojo Sarco, NM: Frontier Education Center, 1998.

Frost, Stephanie S., R. Turner Goins, Rebecca H. Hunter, Steven P. Hooker, Lucinda L. Bryant, Judy Kruger, and Delores Pluto. "Effects of the Built Environment on Physical Activity of Adults Living in Rural Settings." *American Journal of Health Promotion* 24, no. 4 (2010): 267 83.

Frumkin, Howard, Lawrence Frank, and Richard J. Jackson. *Urban Sprawl and Public Health: Designing, Planning, and Building for Healthy Communities*. Washington, DC: Island Press, 2004. https://books.google.com/books?id=Xko6al1sAmUC.

Fuguitt, G. V. "Commuting and the Rural-Urban Hierarchy." *Journal of Rural Studies* 7, no. 4 (1991): 459–66.

Fuguitt, G. V., D. L. Brown, and C. L. Beale. *Rural and Small Town America*. New York: Russell Sage Foundation, 1989. https://books.google.com/books?id=_AW5BgAAQBAJ.

Fuguitt, G. V., and T. B. Heaton. "The Impact of Migration on the Nonmetropolitan Population Age Structure, 1960–1990." *Population Research and Policy Review*, no. 14 (1995): 215–32.

Fullilove, Mindy Thompson. "Promoting Social Cohesion to Improve Health." *Journal of the American Medical Women's Association* 53, no. 2 (1998): 72.

Fulton, Janet E., Jessica L. Shisler, Michelle M. Yore, and Carl J. Caspersen. "Active Transportation to School: Findings from a National Survey." *Research Quarterly for Exercise and Sport* 76, no. 3 (2005): 352–57.

Galea, Sandro, Matthew Riddle, and George A. Kaplan. "Causal Thinking and Complex System Approaches in Epidemiology." *International Journal of Epidemiology* 39, no. 1 (2009): 97–106.

Garcia, Ginny, Thankam S. Sunil, and Pedro Hinojosa. "The Fast Food and Obesity Link: Consumption Patterns and Severity of Obesity." *Obesity Surgery* 22, no. 5 (2012): 810–18.

Garrett, Laurie. *Betrayal of Trust: The Collapse of Global Public Health*. Oxford: Oxford University Press, 2003.

Garrow, John S., and Joan Webster. "Quetelet's Index (W/H2) as a Measure of Fatness." *International Journal of Obesity* 9, no. 2 (1985): 147–53.

Gasana, Janvier, Deepa Dillikar, Angelico Mendy, Erick Forno, and Edgar Ramos Vieira. "Motor Vehicle Air Pollution and Asthma in Children: A Meta-Analysis." *Environmental Research* 117 (2012): 36–45.

Gaston, G., and C. Kreyling. *Shaping the Healthy Community: The Nashville Plan*. Nashville: Vanderbilt University Press, 2015. https://books.google.com/books?id=Qq8XswEACAAJ.

Gatrell, A. C., and S. J. Elliott. *Geographies of Health: An Introduction*. San Francisco: Wiley, 2014. https://books.google.com/books?id=jFyFBQAAQBAJ.

Gesler, W. M., and T. C. Ricketts. *Health in Rural North America: The Geography of Health Care Services and Delivery.* New Brunswick, NJ: Rutgers University Press, 1992. https:// books.google.com/books?id=8Bl-QgAACAAJ.

Getzels, Judith. "Policies and Plans." In *Rural and Small Town Planning,* edited by Judith Getzels and Charles Thurow, 27–38. Chicago, IL: Planners Press, 1979.

Getzels, Judith, and Charles Thurow, eds. *Rural and Small Town Planning.* Chicago: Planners Press, 1979.

Giles-Corti, Billie, Melissa H. Broomhall, Matthew Knuiman, Catherine Collins, Kate Douglas, Kevin Ng, Andrea Lange, and Robert J. Donovan. "Increasing Walking: How Important Is Distance to, Attractiveness, and Size of Public Open Space?" *American Journal of Preventive Medicine* 28, no. 2 (2005): 169–76.

Giles-Corti, Billie, Fiona Bull, Matthew Knuiman, Gavin McCormack, Kimberly Van Niel, Anna Timperio, Hayley Christian, et al. "The Influence of Urban Design on Neighborhood Walking Following Residential Relocation: Longitudinal Results from the Reside Study." *Social Science and Medicine* 77 (2013): 20–30.

Giles-Corti, Billie, Sarah Foster, M. Koohsari, Jacinta Francis, and Paula Hooper. "The Influence of Urban Design and Planning on Physical Activity." In *The Routledge Handbook of Planning for Health and Well-Being-Shaping a Sustainable and Healthy Future,* edited by Hugh Barton, Susan Thompson, Sarah Burgess, and Marcus Grant. New York: Routledge, 2015.

Giles-Corti, Billie, S. Macintyre, J. P. Clarkson, T. Pikora, and R. J. Donovan. "Environmental and Lifestyle Factors Associated with Overweight and Obesity in Perth, Australia." *American Journal of Health Promotion* 18 (2003): 93–102.

Giles-Corti, Billie, K. Ryan, and Sarah Foster. *Increasing Density in Australia: Maximizing the Health Benefits and Minimising Harm. Report to the National Heart Foundation of Australia.* Melbourne, Australia: National Heart Foundation of Australia, 2012.

Giles-Corti, Billie, Anne Vernez-Moudon, Rodrigo Reis, Gavin Turrell, Andrew L. Dannenberg, Hannah Badland, Sarah Foster, et al. "City Planning and Population Health: A Global Challenge." *Lancet* 388, no. 10062 (2016): 2912–24.

Giles-Corti, Billie, Gina Wood, Terri Pikora, Vincent Learnihan, Max Bulsara, Kimberly Van Niel, Anna Timperio, Gavin McCormack, and Karen Villanueva. "School Site and the Potential to Walk to School: The Impact of Street Connectivity and Traffic Exposure in School Neighborhoods." *Health and Place* 17, no. 2 (2011): 545–50.

Ginns, S. E., and A. C. Gatrell. "Respiratory Health Effects of Industrial Air Pollution: A Study in East Lancashire, UK." *Journal of Epidemiology and Community Health* 50 (1996): 631–35.

Glaeser, Edward L., and Bruce Sacerdote. "Why Is There More Crime in Cities?" *Journal of Political Economy* 107, no. S6 (1999): S225–S258.

Glanz, Karen, Ken Resnicow, Jennifer Seymour, Kathy Hoy, Hayden Stewart, Mark Lyons, and Jeanne Goldberg. "How Major Restaurant Chains Plan Their Menus: The Role of Profit, Demand, and Health." *American Journal of Preventive Medicine* 32, no. 5 (2007): 383–88.

Glanz, Karen, Barbara K. Rimer, and Kasisomayajula Viswanath. *Health Behavior and Health Education: Theory, Research, and Practice.* San Francisco: John Wiley and Sons, 2008.

Glasgow, N., E. H. Berry, and J. V. O. Edmund. *Rural Aging in 21st Century America.* Dordrecht: Springer Netherlands, 2012. https://books.google.com/books?id=Zhro DwdDZny4C.

Glasmeier, Amy K., and Tracey Farrigan. "The Economic Impacts of the Prison Development Boom on Persistently Poor Rural Places." *International Regional Science Review* 30, no. 3 (2007): 274–99.

Glasziou, Paul, Iain Chalmers, Douglas G. Altman, Hilda Bastian, Isabelle Boutron, Anne Brice, Gro Jamtvedt, et al. "Taking Healthcare Interventions from Trial to Practice." *British Medical Journal* 341 (2010).

Glazier, Richard H., Maria I. Creatore, Jonathan T. Weyman, Ghazal Fazli, Flora I. Matheson, Peter Gozdyra, Rahim Moineddin, Vered Kaufman Shriqui, and Gillian L. Booth. "Density, Destinations or Both? A Comparison of Measures of Walkability in Relation to Transportation Behaviors, Obesity and Diabetes in Toronto, Canada." *PLoS One* 9, no. 1 (2014): e85295.

Goetz, Stephan J., Yicheol Han, Jill L. Findeis, and Kathryn J. Brasier. "US Commuting Networks and Economic Growth: Measurement and Implications for Spatial Policy." *Growth and Change* 41, no. 2 (2010): 276–302.

Goldberg, Daniel S. "In Support of a Broad Model of Public Health: Disparities, Social Epidemiology and Public Health Causation." *Public Health Ethics* 2, no. 1 (2008): 70–83.

Goldsmith, Victor, Philip G. McGuire, John B. Mollenkopf, and Timothy A. Ross. *Analyzing Crime Patterns: Frontiers of Practice.* Thousand Oaks, CA: Sage Publications, 1999.

Gomez, L. F., D. C. Parra, D. Buchner, R. C. Brownson, O. L. Sarmiento, J. D. Pinzon, M. Ardila, et al. "Built Environment Attributes and Walking Patterns among the Elderly Population in Bogota." *American Journal of Preventive Medicine* 38 (2010): 592–99.

Gonzalez, Richard P., Glenn R. Cummings, Herbert A. Phelan, Madhuri S. Mulekar, and Charles B. Rodning. "Does Increased Emergency Medical Services Prehospital Time Affect Patient Mortality in Rural Motor Vehicle Crashes? A Statewide Analysis." *American Journal of Surgery* 197, no. 1 (2009): 30–34.

Goodman, Anna, Shannon Sahlqvist, David Ogilvie, and iConnect Consortium. "New Walking and Cycling Routes and Increased Physical Activity: One-and 2-Year Findings from the UK iConnect Study." *American Journal of Public Health* 104, no. 9 (2014): e38–e46.

Gordon, Peter, Ajay Kumar, and Harry W. Richardson. "The Influence of Metropolitan Spatial Structure on Commuting Time." *Journal of Urban Economics* 26, no. 2 (1989): 138–51.

Gordon, Peter, and Hung Leung Wong. "The Costs of Urban Sprawl: Some New Evidence." *Environment and Planning A* 17, no. 5 (1985): 661–66.

Gordon-Larsen, P., M. C. Nelson, P. Page, and B. M. Popkin. "Inequality in the Built Environment Underlies Key Health Disparities in Physical Activity and Obesity." *Pediatrics* 117 (2006): 417–24.

Graham, Jay P., Jessica H. Leibler, Lance B. Price, Joachim M. Otte, Dirk U. Pfeiffer, T. Tiensin, and Ellen K. Silbergeld. "The Animal-Human Interface and Infectious Disease in Industrial Food Animal Production: Rethinking Biosecurity and Biocontainment." *Public Health Reports* 123, no. 3 (2008): 282–99.

Graham, Jay P., Lance B. Price, Sean L. Evans, Thaddeus K. Graczyk, and Ellen K. Silbergeld. "Antibiotic Resistant Enterococci and Staphylococci Isolated from Flies Collected near Confined Poultry Feeding Operations." *Science of the Total Environment* 407, no. 8 (2009): 2701–10.

Grahn, P., and U. A. Stigsdotter. "Landscape Planning and Stress." *Urban Forestry and Urban Greening* 2 (2003): 1–18.

Greenberg, Stephanie W., and William M. Rohe. "Neighborhood Design and Crime: A Test of Two Perspectives." *Journal of the American Planning Association* 50, no. 1 (1984): 48–61.

Greenberg, Stephanie W., William M. Rohe, and Jay R. Williams. "Safety in Urban Neighborhoods: A Comparison of Physical Characteristics and Informal Territorial Control in High and Low Crime Neighborhoods." *Population and Environment* 5, no. 3 (1982): 141–65.

Greene, Jay. "Amid Rapid Expansion, Amazon to Shutter Kansas Warehouse." *Seattle Times*, October 1, 2014. https://www.seattletimes.com/business/amid-rapid-expansion-amazon-to-shutter-kansas-warehouse/.

Greene, Margarita. "Housing and Community Consolidation in Informal Settlements: A Case of Movement Economy." Paper presented at the Proceedings of the 4th International Space Syntax Symposium, University College London, 2003.

Grogger, J. "An Economic Model of Recent Trends in Violence." In *The Crime Drop in America*, edited by A. Blumstein and J. Wallman, 266–87. Cambridge, UK: Cambridge University, 2000.

GrowNYC. "Green Market." 2016, accessed August 5, 2020, https://www.grownyc.org/green market.

Haan, M., G. A. Kaplan, and T. Camacho. "Poverty and Health: Prospective Evidence from the Alameda County Study." *American Journal of Epidemiology* 125 (1987): 989–98.

Haines, Andy, R. Sari Kovats, Diarmid Campbell-Lendrum, and Carlos Corvalán. "Climate Change and Human Health: Impacts, Vulnerability and Public Health." *Public Health* 120, no. 7 (2006): 585–96.

Haines, Andy, and Jonathan A. Patz. "Health Effects of Climate Change." *Journal of the American Medical Association* 291, no. 1 (2004): 99–103.

Hajna, Samantha, Nancy A. Ross, Anne-Sophie Brazeau, Patrick Bélisle, Lawrence Joseph, and Kaberi Dasgupta. "Associations between Neighbourhood Walkability and Daily Steps in Adults: A Systematic Review and Meta-Analysis." *BMC Public Health* 15, no. 768 (2015).

Hakim, Simon, George F. Rengert, and Yochanan Shachmurove. "Target Search of Burglars: A Revised Economic Model." *Papers in Regional Science* 80, no. 2 (2001): 121–37.

Hale, Chris. "Fear of Crime: A Review of the Literature." *International Review of Victimology* 4, no. 2 (1996): 79–150.

Hall, Susan A., Jay S. Kaufman, and Thomas C. Ricketts. "Defining Urban and Rural Areas in US Epidemiologic Studies." *Journal of Urban Health* 83, no. 2 (2006): 162–75.

Hallet, Julie, Calvin H. L. Law, Paul J. Karanicolas, Refik Saskin, Ning Liu, and Simron Singh. "Rural-Urban Disparities in Incidence and Outcomes of Neuroendocrine Tumors: A Population-Based Analysis of 6271 Cases." *Cancer* 121, no. 13 (2015): 2214–21.

Halpern, David. *Mental Health and the Planned Environment: More Than Bricks and Mortar?* Bristol: Taylor and Francis, 1995.

Halpern, David. *Social Capital.* Cambridge: Polity, 2005.

Hamer, Mark, and Yoichi Chida. "Active Commuting and Cardiovascular Risk: A Meta-Analytic Review." *Preventive Medicine* 46, no. 1 (January 2008): 9–13. https://doi.org/10.1016/j.ypmed.2007.03.006.

Han, Bing, Deborah Cohen, and Thomas L. McKenzie. "Quantifying the Contribution of Neighborhood Parks to Physical Activity." *Preventive Medicine* 57, no. 5 (2013): 483–87.

Hancock, Trevor. "The Evolution, Impact and Significance of the Healthy Cities/Healthy Communities Movement." *Journal of Public Health Policy* 14, no. 1 (1993): 5–18.

Hancock, Trevor. "The Healthy City from Concept to Application." Chap. 2 in *Healthy Cities: Research and Practice*, edited by John K. Davies and Michael Kelly, 14–24. New York: Routledge, 1993.

Hancock, T., and L. Duhl. "WHO Healthy Cities Paper 1." In *Healthy Cities: Promoting Health in the Urban Context.* Copenhagen: FADL, 1986.

Hancock, Trevor, and F. Perkins. "The Mandala of Health." *Health Education* 24, no. 1 (1985): 8–10.

Handy, Susan L. *Critical Assessment of the Literature on the Relationships among Transportation, Land Use, and Physical Activity.* Washington, DC: Transportation Research Board and the Institute of Medicine Committee on Physical Activity, Health, Transportation, and Land Use, 2005.

Handy, Susan L. "Regional Versus Local Accessibility: Neo-Traditional Development and Its Implications for Non-Work Travel." *Built Environment* 18 (1992): 253–67.

Handy, Susan L. "Understanding the Link between Urban Form and Nonwork Travel Behavior." *Journal of Planning Education and Research* 15, no. 3 (1996): 183–98.

Handy, S., X. Cao, and P. L. Mokhtarian. "Self-Selection in the Relationship between the Built Environment and Walking: Empirical Evidence from Northern California." *Journal of the American Planning Association* 72 (2006): 55–74.

Hanks, Kathy. "Montezuma: A Blend of Culture." *Hutchinson (KS) News*, April 3, 2016. https://www.hutchnews.com/story/news/local/2016/04/03/montezuma-blend-culture /21013643007/.

Hänninen, Otto, Anne B. Knol, Matti Jantunen, Tek-Ang Lim, André Conrad, Marianne Rappolder, Paolo Carrer, et al. "Environmental Burden of Disease in Europe: Assessing Nine Risk Factors in Six Countries." *Environmental Health Perspectives* 122, no. 5 (2014): 439–46.

Hansen, Anush Yousefian, M. Renée Umstattd Meyer, Jennifer D. Lenardson, and David Hartley. "Built Environments and Active Living in Rural and Remote Areas: A Review of the Literature." *Current Obesity Reports* 4, no. 4 (2015): 484–93.

Harries, Keith. "Property Crimes and Violence in United States: An Analysis of the Influence of Population Density." *International Journal of Criminal Justice Sciences* 1, no. 2 (2006): 24–34.

Hart, L. Gary, Eric H. Larson, and Denise M. Lishner. "Rural Definitions for Health Policy and Research." *American Journal of Public Health* 95, no. 7 (2005): 1149–55.

Hart, L. Gary, Edward Salsberg, Debra M. Phillips, and Denise M. Lishner. "Rural Health Care Providers in the United States." *Journal of Rural Health* 18, no. 5 (2002): 211–31.

Hartig, T., G. Evans, L. D. Jamner, D. S. Davis, and T. Garling. "Tracking Restoration in Natural and Urban Field Settings." *Journal of Environmental Psychology* 23 (2003): 109–23.

Hartley, David. "Rural Health Disparities, Population Health, and Rural Culture." *American Journal of Public Health* 94, no. 10 (2004): 1675–78.

Harvard Medical School. "National Comorbidity Survey (NCS)." 2005. https://www.hcp.med .harvard.edu/ncs/.

Haukka, Jari, J. Suvisaari, T. Varilo, and J. Lönnqvist. "Regional Variation in the Incidence of Schizophrenia in Finland: A Study of Birth Cohorts Born from 1950 to 1969." *Psychological Medicine* 31, no. 6 (2001): 1045.

Head, Brian W. "Community Engagement: Participation on Whose Terms?" *Australian Journal of Political Science* 42, no. 3 (2007): 441–54.

Healy, Genevieve N., David W. Dunstan, J. O. Salmon, Jonathan E. Shaw, Paul Z. Zimmet, and Neville Owen. "Television Time and Continuous Metabolic Risk in Physically Active Adults." *Medicine and Science in Sports and Exercise* 40, no. 4 (2008): 639–45.

Heaton, Tim B., Daniel T. Lichter, and Acheampong Amoateng. "The Timing of Family Formation: Rural-Urban Differentials in First Intercourse, Childbirth, and Marriage." *Rural Sociology* 54, no. 1 (1989): 1.

Heaviside, Clare, Helen Macintyre, and Sotiris Vardoulakis. "The Urban Heat Island: Implications for Health in a Changing Environment." *Current Environmental Health Reports* 4, no. 3 (2017): 296–305.

Heilman, Matt. "Medical Center Marks Diabetes Month." *Ark Valley (KS) News*, November 15, 2012. http://www.arkvalleynews.com/web/isite.dll?1353019293703~health.

Hendrickson, Deja, Chery Smith, and Nicole Eikenberry. "Fruit and Vegetable Access in Four Low-Income Food Deserts Communities in Minnesota." *Agriculture and Human Values* 23, no. 3 (2006): 371–83.

Hennessy, Erin, Vivica I. Kraak, Raymond R. Hyatt, Julia Bloom, Mark Fenton, Colby Wagoner, and Christina D. Economos. "Active Living for Rural Children: Community Perspectives Using Photovoice." *American Journal of Preventive Medicine* 39, no. 6 (2010): 537–45.

Henning-Smith, Carrie, Alex Evenson, Amanda Corbett, Katy Kozhimannil, and Ira Moscovice. *Rural Transportation: Challenges and Opportunities, Policy Brief.* Minneapolis: University of Minnesota Rural Health Research Center, 2017. http://rhrc.umn.edu/wp-content/files_mf/1518734252UMRHRCTransportationChallenges.pdf.

Heritage, Zoë, and Mark Dooris. "Community Participation and Empowerment in Healthy Cities." *Health Promotion International* 24, no. S1 (2009): i45–i55.

Hewitt, Maria Elizabeth. *Defining 'Rural' Areas: Impact on Health Care Policy and Research.* Washington, DC: Health Program, Office of Technology Assessment, Congress of the United States, 1989.

Hicks, G., R. Powers, and W. F. Broderick. *Small Town.* New York: Fordham University Press, 2004. https://books.google.com/books?id=hTK3CwAAQBAJ.

Hillier, Amy, Tony Smith, Carolyn C. Cannuscio, Allison Karpyn, and Karen Glanz. "A Discrete Choice Approach to Modeling Food Store Access." *Environment and Planning B: Planning and Design* 42, no. 2 (2015): 263–78.

Hillier, Bill. "The Art of Place and the Science of Space." *World Architecture* 185 (2005): 96–102.

Hillier, Bill. "Can Streets Be Made Safe?" *Urban Design International* 9, no. 1 (2004): 31–45.

Hillier, Bill. *Space Is the Machine: A Configurational Theory of Architecture.* London: Space Syntax, 2007. First published 1996.

Hillier, Bill. "Studying Cities to Learn about Minds: Some Possible Implications of Space Syntax for Spatial Cognition." *Environment and Planning B: Planning and Design* 39, no. 1 (2012): 12–32.

Hillier, Bill. "A Theory of the City as Object: Or, How Spatial Laws Mediate the Social Construction of Urban Space." *Urban Design International* 7, no. 3–4 (2002): 153–79.

Hillier, Bill, and Julienne Hanson. *The Social Logic of Space.* Cambridge: Cambridge University Press, 1984.

Hillier, Bill, and Shinichi Iida. "Network and Psychological Effects in Urban Movement." Paper presented at the International Conference on Spatial Information Theory, 2005.

Hillier, Bill, and Alan Penn. "Rejoinder to Carlo Ratti." *Environment and Planning B: Planning and Design* 31, no. 4 (2004): 501–11.

Hillier, Bill, Alan Penn, Julienne Hanson, Tadeusz Grajewski, and Jianming Xu. "Natural Movement: Or, Configuration and Attraction in Urban Pedestrian Movement." *Environment and Planning B: Planning and Design* 20, no. 1 (1993): 29–66.

Hillier, Bill, and Ozlem Sahbaz. "Safety in Numbers: High-Resolution Analysis of Crime in Street Networks." In *The Urban Fabric of Crime and Fear*, edited by V. Ceccato, 111–37. Dordrecht: Springer, 2011.

Hilmers, Angela, David C. Hilmers, and Jayna Dave. "Neighborhood Disparities in Access to Healthy Foods and Their Effects on Environmental Justice." *American Journal of Public Health* 102, no. 9 (2012): 1644–54.

Hirsch, J. A., A. V. Diez-Roux, D. A. Rodriguez, S. J. Brines, and K. A. Moore. "Discrete Land Uses and Transportation Walking in Two U.S. Cities: The Multi-Ethnic Study of Atherosclerosis." *Health and Place*, no. 24 (2013): 196–202.

Hittle, Shaun. "Losing the Meth War." *Lawrence (KS) Journal-World*, March 4, 2021. https://www2.ljworld.com/news/2012/mar/04/losing-meth-war/.

Hofferth, Sandra L., and John Iceland. "Social Capital in Rural and Urban Communities." *Rural Sociology* 63, no. 4 (1998): 574–98.

Hoffman, Ryan A. *Commission Staff's Report and Recommendation Docket No. 15-Cons-770-Cmsc.* Wichita: Conservation Division, State Corporation Commission of the State of Kansas, 2017.

Hoffmann, Rasmus. *Socioeconomic Differences in Old Age Mortality.* The Springer Series on

Demographic Methods and Population Analysis. Vol. 25. N.p.: Springer Science and Business Media, 2008.

Hollingshead, A. B. "The Life Cycle of Nebraska Rural Churches." *Rural Sociology* 2, no. 2 (1937): 180–91.

Holt-Lunstad, Julianne, Timothy B. Smith, Mark Baker, Tyler Harris, and David Stephenson. "Loneliness and Social Isolation as Risk Factors for Mortality: A Meta-Analytic Review." *Perspectives on Psychological Science* 10, no. 2 (2015): 227–37.

Holt-Lunstad, Julianne, Timothy B. Smith, and J. Bradley Layton. "Social Relationships and Mortality Risk: A Meta Analytic Review." *PLoS Medicine* 7, no. 7 (2010): e1000316.

Hooks, Gregory, Clayton Mosher, Shaun Genter, Thomas Rotolo, and Linda Lobao. "Revisiting the Impact of Prison Building on Job Growth: Education, Incarceration, and County-Level Employment, 1976–2004." *Social Science Quarterly* 91, no. 1 (2010): 228–44.

Housing Assistance Council. "Race and Ethnicity in Rural America." Rural Research Briefs, 2012. http://www.ruralhome.org/storage/research_notes/rrn-race-and-ethnicity-web.pdf.

Howden-Chapman, P. "Housing Standards: A Glossary of Housing and Health." *Journal of Epidemiology and Community Health* 58, no. 3 (2004): 162–68.

Huang, Sheu-Jen, Wen-Chi Hung, Patricia A. Sharpe, and Jackson P. Wai. "Neighborhood Environment and Physical Activity among Urban and Rural Schoolchildren in Taiwan." *Health and Place* 16 (2010): 470–76.

Hughes, Georgina, Kate M. Bennett, and Marion M. Hetherington. "Old and Alone: Barriers to Healthy Eating in Older Men Living on Their Own." *Appetite* 43, no. 3 (2004): 269–76.

Human, Jeffrey, and Cathy Wasem. "Rural Mental Health in America." *American Psychologist* 46, no. 3 (1991): 232.

Hummer, Robert A., and Joseph T. Lariscy. "Educational Attainment and Adult Mortality." In *International Handbook of Adult Mortality*, edited by R. G. Rogers and E. M. Crimmins, 241–61. N.p.: Springer, 2011.

Humphreys, Keith, and Roy Carr-Hill. "Area Variations in Health Outcomes: Artefact or Ecology." *International Journal of Epidemiology* 20, no. 1 (1991): 251–58.

Huttlinger, Kathleen. "Research and Collaboration in Rural Community Health." *Online Journal of Rural Nursing and Health Care* 4, no. 1 (2004): 22–36.

Hynes, H. P., and R. Lopez. *Urban Health: Readings in the Social, Built, and Physical Environments of U.S. Cities.* Sudbury, MA: Jones and Bartlett Publishers, 2009. https://books.google.com/books?id=Kc8ITLziv1YC.

Iceland, John, Daniel H. Weinberg, and Erika Steinmetz. *Racial and Ethnic Residential Segregation in the United States 1980–2000.* Vol. 8. Washington, DC: Government Printing Office, 2002.

Inagami, S., D. A. Cohen, B. K. Finch, and S. M. Asch. "You Are Where You Shop: Grocery Store Locations, Weight, and Neighborhoods." *American Journal of Preventive Medicine* 31 (2006): 10–17.

Ingram, Deborah D., and Sheila J. Franco. *2013 NCHS Urban-Rural Classification Scheme for Counties, National Center for Vital Health Statistics 2 (166).* Hyattsville, MD: US Department of Health and Human Services, Centers for Disease Control and Prevention, 2014.

Institute of Medicine. *Rebuilding the Unity of Health and the Environment in Rural America: Workshop Summary.* Edited by J. Merchant, C. Coussens and D. Gilbert. Washington, DC: National Academies Press, 2006. https://doi.org/10.17226/11596.

Institute of Medicine, Committee for the Study of the Future of Public Health, and Richard D. Remington. *The Future of Public Health.* Washington, DC: National Academies Press, 1988.

Intergovernmental Panel on Climate Change. *Climate Change 2014: Impacts, Adaptation and Vulnerability.* Geneva: IPCC, 2014. www.ipcc.ch/report/ar5/wg2.

International Council for Science. *Report of the ICSU Planning Group on Health and Wellbeing in the Changing Urban Environment: A Systems Analysis Approach*. Paris: International Council for Science, 2012.

Isalgue, Antonio, Helena Coch, and Rafael Serra. "Scaling Laws and the Modern City." *Physica A: Statistical Mechanics and Its Applications* 382, no. 2 (2007): 643–49.

Ising, Hartmut, and Barbara Kruppa. "Health Effects Caused by Noise: Evidence in the Literature from the Past 25 Years." *Noise and Health* 6, no. 22 (2004): 5.

Isserman, Andrew M. "In the National Interest: Defining Rural and Urban Correctly in Research and Public Policy." *International Regional Science Review* 28, no. 4 (2005): 465–99.

Jackson, J. Elizabeth, Mark P. Doescher, Anthony F. Jerant, and L. Gary Hart. "A National Study of Obesity Prevalence and Trends by Type of Rural County." *Journal of Rural Health* 21, no. 2 (2005): 140–48.

Jackson, Richard J., Andrew L. Dannenberg, and Howard Frumkin. "Health and the Built Environment: 10 Years After." *American Journal of Public Health* 103, no. 9 (2013): 1542–44.

Jackson, R. J., and S. Sinclair. *Designing Healthy Communities*. San Francisco: Jossey-Bass, 2011.

Jackson-Smith, Douglas B., and Eric Jensen. "Finding Farms: Comparing Indicators of Farming Dependence and Agricultural Importance in the United States." *Rural Sociology* 74, no. 1 (2009): 37–55.

Jacobson, Dawn Marie, and Steven Teutsch. *An Environmental Scan of Integrated Approaches for Defining and Measuring Total Population Health*. Washington, DC: National Quality Forum, 2012.

James, Wesley L. "All Rural Places Are Not Created Equal: Revisiting the Rural Mortality Penalty in the United States." *American Journal of Public Health* 104, no. 11 (2014): 2122–29.

Jekanowski, Mark D., James K. Binkley, and James Eales. "Convenience, Accessibility, and the Demand for Fast Food." *Journal of Agricultural and Resource Economics* 26, no. 1 (2001): 58–74.

Jemal, Ahmedin, Elizabeth Ward, Yongping Hao, and Michael Thun. "Trends in the Leading Causes of Death in the United States, 1970–2002." *Journal of the American Medical Association* 294, no. 10 (2005): 1255–59.

Jephcote, Calvin, and Haibo Chen. "Environmental Injustices of Children's Exposure to Air Pollution from Road-Transport within the Model British Multicultural City of Leicester: 2000–09." *Science of the Total Environment* 414 (2012): 140–51.

Jiang, Bin, and Chengke Liu. "Street-Based Topological Representations and Analyses for Predicting Traffic Flow in GIS." *International Journal of Geographical Information Science* 23, no. 9 (2009): 1119–37.

Jiao, Junfeng, Anne V. Moudon, Jared Ulmer, Philip M. Hurvitz, and Adam Drewnowski. "How to Identify Food Deserts: Measuring Physical and Economic Access to Supermarkets in King County, Washington." *American Journal of Public Health* 102, no. 10 (2012): e32–e39.

Jilcott, Stephanie B., Kelly R. Evenson, Barbara A. Laraia, and Alice S. Ammerman. "Association between Physical Activity and Proximity to Physical Activity Resources among Low-Income, Midlife Women." *Preventing Chronic Disease* 4, no. 1 (2007).

Jobes, Patrick C. "Residential Stability and Crime in Small Rural Agricultural and Recreational Towns." *Sociological Perspectives* 42, no. 3 (1999): 499–524.

Joens-Matre, Roxane R., Gregory J. Welk, Miguel A. Calabro, Daniel W. Russell, Elizabeth Nicklay, and Larry D. Hensley. "Rural-Urban Differences in Physical Activity, Physical Fitness, and Overweight Prevalence of Children." *Journal of Rural Health* 24, no. 1 (2008): 49–54.

Johansen, H. E., and G. V. Fuguitt. *The Changing Rural Village in America: Demographic and Economic Trends since 1950*. Cambridge, MA: Ballinger, 1984.

Johns, Susan, Sue Kilpatrick, and Jessica Whelan. "Our Health in Our Hands: Building Effective Community Partnerships for Rural Health Service Provision." *Rural Society* 17, no. 1 (2007): 50–65.

Johnson, K. M. *Demographic Trends in Rural and Small Town America*. Durham: Casey Institute, University of New Hampshire, 2006.

Johnson, K. M. "Recent Population Redistribution Trends in Nonmetropolitan America." *Rural Sociology* 54, no. 3 (1989): 301 26.

Johnson, K. M., and C. L. Beale. "Nonmetro Recreation Counties: Their Identification and Rapid Growth." *Rural America* 17, no. 4 (2003): 12–19.

Johnson, K. M., and J. B. Cromartie. "The Rural Rebound and Its Aftermath: Changing Demographic Dynamics and Regional Contrasts." In *Population Change and Rural Society*, edited by W. Kandel and D. L. Brown. Dordrect, Netherlands: Springer, 2006.

Johnson, K. M., and G. V. Fuguitt. "Continuity and Change in Rural Migration Patterns, 1950–1995." *Rural Sociology* 65, no. 1 (2000): 27–49.

Johnson, K. M., and D. T. Lichter. "Natural Increase: A New Source of Population Growth in Emerging Hispanic Destinations." *Population and Development Review* 34, no. 2 (2008): 327–46.

Johnson, Kenneth M., John P. Pelissero, David B. Holian, and Michael T. Maly. "Local Government Fiscal Burden in Nonmetropolitan America." *Rural Sociology* 60, no. 3 (1995): 381–98.

Johnson, K. M., and S. I. Stewart. "Amenity Migration to Urban Proximate Counties." In *Amenities and Rural Development: Theory, Methods and Public Policy*, edited by G. P. Green, D. Marcouiller and S. Deller. Northampton, MA: Edward Elgar Publishing, 2006.

Johnson, K. M., P. R. Voss, R. B. Hammer, G. V. Fuguitt, and S. McNiven. "Temporal and Spatial Variation in Age-Specific Net Migration in the United States." *Demography* 42, no. 4 (2005): 751–812.

Johnson, Mark E., Christiane Brems, Teddy D. Warner, and Laura Weiss Roberts. "Rural-Urban Health Care Provider Disparities in Alaska and New Mexico." *Administration and Policy in Mental Health and Mental Health Services Research* 33, no. 4 (2006): 504–07.

Johnson, S., and K. Bowers. "Permeability and Burglary Risk: Are Cul-de-Sacs Safer?" *Quantitative Journal of Criminology* 26, no. 1 (2010): 89–111.

Johnson-Lawrence, Vicki, Anna Zajacova, and Rodlescia Sneed. "Education, Race/Ethnicity, and Multimorbidity among Adults Aged 30–64 in the National Health Interview Survey." *SSM-Population Health* 3 (2017): 366–72.

Jolliffe, D. *Rural Poverty at a Glance*. Washington, DC: Economic Research Service, USDA, 2004.

Jones, Carol Adaire. "Rural Populations Have Higher Rates of Chronic Disease." *Amber Waves* 8, no. 2 (2010): 5.

Jones, Carol A., William Kandel, and Timothy Parker. "Population Dynamics Are Changing the Profile of Rural Areas." *Amber Waves*, April 2007. https://www.ers.usda.gov/amber -waves/2007/April/population-dynamics-are-changing-the-profile-of-rural-areas.

Jones, Elvyn. "Top-Five Stories of Baldwin City for 2014." *Baldwin City (KS) Signal*, December 30, 2014. http://signal.baldwincity.com/news/2014/dec/30/top-five-stories-baldwin-city -2014/.

Jones, Elvyn. "Volunteers See Community Benefits to Baldwin City of Foot Trail Being Built at Douglas County State Lake." *Baldwin City (KS) Signal*, June 4, 2014. http://signal.baldwin city.com/news/2014/jun/04/volunteers-see-community-benefits-baldwin-city-foo/.

Jones, Elvyn. "Walmart Withdraws Plans for Store at Eisenhower Avenue/U.S. 56." *Baldwin*

City (KS) Signal, August 1, 2014. http://signal.baldwincity.com/news/2014/aug/01/wal-mart
-withdraws-plans-store-eisenhower-avenueus/.

Jones, Kelvyn, and Craig Duncan. "Individuals and Their Ecologies: Analysing the Geography
of Chronic Illness within a Multilevel Modelling Framework." *Health and Place* 1, no. 1
(1995): 27–40.

Joynt, Karen E., Yael Harris, E. John Orav, and Ashish K. Jha. "Quality of Care and Patient
Outcomes in Critical Access Rural Hospitals." *Journal of the American Medical Association*
306, no. 1 (2011): 45–52.

Kaczynski, Andrew T., Amanda J. Johnson, and Brian E. Saelens. "Neighborhood Land Use
Diversity and Physical Activity in Adjacent Parks." *Health and Place* 16, no. 2 (2010):
413–15.

Kaczynski, Andrew T., Luke R. Potwarka, and Brian E. Saelens. "Association of Park Size,
Distance, and Features with Physical Activity in Neighborhood Parks." *American Journal
of Public Health* 98, no. 8 (2008): 1451–56.

Kandel, William, and John Cromartie. *New Patterns of Hispanic Settlement in Rural America.*
Rural Development Research Report, Number 99. Washington, DC: Economic Research
Service, USDA, 2004. https://www.ers.usda.gov/publications/pub-details/?pubid=47091.

Kansas Behavioral Risk Factor Surveillance System. *Health Risk Behaviors of Kansans 2018.*
Topeka: Kansas Department of Health and Environment, 2020. https://www.kdheks.gov
/brfss/PDF/2018_Kansas_BRFSS_Report.pdf.

Kansas Bureau of Investigation. "Statistics." Accessed August 3, 2020, http://www.kansas.gov
/kbi/stats/stats.shtml.

Kansas Care Planning Council. "Kansas Adult Day Services." 2013, accessed September 18,
2021. https://www.carekansas.org/list06_kansas_adult_day_care.htm.

Kansas Health Institute. "Kickapoo in a Race to Stem the Tide of Diabetes: Effort Part of
CDC-Funded Initiative to Slow Spread of the Disease among American Indians." September 2, 2014. https://www.khi.org/news/article/kickapoo-race-stem-tide-diabetes.

Kansas Health Matters. "Kansas Health Matters." 2020, accessed August 3, 2020, https://www
.kansashealthmatters.org/.

Kansas Hospital Association. "All Drugs-Related Poisoning Hospital Discharges by County."
2016 January, accessed September 18, 2021, https://www.kdheks.gov/idp/download/HDD
2005_2014.pdf.

Kansas Hospital Association. "Opioid Crisis." Accessed September 18, 2021. https://www.kha
-net.org/CriticalIssues/BehavioralHealthandSubstanceAbuse/opioid-crisis/.

Kansas Information for Communities. "2013–2017 Vital Statistics Data." Bureau of Epidemiology and Public Health Informatics KDHE, 2020. http://kic.kdheks.gov/death_new.php.

Kansas Injury and Violence Prevention Program. *Kansas Trends in Drug Poisoning Deaths,
Special Emphasis Report: Drug Poisoning Deaths, 2005–2016.* Topeka: Bureau of Health
Promotion, Kansas Department of Health and Environment, 2017. https://www.kdheks
.gov/pdomp/download/2017_KS_SER_Drug_Poisoning.pdf.

Kansas Office of Revisor of Statutes. "Kansas Statutes." Accessed September 14, 2021. https://
www.ksrevisor.org/ksa.html.

Kansas Prevention Collaborative. *Kansas Suicide Prevention Plan 2021–25.* Topeka: Kansas
Department of Aging and Disability Services, 2020. https://kansaspreventioncollaborative
.org/wp-content/uploads/2020/12/Kansas-suicide-prevention-Plan.pdf.

Kansas State University. "Rural Grocery Initiative." Accessed September 19, 2021. https://www
.ruralgrocery.org/.

Kansas Violent Death Reporting System. *Suicide Statistics in Kansas (2015–2017): An Analysis
from the Kansas Violent Death Reporting System.* Topeka: Kansas Department of Health
and Environment, n.d. https://www.kdheks.gov/idp/download/Suicide_Infographic.pdf.

Kansas Violent Death Reporting System. *2015–2017 Death Circumstances Data*. Topeka: Injury and Disability Programs, Bureau of Health Promotion, Kansas Department of Health and Environment, 2019.

Kaplan, George A., John W. Lynch, Richard D. Cohen, Jennifer L. Balfour, and Elsie R. Pamuk. "Income and Mortality in the United States." *BMJ* 313, no. 7066 (1996): 1207.

Kaplan, George A., Elsie R. Pamuk, John W. Lynch, Richard D. Cohen, and Jennifer L. Balfour. "Inequality in Income and Mortality in the United States: Analysis of Mortality and Potential Pathways." *BMJ* 312, no. 7037 (1996): 999–1003.

Kaplan, Stephen. "Aesthetics, Affect, and Cognition: Environmental Preference from an Evolutionary Perspective." *Environment and Behavior* 19, no. 1 (1987): 3–32.

Kawachi, Ichiro, and Bruce P. Kennedy. "Socioeconomic Determinants of Health: Health and Social Cohesion: Why Care About Income Inequality?" *BMJ* 314, no. 7086 (1997): 1037.

Kawachi, Ichiro, Bruce P. Kennedy, Kimberly Lochner, and Deborah Prothrow-Stith. "Social Capital, Income Inequality, and Mortality." *American Journal of Public Health* 87, no. 9 (1997): 1491–98.

Kazi, Ambreen, Myanna Duncan, Stacy Clemes, and Cheryl Haslam. "A Survey of Sitting Time among UK Employees." *Occupational Medicine* 64, no. 7 (2014): 497–502.

Keller, Suzanne. *Community: Pursuing the Dream, Living the Reality*. Princeton, NJ: Princeton University Press, 2003.

Kellett, J. M. "Crowding and Mortality in London Boroughs." In *Unhealthy Housing: Research, Remedies and Reforms*, edited by R. Burridge and D. Ormandy. London: Chapman and Hall, 1993.

Kelly, Bridget, Victoria M. Flood, and Heather Yeatman. "Measuring Local Food Environments: An Overview of Available Methods and Measures." *Health and Place* 17, no. 6 (2011): 1284–93.

Kelly, Cheryl, Jeffrey S. Wilson, Mario Schootman, Morgan Clennin, Elizabeth A. Baker, and Douglas K. Miller. "The Built Environment Predicts Observed Physical Activity." *Frontiers in Public Health* 2, no. 52 (2014). https://doi.org/10.3389/fpubh.2014.00052.

Kennedy, Bruce P., Ichiro Kawachi, and Deborah Prothrow-Stith. "Income Distribution and Mortality: Cross Sectional Ecological Study of the Robin Hood Index in the United States." *BMJ* 312, no. 7037 (1996): 1004–07.

Kennedy, Christopher A., Iain Stewart, Angelo Facchini, Igor Cersosimo, Renata Mele, Bin Chen, Mariko Uda, et al. "Energy and Material Flows of Megacities." *Proceedings of the National Academy of Sciences* 112, no. 19 (2015): 5985–90.

Kenney, Mary Kay, Jing Wang, and Ron Iannotti. "Residency and Racial/Ethnic Differences in Weight Status and Lifestyle Behaviors among US Youth." *Journal of Rural Health* 30, no. 1 (2014): 89–100.

Kenny, Amanda, Jane Farmer, Virginia Dickson-Swift, and Nerida Hyett. "Community Participation for Rural Health: A Review of Challenges." *Health Expectations* 18, no. 6 (2015): 1906–17.

Kenny, Amanda, Nerida Hyett, John Sawtell, Virginia Dickson-Swift, Jane Farmer, and Peter O'Meara. "Community Participation in Rural Health: A Scoping Review." *BMC Health Services Research* 13, no. 1 (2013): 1–8.

Kent, Jennifer, Susan Thompson, and Bin Jalaludin. *Healthy Built Environments: A Review of the Literature*. Sydney: Healthy Built Environments Program, City Futures Research Centre, University of New South Wales, 2011.

Kerr, Jacqueline, Lawrence Frank, James F. Sallis, and Jim Chapman. "Urban Form Correlates of Pedestrian Travel in Youth: Differences by Gender, Race-Ethnicity and Household Attributes." *Transportation Research Part D: Transport and Environment* 12, no. 3 (2007): 177–82.

Kerr, Jacqueline, Dori Rosenberg, James F. Sallis, Brian E. Saelens, Lawrence D. Frank, and Terry L. Conway. "Active Commuting to School: Associations with Environment and Parental Concerns." *Medicine and Science in Sports and Exercise* 38, no. 4 (2006): 787–93.

Kickbusch, Ilona. *Good Planets Are Hard to Find*. Geneva: World Health Organization, 1989.

Kickbusch, Ilona. "Healthy Cities: A Working Project and a Growing Movement." *Health Promotion International* 4, no. 2 (1989): 77–82.

Kidd, Susan, Amanda Kenny, and Ruth Endacott. "Consumer Advocate and Clinician Perceptions of Consumer Participation in Two Rural Mental Health Services." *International Journal of Mental Health Nursing* 16, no. 3 (2007): 214–22.

Kidder, Ben. *The Challenges of Rural Transportation*. Logan: Western Rural Development Center, Utah State University, 2006.

Kilpatrick, Sue. "Multi-Level Rural Community Engagement in Health." *Australian Journal of Rural Health* 17, no. 1 (2009): 39–44.

Kim, Chansung. "Commuting Time Stability: A Test of a Co-Location Hypothesis." *Transportation Research Part A: Policy and Practice* 42, no. 3 (2008): 524–44.

Kim, Hyung Jin, and Katie M. Heinrich. "Built Environment Factors Influencing Walking to School Behaviors: A Comparison between a Small and Large US City." *Frontiers in Public Health* 4 (2016): 77.

Kim, Young Ook. "The Role of Spatial Configuration in Spatial Cognition." Paper presented at the Proceedings of the 3rd International Space Syntax Symposium, Georgia Tech, Atlanta, 2001.

Kindig, David, and Greg Stoddart. "What Is Population Health?" *American Journal of Public Health* 93, no. 3 (2003): 380–83.

King, Gary, Alan J. Flisher, Robyn Mallett, John Graham, Carl Lombard, Tanya Rawson, Neo K. Morojele, and Martie Muller. "Smoking in Cape Town: Community Influences on Adolescent Tobacco Use." *Preventive Medicine* 36, no. 1 (2003): 114–23.

King-Shier, K. M., C. Mather, and P. LeBlanc. "Understanding the Influence of Urban- or Rural-Living on Cardiac Patients' Decisions about Diet and Physical Activity: Descriptive Decision Modeling." *International Journal of Nursing Studies* 50, no. 11 (2013): 1513–23.

Kitagawa, Evelyn M., and Philip M. Hauser. *Differential Mortality in the United States: A Study in Socioeconomic Epidemiology*. Cambridge, MA: Harvard University Press, 2013.

Kley, A., and H. Paul. *Rural America*. Heidelberg: Universitätsverlag Winter, 2015. https://books.google.com/books?id=6RHQoQEACAAJ.

Kligerman, Morton, James F. Sallis, Sherry Ryan, Lawrence D. Frank, and Philip R. Nader. "Association of Neighborhood Design and Recreation Environment Variables with Physical Activity and Body Mass Index in Adolescents." *American Journal of Health Promotion* 21, no. 4 (2007): 274–77.

Knave, Bengt. "Electric and Magnetic Fields and Health Outcomes—an Overview." *Scandinavian Journal of Work, Environment and Health* 20 (1994): 78–89.

Kocken, Paul L., Jennifer Eeuwijk, Nicole M. C. Van Kesteren, Elise Dusseldorp, Goof Buijs, Zeina Bassa-Dafesh, and Jeltje Snel. "Promoting the Purchase of Low-Calorie Foods from School Vending Machines: A Cluster-Randomized Controlled Study." *Journal of School Health* 82, no. 3 (2012): 115–22.

Koh, Howard K., Garth Graham, and Sherry A. Glied. "Reducing Racial and Ethnic Disparities: The Action Plan from the Department of Health and Human Services." *Health Affairs* 30, no. 10 (2011): 1822–29.

Koohsari, Mohammad Javad, Takemi Sugiyama, Shannon Sahlqvist, Suzanne Mavoa, Nyssa Hadgraft, and Neville Owen. "Neighborhood Environmental Attributes and Adults' Sedentary Behaviors: Review and Research Agenda." *Preventive Medicine* 77 (2015): 141–49.

Krannich, Richard, and Peggy Petrzelka. "Tourism and Natural Amenity Development: Real Opportunities." In *Challenges for Rural America in the Twenty-First Century*, edited by David L. Brown and Louis E. Swanson, 190–99. University Park: Pennsylvania State University Press, 2003.

Krishna, Santosh, Kathleen N. Gillespie, and Timothy M. McBride. "Diabetes Burden and Access to Preventive Care in the Rural United States." *Journal of Rural Health* 26, no. 1 (2010): 3–11.

Križan, František, Kristína Bilková, Pavol Kita, and Marcel Horňák. "Potential Food Deserts and Food Oases in a Post-Communist City: Access, Quality, Variability and Price of Food in Bratislava-Petržalka." *Applied Geography* 62 (2015): 8–18.

Krout, John A. "Rural versus Urban Differences in Health Dependence among the Elderly Population." *International Journal of Aging and Human Development* 28, no. 2 (1989): 141–56.

Kuczmarski, Robert J., Katherine M. Flegal, Stephen M. Campbell, and Clifford L. Johnson. "Increasing Prevalence of Overweight among US Adults: The National Health and Nutrition Examination Surveys, 1960 to 1991." *Journal of the American Medical Association* 272, no. 3 (1994): 205–11.

Kühnert, Christian, Dirk Helbing, and Geoffrey B. West. "Scaling Laws in Urban Supply Networks." *Physica A: Statistical Mechanics and Its Applications* 363, no. 1 (2006): 96–103.

Kulig, Judith C., and Allison M. Williams. *Health in Rural Canada*. Vancouver: University of British Columbia Press, 2011.

Künzli, Nino, Reinhard Kaiser, Sylvia Medina, Michael Studnicka, Olivier Chanel, Paul Filliger, Max Herry, et al. "Public-Health Impact of Outdoor and Traffic-Related Air Pollution: A European Assessment." *Lancet* 356, no. 9232 (2000): 795–801.

Kuo, Ming. "How Might Contact with Nature Promote Human Health? Promising Mechanisms and a Possible Central Pathway." *Frontiers in Psychology* 6 (2015): 1093.

Kurtz, Hilda E. "Scale Frames and Counter-Scale Frames: Constructing the Problem of Environmental Injustice." *Political Geography* 22, no. 8 (2003): 887–916.

Lachapelle, Ugo, and Robert B. Noland. "Inconsistencies in Associations between Crime and Walking: A Reflection of Poverty and Density." *International Journal of Sustainable Transportation* 9, no. 2 (2015): 103–15.

Lachowycz, Kate, and Andy P. Jones. "Greenspace and Obesity: A Systematic Review of the Evidence." *Obesity Reviews* 12, no. 5 (2011): e183–e89.

Ladbrook, Denis A. "Why Are Crime Rates Higher in Urban Than in Rural Areas? Evidence from Japan." *Australian and New Zealand Journal of Criminology* 21, no. 2 (1988): 81–103.

Landsbergis, Paul A., Peter L. Schnall, Karen L. Belkić, Dean Baker, Joseph E. Schwartz, and Thomas G. Pickering. "The Workplace and Cardiovascular Disease: Relevance and Potential Role for Occupational Health Psychology." In *Handbook of Occupational Health Psychology*, 265–87. Washington, DC: American Psychological Association, 2003.

Lang, Thierry, Christiane Fouriaud, and Marie-Christine Jacquinet-Salord. "Length of Occupational Noise Exposure and Blood Pressure." *International Archives of Occupational and Environmental Health* 63, no. 6 (1992): 369–72.

Larsen, Kristian, Brian Cook, Michelle R. Stone, and Guy E. J. Faulkner. "Food Access and Children's BMI in Toronto, Ontario: Assessing How the Food Environment Relates to Overweight and Obesity." *International Journal of Public Health* 60, no. 1 (2015): 69–77.

Larsen, Kristian, and Jason Gilliland. "A Farmers' Market in a Food Desert: Evaluating Impacts on the Price and Availability of Healthy Food." *Health and Place* 15, no. 4 (2009): 1158–62.

Larson, James S. "The Conceptualization of Health." *Medical Care Research and Review* 56, no. 2 (1999): 123–36.

Larson, Nicole, Dianne Neumark-Sztainer, Melissa Nelson Laska, and Mary Story. "Young Adults and Eating Away from Home: Associations with Dietary Intake Patterns and Weight Status Differ by Choice of Restaurant." *Journal of the American Dietetic Association* 111, no. 11 (2011): 1696–703.

Larson, N. I., M. T. Story, and M. C. Nelson. "Neighborhood Environments: Disparities in Access to Healthy Foods in the U.S." *American Journal of Preventive Medicine* 36, no. 1 (2009): 74–81. https://doi.org/10.1016/j.amepre.2008.09.025.

Lasley, J. *Designing Out Gang Homicides and Street Assaults.* Washington, DC: National Institute of Justice, 1998.

Laverack, Glenn. "Improving Health Outcomes through Community Empowerment: A Review of the Literature." *Journal of Health, Population and Nutrition* 24, no. 1 (2006): 113–20.

Law, Stephen, Alain Chiaradia, and Christian Schwander. "Towards a Multimodal Space Syntax Analysis: A Case Study of the London Street and Underground Network." Paper presented at the Proceedings of the 8th International Space Syntax Symposium, Santiago de Chile, Chile, 2012.

Lawlor, Debbie A., Li Benfield, Jennifer Logue, Kate Tilling, Laura D. Howe, Abigail Fraser, Lynne Cherry, et al. "Association between General and Central Adiposity in Childhood, and Change in These, with Cardiovascular Risk Factors in Adolescence: Prospective Cohort Study." *BMJ* 341 (2010).

Lawrence, Elizabeth M. "Why Do College Graduates Behave More Healthfully Than Those Who Are Less Educated?" *Journal of Health and Social Behavior* 58, no. 3 (2017): 291–306.

Learnihan, V., K. P. Van Niel, B. Giles-Corti, and M. Knuiman. "Effect of Scale on the Links between Walking and Urban Design." *Geographical Research* 49, no. 2 (2011): 183–91.

Lee, Chanam, and Anne Vernez Moudon. "Correlates of Walking for Transportation or Recreation Purposes." *Journal of Physical Activity and Health* 3, no. s1 (2006): S77–S98.

Lee, Chanam, and Anne Vernez Moudon. "The 3Ds+ R: Quantifying Land Use and Urban Form Correlates of Walking." *Transportation Research Part D: Transport and Environment* 11, no. 3 (2006): 204–15.

Lee, I-Min, and Ralph S. Paffenbarger Jr. "Associations of Light, Moderate, and Vigorous Intensity Physical Activity with Longevity: The Harvard Alumni Health Study." *American Journal of Epidemiology* 151, no. 3 (2000): 293–99.

Lee, I-Min, Eric J. Shiroma, Felipe Lobelo, Pekka Puska, Steven N. Blair, Peter T. Katzmarzyk, and Lancet Physical Activity Series Working Group. "Effect of Physical Inactivity on Major Non-Communicable Diseases Worldwide: An Analysis of Burden of Disease and Life Expectancy." *Lancet* 380, no. 9838 (2012): 219–29.

Lee, Matthew R., and Graham C. Ousey. "Size Matters: Examining the Link between Small Manufacturing, Socioeconomic Deprivation, and Crime Rates in Nonmetropolitan Communities." *Sociological Quarterly* 42, no. 4 (2001): 581–602.

Lee, Seungjae, and Seungkyu Ryu. "Multiple Path-Finding Models Using Kalman Filtering and Space Syntax Techniques." *Transportation Research Record: Journal of the Transportation Research Board*, no. 2029 (2007): 87–95.

Leech, J. A., W. C. Nelson, R. T. Burnett, S. Aaron, and M. E. Raizenne. "It's About Time: A Comparison of Canadian and American Time-Activity Patterns." *Journal of Exposure Science and Environmental Epidemiology* 12, no. 6 (2002): 427–32.

Leigh-Preston, Nancey. *The Nation's Changing Earning Distribution from 1967 to 1986: What Has Happened to the Middle?* Berkeley: Institute of Urban and Regional Development, University of California at Berkeley, 1988.

Lenardson, Jennifer D., Erika C. Ziller, David Lambert, Melanie M. Race, and Anush Yousefian. *Access to Mental Health Services and Family Impact of Rural Children with Mental Health Problems.* Portland: Maine Rural Health Research Center, 2010.

Lensmire, T. J. *White Folks: Race and Identity in Rural America*. New York: Taylor and Francis, 2017. https://books.google.com/books?id=pgkqDwAAQBAJ.

Leslie, Eva, and Ester Cerin. "Are Perceptions of the Local Environment Related to Neighborhood Satisfaction and Mental Health in Adults?" *Preventive Medicine* 47, no. 3 (2008): 273–78.

Levin, Kate A., and Alastair H. Leyland. "Urban/Rural Inequalities in Suicide in Scotland, 1981–1999." *Social Science and Medicine* 60, no. 12 (2005): 2877–90.

Leyden, Kevin M. "Social Capital and the Built Environment: The Importance of Walkable Neighborhoods." *American Journal of Public Health* 93, no. 9 (2003): 1546–51.

Li, Chuo, Guangqing Chi, and Robert Jackson. "Perceptions and Barriers to Walking in the Rural South of the United States: The Influence of Neighborhood Built Environment on Pedestrian Behaviors." *Urban Design International* 20, no. 4 (2015): 255–73.

Li, Fuzhong, K. John Fisher, Adrian Bauman, Marcia G. Ory, Wojtek Chodzko-Zajko, Peter Harmer, Mark Bosworth, and Minot Cleveland. "Neighborhood Influences on Physical Activity in Middle-Aged and Older Adults: A Multilevel Perspective." *Journal of Aging and Physical Activity* 13, no. 1 (2005): 87–114.

Li, Fuzhong, Peter A. Harmer, Bradley J. Cardinal, Mark Bosworth, Alan Acock, Deborah Johnson-Shelton, and Jane M. Moore. "Built Environment, Adiposity, and Physical Activity in Adults Aged 50–75." *American Journal of Preventive Medicine* 35, no. 1 (2008): 38–46.

Li, Fuzhong, Peter Harmer, Bradley J. Cardinal, and Naruepon Vongjaturapat. "Built Environment and Changes in Blood Pressure in Middle Aged and Older Adults." *Preventive Medicine* 48, no. 3 (2009): 237–41.

Liberato, Selma C., Ross Bailie, and Julie Brimblecombe. "Nutrition Interventions at Point-of-Sale to Encourage Healthier Food Purchasing: A Systematic Review." *BMC Public Health* 14, no. 1 (2014): 1–14.

Lichter, Daniel T. "Immigration and the New Racial Diversity in Rural America." *Rural Sociology* 77, no. 1 (2012): 3–35.

Lichter, Daniel T. "Race and Underemployment: Black Employment Hardship in the Rural South." In *The Rural South in Crisis*, edited by L. J. Beaulieu, 181–97. Boulder, CO: Westview Press, 1988.

Lichter, Daniel T. "Race, Employment Hardship, and Inequality in the American Nonmetropolitan South." *American Sociological Review* 54, no. 3 (1989): 436–46.

Lichter, Daniel T., and David L. Brown. "Rural America in an Urban Society: Changing Spatial and Social Boundaries." *Annual Review of Sociology* 37 (2011): 565–92.

Lichter, Daniel T., and Kenneth M. Johnson. "Emerging Rural Settlement Patterns and the Geographic Redistribution of America's New Immigrants." *Rural Sociology* 71, no. 1 (2006): 109–31.

Lichter, Daniel T., D. K. McLaughlin, and G. T. Cornwell. "Migration and the Loss of Human Resources in Rural America." In *Investing in People: The Human Capital Needs of Rural America*, edited by L. J. Beaulieu and D. Mulkay, 235–56. Boulder, CO: Westview, 1995.

Lichter, Daniel T., Domenico Parisi, Michael C. Taquino, and Steven Michael Grice. "Residential Segregation in New Hispanic Destinations: Cities, Suburbs, and Rural Communities Compared." *Social Science Research* 39, no. 2 (2010): 215–30.

Liese, Angela D., Kristina E. Weis, Delores Pluto, Emily Smith, and Andrew Lawson. "Food Store Types, Availability, and Cost of Foods in a Rural Environment." *Journal of the American Dietetic Association* 107, no. 11 (2007): 1916–23.

Liffman, M. *Power for the Poor—Family Centre Project: An Experience in Self-Help?* London: George Allen and Unwin, 1978.

Lim, Stephen S., Theo Vos, Abraham D. Flaxman, Goodarz Danaei, Kenji Shibuya, Heather Adair-Rohani, Mohammad A. AlMazroa, et al. "A Comparative Risk Assessment of

Burden of Disease and Injury Attributable to 67 Risk Factors and Risk Factor Clusters in 21 Regions, 1990–2010: A Systematic Analysis for the Global Burden of Disease Study 2010." *Lancet* 380, no. 9859 (2012): 2224–60.

Link, Rachael. "What's Wrong with Factory Farming?" Nutrition Stripped, August 23, 2019. https://nutritionstripped.com/whats-wrong-with-factory-farming/.

Listerborn, Carina. "Women's Fear and Space Configurations." Paper presented at the Proceedings of the 2nd International Symposium on Space Syntax, University of Brasilia, Brazil, March 29–April 2, 1999.

Litman, Todd, and MacPherson Hughes-Cromwick. *Public Transportation's Impact on Rural and Small Towns: A Vital Mobility Link.* Washington, DC: American Public Transportation Association, 2017.

Liu, Ji-Hong, Sonya J. Jones, Han Sun, Janice C. Probst, Anwar T. Merchant, and Philip Cavicchia. "Diet, Physical Activity, and Sedentary Behaviors as Risk Factors for Childhood Obesity: An Urban and Rural Comparison." *Childhood Obesity (Formerly Obesity and Weight Management)* 8, no. 5 (2012): 440–48.

Lobao, Linda. "Continuity and Change in Place Stratification: Spatial Inequality and Middle-Range Territorial Units." *Rural Sociology* 69, no. 1 (2004): 1–30.

Lobao, Linda, and Katherine Meyer. "The Great Agricultural Transition: Crisis, Change, and Social Consequences of Twentieth Century US Farming." *Annual Review of Sociology* 27, no. 1 (2001): 103–24.

Locher, Julie L., Christine S. Ritchie, David L. Roth, Patricia Sawyer Baker, Eric V. Bodner, and Richard M. Allman. "Social Isolation, Support, and Capital and Nutritional Risk in an Older Sample: Ethnic and Gender Differences." *Social Science and Medicine* 60, no. 4 (2005): 747–61.

Lock, Karen, Joceline Pomerleau, Louise Causer, Dan R. Altmann, and Martin McKee. "The Global Burden of Disease Attributable to Low Consumption of Fruit and Vegetables: Implications for the Global Strategy on Diet." *Bulletin of the World Health Organization* 83 (2005): 100–08.

Long, Kathleen Ann, and Clarann Weinert. "Rural Nursing: Developing the Theory Base." In *Rural Nursing: Concepts, Theory, and Practice,* edited by Helen J. Lee and Charlene A. Winters, 3–16. New York: Springer, 2006.

Long, Larry, and Alfred Nucci. "Accounting for Two Population Turnarounds in Nonmetropolitan America." *Research in Rural Sociology and Development* 7 (1998): 47–70.

Long, Yixiang. "The Relationships between Objective and Subjective Evaluations of the Urban Environment: Space Syntax, Cognitive Maps, and Urban Legibility." PhD diss., North Carolina State University, 2007. ProQuest.

Lopez, R. *The Built Environment and Public Health.* San Francisco: Wiley, 2012. https://books.google.com/books?id=ffnSgk3f1cYC.

Lorenc, Theo, Stephen Clayton, David Neary, Margaret Whitehead, Mark Petticrew, Hilary Thomson, Steven Cummins, Amanda Sowden, and Adrian Renton. "Crime, Fear of Crime, Environment, and Mental Health and Wellbeing: Mapping Review of Theories and Causal Pathways." *Health and Place* 18, no. 4 (2012): 757–65.

Loucaides, Constantinos A., Ronald C. Plotnikoff, and Kim Bercovitz. "Differences in the Correlates of Physical Activity between Urban and Rural Canadian Youth." *Journal of School Health* 77, no. 4 (2007): 164–70.

Loukaitou-Sideris, Anastasia. "Hot Spots of Bus Stop Crime: The Importance of Environmental Attributes." *Journal of the American Planning Association* 65, no. 4 (1999): 395–411.

Lovasi, Gina S., Malo A. Hutson, Monica Guerra, and Kathryn M. Neckerman. "Built Environments and Obesity in Disadvantaged Populations." *Epidemiologic Reviews* 31, no. 1 (2009): 7–20.

Lovell, Sarah Taylor. "Multifunctional Urban Agriculture for Sustainable Land Use Planning in the United States." *Sustainability* 2, no. 8 (2010): 2499–522.

Luedtke, G., and Associates. *Crime and the Physical City: Neighborhood Design Techniques for Crime Reduction*. Washington, DC, 1970.

Lund, Hollie. "Pedestrian Environments and Sense of Community." *Journal of Planning Education and Research* 21, no. 3 (2002): 301–12.

Lutfiyya, May Nawal, Deepa K. Bhat, Seema R. Gandhi, Catherine Nguyen, Vicki L. Weidenbacher Hoper, and Martin S. Lipsky. "A Comparison of Quality of Care Indicators in Urban Acute Care Hospitals and Rural Critical Access Hospitals in the United States." *International Journal for Quality in Health Care* 19, no. 3 (2007): 141–49.

Lutfiyya, May Nawal, Linda F. Chang, and Martin S. Lipsky. "A Cross-Sectional Study of US Rural Adults' Consumption of Fruits and Vegetables: Do They Consume at Least Five Servings Daily?" *BMC Public Health* 12, no. 1 (2012): 280.

Lutfiyya, May Nawal, Martin S. Lipsky, Jennifer Wisdom-Behounek, and Melissa Inpanbutr-Martinkus. "Is Rural Residency a Risk Factor for Overweight and Obesity for US Children?" *Obesity* 15, no. 9 (2007): 2348–56.

Lutfiyya, May Nawal, Joel Emery McCullough, Irina V. Haller, Stephen C. Waring, Joseph A. Bianco, and Martin Stephen Lipsky. "Rurality as a Root or Fundamental Social Determinant of Health." *Disease-a-Month* 58, no. 11 (2012): 620–28.

Lutfiyya, May Nawal, Joel Emery McCullough, and Martin Stephen Lipsky. "A Population-Based Study of Health Service Deficits for US Adults with Asthma." *Journal of Asthma* 48, no. 9 (2011): 931–44.

Lutfiyya, May Nawal, Joel E. McCullough, Lori Mitchell, L. Scott Dean, and Martin S. Lipsky. "Adequacy of Diabetes Care for Older US Rural Adults: A Cross-Sectional Population Based Study Using 2009 BRFSS Data." *BMC Public Health* 11, no. 1 (2011): 940.

Lutfiyya, May Nawal, Yogi R. Patel, John B. Steele, Beatrice S. Tetteh, Linda Chang, Carlos Aguero, Om Prakash, and Martin S. Lipsky. "Are There Disparities in Diabetes Care? A Comparison of Care Received by US Rural and Non-Rural Adults with Diabetes." *Primary Health Care Research and Development* 10, no. 4 (2009): 320–31.

Lutfiyya, May Nawal, K. K. Shah, M. Johnson, R. W. Bales, I. Cha, C. McGrath, L. Serpa, and M. Lipsky. "Adolescent Daily Cigarette Smoking: Is Rural Residency a Risk Factor?" *Rural and Remote Health* 8 (2008): 875.

Lynch, John W., George A. Kaplan, Elsie R. Pamuk, Richard D. Cohen, Katherine E. Heck, Jennifer L. Balfour, and Irene H. Yen. "Income Inequality and Mortality in Metropolitan Areas of the United States." *American Journal of Public Health* 88, no. 7 (1998): 1074–80.

Lynch, John W., George Davey Smith, George A. Kaplan, and James S. House. "Income Inequality and Mortality: Importance to Health of Individual Income, Psychosocial Environment, or Material Conditions." *BMJ* 320, no. 7243 (2000): 1200–04.

Lyson, Thomas A. "Big Business and Community Welfare: Revisiting a Classic Study by C. Wright Mills and Melville Ulmer." *American Journal of Economics and Sociology* 65, no. 5 (2006): 1001–23.

Lyson, T. "Entry into Farming: Implications of a Dual Agricultural Structure." In *Agricultural Change*, edited by J. Molnar, 155–76. Boulder, CO: Westview Press, 1986.

Maas, Jolanda, Robert A. Verheij, Sjerp de Vries, Peter Spreeuwenberg, Francois G. Schellevis, and Peter P. Groenewegen. "Morbidity Is Related to a Green Living Environment." *Journal of Epidemiology and Community Health* 63, no. 12 (2009): 967–73.

Maas, Jolanda, Robert A. Verheij, Peter P. Groenewegen, Sjerp De Vries, and Peter Spreeuwenberg. "Green Space, Urbanity, and Health: How Strong Is the Relation?" *Journal of Epidemiology and Community Health* 60, no. 7 (2006): 587–92.

Macdonald, Laura, Anne Ellaway, and Sally Macintyre. "The Food Retail Environment and

Area Deprivation in Glasgow City, UK." *International Journal of Behavioral Nutrition and Physical Activity* 6, no. 52 (2009). https://link.springer.com/article/10.1186/1479-5868-6-52.

Macintyre, Sally. "The Black Report and Beyond What Are the Issues?" *Social Science and Medicine* 44, no. 6 (1997): 723–45.

Macintyre, Sally, and Anne Ellaway. "Ecological Approaches: Rediscovering the Role of the Physical and Social Environment." *Social Epidemiology* 9, no. 5 (2000): 332–48.

Macintyre, Sally, and Anne Ellaway. "Neighborhoods and Health: An Overview." In *Neighborhoods and Health*, edited by Ichiro Kawachi and Lisa F. Berkman, 20–42. Oxford: Oxford University Press, 2003.

Macintyre, Sally, Anne Ellaway, and Steven Cummins. "Place Effects on Health: How Can We Conceptualise, Operationalise and Measure Them?" *Social Science and Medicine* 55, no. 1 (2002): 125–39.

Macintyre, Sally, Sheila Maciver, and Anne Sooman. "Area, Class and Health: Should We Be Focusing on Places or People?" *Journal of Social Policy* 22, no. 2 (1993): 213–34.

Mackenbach, Joreintje D., Harry Rutter, Sofie Compernolle, Ketevan Glonti, Jean-Michel Oppert, Helene Charreire, Ilse De Bourdeaudhuij, et al. "Obesogenic Environments: A Systematic Review of the Association between the Physical Environment and Adult Weight Status, the Spotlight Project." *BMC Public Health* 14, no. 1 (2014): 233.

MacKinney, A. Clinton, Keith J. Mueller, and Timothy D. McBride. "The March to Accountable Care Organizations—How Will Rural Fare?" *Journal of Rural Health* 27, no. 1 (2011): 131–37.

Maley, Mary, Barbour S. Warren, and Carol M. Devine. "Perceptions of the Environment for Eating and Exercise in a Rural Community." *Journal of Nutrition Education and Behavior* 42, no. 3 (2010): 185–91.

Marcelis, Machteld, F. Navarro-Mateu, Robin Murray, Jean-Paul Selten, and Jim van Os. "Urbanization and Psychosis: A Study of 1942–1978 Birth Cohorts in the Netherlands." *Psychological Medicine* 28, no. 4 (1998): 871–79.

Marcelis, Machteld, N. Takei, and Jim van Os. "Urbanization and Risk for Schizophrenia: Does the Effect Operate before or around the Time of Illness Onset?" *Psychological Medicine* 29, no. 5 (1999): 1197–203.

Marmot, Michael. *Status Syndrome: How Your Social Standing Directly Affects Your Health.* London: Bloomsbury, 2005.

Marmot, Michael, Jessica Allen, Ruth Bell, Ellen Bloomer, and Peter Goldblatt. "WHO European Review of Social Determinants of Health and the Health Divide." *Lancet* 380, no. 9846 (2012): 1011–29.

Marmot, Michael, Jessica Allen, Ruth Bell, and Peter Goldblatt. "Building of the Global Movement for Health Equity: From Santiago to Rio and Beyond." *Lancet* 379, no. 9811 (2012): 181–88.

Marmot, Michael, Sharon Friel, Ruth Bell, Tanja Houweling, and Sebastian Taylor. "Closing the Gap in a Generation: Health Equity through Action on the Social Determinants of Health." *Lancet* 372, no. 9650 (2008): 1661–69.

Martin, Claudia J., Stephen D. Platt, and Sonja M. Hunt. "Housing Conditions and Ill Health." *British Medical Journal (Clinical Research Edition)* 294, no. 6580 (1987): 1125–27.

Martin, Linda G., Robert F. Schoeni, and Patricia M. Andreski. "Trends in Health of Older Adults in the United States: Past, Present, Future." *Demography* 47, no. 1 (2010): S17–S40.

Martin, Sarah Levin, Gregory J. Kirkner, Kelly Mayo, Charles E. Matthews, J. Larry Durstine, and James R. Hebert. "Urban, Rural, and Regional Variations in Physical Activity." *Journal of Rural Health* 21, no. 3 (2005): 239–44.

Mason, Phil, Ade Kearns, and Mark Livingston. "'Safe Going': The Influence of Crime Rates and Perceived Crime and Safety on Walking in Deprived Neighborhoods." *Social Science and Medicine* 91 (2013): 15–24.

Massey, Douglas S., ed. *New Faces in New Places: The Changing Geography of American Immigration.* New York: Russell Sage Foundation, 2008.

Massey, Douglas S., and Nancy A. Denton. *American Apartheid: Segregation and the Making of the Underclass.* Cambridge, MA: Harvard University Press, 1993.

Maxouris, Christina. "For Months, a Rural Kansas Community Watched the Covid-19 Pandemic Unfold from Afar. Then, a Deadly Outbreak Landed Right on Their Doorstep." CNN, November 28, 2020, https://www.cnn.com/2020/11/28/us/rural-america-covid-norton-kansas/index.html.

Mayer, Amy. "Across Midwest Farm Fields, Pesticide Exposure Is Tracked Unevenly or Not at All." Illinois Public Media, May 14, 2019, https://will.illinois.edu/news/story/across-midwest-farm-fields-pesticide-exposure-is-tracked-unevenly-or-not-at.

Mayer, Leo V. "Agricultural Change and Rural America." *Annals of the American Academy of Political and Social Science* 529, no. 1 (1993): 80–91.

Mayer, Susan, and Christopher Jencks. "War on Poverty: No Apologies, Please." *New York Times,* November 9, 1995.

McCahill, Chris, and Norman Garrick. "The Applicability of Space Syntax to Bicycle Facility Planning." *Transportation Research Record: Journal of the Transportation Research Board,* no. 2074 (2008): 46–51.

McCann, B., and Reid Ewing. *Measuring the Health Effects of Sprawl: A National Analysis of Physical Activity, Obesity and Chronic Disease.* Washington, DC: Surface Transportation Policy Project, 2003.

McConnell, Eileen Diaz, and Faranak Miraftab. "Sundown Town to 'Little Mexico': Old-Timers and Newcomers in an American Small Town." *Rural Sociology* 74, no. 4 (2009): 605–29.

McCormack, Gavin R., Billie Giles-Corti, and Max Bulsara. "Correlates of Using Neighborhood Recreational Destinations in Physically Active Respondents." *Journal of Physical Activity and Health* 4, no. 1 (2007): 39–53.

McCormack, Gavin R., and Alan Shiell. "In Search of Causality: A Systematic Review of the Relationship between the Built Environment and Physical Activity among Adults." *International Journal of Behavioral Nutrition and Physical Activity* 8, no. 125 (2011). https://link.springer.com/article/10.1186/1479-5868-8-125.

McDowell, I., and C. Newell. *Measuring Health: A Guide to Rating Scales and Questionnaires.* New York: Oxford University Press, 1987.

McEachran, Andrew D., Brett R. Blackwell, J. Delton Hanson, Kimberly J. Wooten, Gregory D. Mayer, Stephen B. Cox, and Philip N. Smith. "Antibiotics, Bacteria, and Antibiotic Resistance Genes: Aerial Transport from Cattle Feed Yards via Particulate Matter." *Environmental Health Perspectives* 123, no. 4 (2015): 337–43.

McEntire, K. "Kansas's 20 Safest Cities of 2021." SafeWise, March 2021, accessed September 19, 2021, https://www.safewise.com/blog/safest-cities-kansas/.

McGranahan, David A. *Natural Amenities Drive Rural Population Change.* Washington, DC: Department of Agriculture, Economic Research Service, 1999.

McGrath, John, Sukanta Saha, Joy Welham, Ossama El Saadi, Clare MacCauley, and David Chant. "A Systematic Review of the Incidence of Schizophrenia: The Distribution of Rates and the Influence of Sex, Urbanicity, Migrant Status and Methodology." *BMC Medicine* 2 (April 2004).

McKenzie, Brian S. "Access to Supermarkets among Poorer Neighborhoods: A Comparison of Time and Distance Measures." *Urban Geography* 35, no. 1 (January 2014): 133–51. https://doi.org/10.1080/02723638.2013.856195.

McKinnon, Robin A., Jill Reedy, Meredith A. Morrissette, Leslie A. Lytle, and Amy L. Yaroch. "Measures of the Food Environment: A Compilation of the Literature, 1990–2007." *American Journal of Preventive Medicine* 36, no. 4 (2009): S124–S33.

McLean, Jim. "'Get Big or Get out' Farming Has Left Kansas Towns Struggling for Survival." KCUR, October 18, 2019. https://www.kcur.org/agriculture/2019-10-18/get-big-or-get-out-farming-has-left-kansas-towns-struggling-for-survival.

McLeroy, Kenneth R., Daniel Bibeau, Allan Steckler, and Karen Glanz. "An Ecological Perspective on Health Promotion Programs." *Health Education Quarterly* 15, no. 4 (1988): 351–77.

McMichael, Anthony J., Rosalie E. Woodruff, and Simon Hales. "Climate Change and Human Health: Present and Future Risks." *Lancet* 367, no. 9513 (2006): 859–69.

McMichael, Philip. "The Impact of Global Economic Practices on American Farming." In *Challenges for Rural America in the Twenty-First Century*, edited by D. L. Brown and L. E. Swanson, 375–84. University Park: Pennsylvania State University Press, 2003.

McNeill, J. R. *Something New Under the Sun: An Environmental History of the Twentieth Century*. New York: Norton, 2000.

Meara, Ellen R., Seth Richards, and David M. Cutler. "The Gap Gets Bigger: Changes in Mortality and Life Expectancy, by Education, 1981–2000." *Health Affairs* 27, no. 2 (2008): 350–60.

Medicare Learning Network. *Critical Access Hospital*. Washington, DC: Centers for Medicare and Medicaid Services, US Department of Health and Human Services, 2021. https://www.cms.gov/Outreach-and-Education/Medicare-Learning-Network-MLN/MLNProducts/downloads/CritAccessHospfctsht.pdf.

Mehta, Neil K., and Virginia W. Chang. "Weight Status and Restaurant Availability: A Multilevel Analysis." *American Journal of Preventive Medicine* 34, no. 2 (2008): 127–33.

Meit, Michael, Alana Knudson, Tess Gilbert, Amanda Tzy-Chyi Yu, Erin Tanenbaum, Elizabeth Ormson, Shannon TenBroeck, Alycia Bayne, and Shena Popat. *The 2014 Update of the Rural-Urban Chartbook*. Bethesda, MD: Rural Health Reform Policy Research Center and Walsh Center for Rural Health Analysis, 2014. https://ruralhealth.und.edu/projects/health-reform-policy-research-center/pdf/2014-rural-urban-chartbook-update.pdf.

Melia, Steve, Graham Parkhurst, and Hugh Barton. "The Paradox of Intensification." *Transport Policy* 18, no. 1 (2011): 46–52.

Melosi, M. *The Sanitary City: Urban Infrastructure in America from Colonial Times to the Present*. Baltimore: Johns Hopkins University Press, 2000.

Merlo, Juan. "Multilevel Analytical Approaches in Social Epidemiology: Measures of Health Variation Compared with Traditional Measures of Association." *Journal of Epidemiology and Community Health* 57 (2003): 550–52.

Messick, Taylor. "Bel Aire Residents Want Good Roadways." *Ark Valley (KS) News*, February 24, 2017. http://www.arkvalleynews.com/web/isite.dll?1487889999333~health.

Messick, Taylor. "Park City Hoping to Improve Sidewalks." *Ark Valley (KS) News*, May 25, 2017. http://www.arkvalleynews.com/web/isite.dll?1495746450962~health.

Mexican American Legal Defense and Educational Fund. "Immigrants' Rights." Accessed September 30, 2021, https://www.maldef.org/category/immigrants-rights/.

Michael, Yvonne L., Leslie A. Perdue, Eric S. Orwoll, Marcia L. Stefanick, Lynn M. Marshall, and Osteoporotic Fractures in Men Study Group. "Physical Activity Resources and Changes in Walking in a Cohort of Older Men." *American Journal of Public Health* 100, no. 4 (2010): 654–60.

Michimi, Akihiko, and Michael C. Wimberly. "Associations of Supermarket Accessibility with Obesity and Fruit and Vegetable Consumption in the Conterminous United States." *International Journal of Health Geographics* 9, no. 49 (2010).

Miethe, Terance D., Michael Hughes, and David McDowall. "Social Change and Crime Rates: An Evaluation of Alternative Theoretical Approaches." *Social Forces* 70, no. 1 (1991): 165–85.

Milio, N. "Healthy Cities: The New Public Health and Supportive Research." *Health Promotion International* 5, no. 4 (1990): 291–97.

Miller, Michael K., and Albert E. Luloff. *Who Is Rural? A Typological Approach to the Examination of Rurality.* Fayetteville: Arkansas Agricultural Experiment Station, 1980.

Mirowsky, John, and Catherine E. Ross. "Education and Self-Rated Health: Cumulative Advantage and Its Rising Importance." *Research on Aging* 30, no. 1 (2008): 93–122.

Mirowsky, John, and Catherine E. Ross. *Education, Social Status, and Health.* New York: Routledge, 2017.

Mitchell, Richard, and Frank Popham. "Effect of Exposure to Natural Environment on Health Inequalities: An Observational Population Study." *Lancet* 372, no. 9650 (2008): 1655–60.

Mitton, Craig, Neale Smith, Stuart Peacock, Brian Evoy, and Julia Abelson. "Public Participation in Health Care Priority Setting: A Scoping Review." *Health Policy* 91, no. 3 (2009): 219–28.

Mobley, Lee R., Elisabeth D. Root, Eric A. Finkelstein, Olga Khavjou, Rosanne P. Farris, and Julie C. Will. "Environment, Obesity, and Cardiovascular Disease Risk in Low-Income Women." *American Journal of Preventive Medicine* 30, no. 4 (2006): 327–32.

Mohatt, Dennis F., Mimi M. Bradley, Scott J. Adams, and Chad D. Morris. *Mental Health and Rural America: 1994–2005. An Overview and Annotated Bibliography.* Washington, DC: Department of Health and Human Services; Health Resources and Services Administration, Office of Rural Health Policy, 2006.

Mohnen, Sigrid M., Peter P. Groenewegen, Beate Völker, and Henk Flap. "Neighborhood Social Capital and Individual Health." *Social Science and Medicine* 72, no. 5 (2011): 660–67.

Mokdad, Ali H., Barbara A. Bowman, Earl S. Ford, Frank Vinicor, James S. Marks, and Jeffrey P. Koplan. "The Continuing Epidemics of Obesity and Diabetes in the United States." *Journal of the American Medical Association* 286, no. 10 (2001): 1195–200.

Mokdad, Ali H., Mary K. Serdula, William H. Dietz, Barbara A. Bowman, James S. Marks, and Jeffrey P. Koplan. "The Spread of the Obesity Epidemic in the United States, 1991–1998." *Journal of the American Medical Association* 282, no. 16 (1999): 1519–22. https://doi.org/10.1001/jama.282.16.1519.

Molnar, J., ed. *Agricultural Change.* Boulder, CO: Westview Press, 1986.

Molnar, Joseph J. "Climate Change and Societal Response: Livelihoods, Communities, and the Environment." *Rural Sociology* 75, no. 1 (2010): 1–16.

Montez, Jennifer Karas, and Anna Zajacova. "Trends in Mortality Risk by Education Level and Cause of Death among US White Women from 1986 to 2006." *American Journal of Public Health* 103, no. 3 (2013): 473–79.

Montoya, Michael J., and Erin E. Kent. "Dialogical Action: Moving from Community-Based to Community-Driven Participatory Research." *Qualitative Health Research* 21, no. 7 (2011): 1000–1011.

Moonshadow Mobile. "Censusviewer." n.d., accessed September 26, 2021, http://censusviewer.com/.

Moore, Justin B., Jason Brinkley, Thomas W. Crawford, Kelly R. Evenson, and Ross C. Brownson. "Association of the Built Environment with Physical Activity and Adiposity in Rural and Urban Youth." *Preventive Medicine* 56, no. 2 (2013): 145–48.

Moore, R. M. *The Hidden America: Social Problems in Rural America for the Twenty-First Century.* Selinsgrove, PA: Susquehanna University Press, 2001. https://books.google.com/books?id=kQkquC4-xloC.

Morland, Kimberly, Ana V. Diez-Roux, and Steve Wing. "Supermarkets, Other Food Stores, and Obesity: The Atherosclerosis Risk in Communities Study." *American Journal of Preventive Medicine* 30, no. 4 (2006): 333–39.

Morland, Kimberly B., and Kelly R. Evenson. "Obesity Prevalence and the Local Food Environment." *Health and Place* 15, no. 2 (2009): 491–95.

Morland, Kimberly, Steve Wing, Ana Diez-Roux, and Charles Poole. "Neighborhood Characteristics Associated with the Location of Food Stores and Food Service Places." *American Journal of Preventive Medicine* 22, no. 1 (2002): 23–29.

Morris, Frank. "A Thriving Rural Town's Winning Formula Faces New Threats under Trump Administration." NPR, February 19, 2017. https://www.npr.org/2017/02/19/516016940/a-thriving-rural-towns-winning-formula-faces-new-threats-under-trump-administrat.

Morris, J. N., D. B. Blane, and I. R. White. "Levels of Mortality, Education, and Social Conditions in the 107 Local Education Authority Areas of England." *Journal of Epidemiology and Community Health* 50, no. 1 (1996): 15–17.

Morris, Jeremiah N., J. A. Heady, P. A. B. Raffle, C. G. Roberts, and J. W. Parks. "Coronary Heart-Disease and Physical Activity of Work." *Lancet* 262, no. 6796 (1953): 1111–20.

Morton, Lois Wright, Ella Annette Bitto, Mary Jane Oakland, and Mary Sand. "Solving the Problems of Iowa Food Deserts: Food Insecurity and Civic Structure." *Rural Sociology* 70, no. 1 (2005): 94–112.

Moudon, Anne Vernez. "Real Noise from the Urban Environment: How Ambient Community Noise Affects Health and What Can Be Done About It." *American Journal of Preventive Medicine* 37, no. 2 (2009): 167–71.

Murayama, Hiroshi, Yoshinori Fujiwara, and Ichiro Kawachi. "Social Capital and Health: A Review of Prospective Multilevel Studies." *Journal of Epidemiology* 22, no. 3 (2012).

Muro, Mark, and Robert Puentes. *Investing in a Better Future: A Review of the Fiscal and Competitive Advantages of Smarter Growth Development Patterns.* Washington, DC: Center on Urban and Metropolitan Policy, Brookings Institution, 2004.

Murphy, Sherry L., Jiaquan Xu, and Kenneth D. Kochanek. "Deaths: Final Data for 2010." In *National Vital Statistics Reports, Vol. 61 No. 4.* Hyattsville, MD: National Center for Health Statistics, 2013. http://www.cdc.gov/nchs/data/nvsr/nvsr61/nvsr61_04.pdf.

Murray, Christopher J. L., Sandeep C. Kulkarni, Catherine Michaud, Niels Tomijima, Maria T. Bulzacchelli, Terrell J. Iandiorio, and Majid Ezzati. "Eight Americas: Investigating Mortality Disparities across Races, Counties, and Race-Counties in the United States." *PLoS Med* 3, no. 9 (2006): e260. https://doi.org/10.1371/journal.pmed.0030260.

Must, Aviva, Jennifer Spadano, Eugenie H. Coakley, Alison E. Field, Graham Colditz, and William H. Dietz. "The Disease Burden Associated with Overweight and Obesity." *Journal of the American Medical Association* 282, no. 16 (1999): 1523–29.

Nadimpalli, Maya, Jessica L. Rinsky, Steve Wing, Devon Hall, Jill Stewart, Jesper Larsen, Keeve E. Nachman, et al. "Persistence of Livestock-Associated Antibiotic-Resistant Staphylococcus Aureus among Industrial Hog Operation Workers in North Carolina over 14 Days." *Occupational and Environmental Medicine* 72, no. 2 (2015): 90–99.

Nagel, Corey L., Nichole E. Carlson, Mark Bosworth, and Yvonne L. Michael. "The Relation between Neighborhood Built Environment and Walking Activity among Older Adults." *American Journal of Epidemiology* 168, no. 4 (2008): 461–68.

Nasar, Jack L., and David A. Julian. "The Psychological Sense of Community in the Neighborhood." *Journal of the American Planning Association* 61, no. 2 (1995): 178–84.

National Agricultural Statistics Service. "Kansas Farm Facts." Department of Agriculture, 2000, accessed July 17, 2019. https://quickstats.nass.usda.gov/.

National Center for Health Statistics. *Health, United States, 2011: With Special Feature on Socioeconomic Status and Health (Trend Tables).* Hyattsville, MD: National Center for Health Statistics, 2012. http://www.cdc.gov/nchs/data/hus/hus11.pdf.

National Center for Health Statistics. "Health, United States, 2012: With Special Feature on Emergency Care (Table 114)." In *DHHS Publication No. 2013–1232*. Hyattsville, MD: National Center for Health Statistics, 2013. http://www.cdc.gov/nchs/data/hus/hus12.pdf.

National Center for Health Statistics. *Health, United States, 2013: With Special Feature on Prescription Drugs*. Hyattsville, MD: National Center for Health Statistics, 2014.

National Center for Health Statistics. *Urban Rural Health Chart Book. Health, United States 2001*. Hyattsville, MD: National Center for Health Statistics, 2001.

National Hog Farmer. "FDA Announces Implementation of GFI #213, Outlines Continuing Efforts to Address Antimicrobial Resistance." January 6, 2017. https://www.nationalhog farmer.com/animal-health/fda-concludes-medically-important-antimicrobials-transition -process.

National Institutes of Health. "National Institute on Drug Abuse." Accessed September 24, 2021, https://www.drugabuse.gov/.

National Policy and Legal Analysis Network to Prevent Childhood Obesity and ChangeLab Solutions. *Ground Rules: A Legal Toolkit for Community Gardens*. Oakland, CA: ChangeLab Solutions, 2012.

Needham, Catherine. "Realizing the Potential of Co-Production: Negotiating Improvements in Public Services." *Social Policy and Society* 7, no. 2 (2008): 221–31.

Neff, R. *Introduction to the US Food System: Public Health, Environment, and Equity*. San Francisco: Wiley, 2014. https://books.google.com/books?id=aaTHBAAAQBAJ.

Nelson, Melissa C., Penny Gordon-Larsen, Yan Song, and Barry M. Popkin. "Built and Social Environments: Associations with Adolescent Overweight and Activity." *American Journal of Preventive Medicine* 31, no. 2 (2006): 109–17.

Nelson, Peter B., Ahn Wei Lee, and Lise Nelson. "Linking Baby Boomer and Hispanic Migration Streams into Rural America—a Multi-Scaled Approach." *Population, Space and Place* 15, no. 3 (2009): 277–93.

Newill, Cody. "For This Kansas Town, Being the Geographic Center of the U.S. May Be a Lifeline." KCUR, October 13, 2016. https://www.kcur.org/show/central-standard/2016-10 -13/for-this-kansas-town-being-the-geographic-center-of-the-u-s-may-be-a-lifeline.

Newman, Oscar. *Defensible Space*. New York: Macmillan, 1972.

Newman, Oscar. *Defensible Space: Crime Prevention through Urban Design*. New York: Collier Books, 1973.

Newman, Oscar. "Defensible Space: A New Physical Planning Tool for Urban Revitalization." *Journal of the American Planning Association* 61, no. 2 (1995): 149–55.

Newman, Oscar. *Defensible Space: People and Design in the Violent City*. London: Architectural Press, 1973.

News Staff. "'Biggest Loser' Father and Son Bringing Message of Healthy Living to Valley Center." *Ark Valley (KS) News*, September 13, 2012. http://www.arkvalleynews.com/web /isite.dll?1347541578430~health.

News Staff. "Community Health Fair Set." *Ark Valley (KS) News*, April 14, 2016. http://www .arkvalleynews.com/web/isite.dll?1460668068203~health.

New York City Department of Transportation. *Measuring the Street: New Metrics for 21st Century Streets*. New York: NYCDOT, 2012.

New York City Departments of Design and Construction, Health and Mental Hygiene, Transportation, and City Planning. *Active Design Guidelines: Promoting Physical Activity and Health in Design*. New York: City of New York, 2010.

Ng, Marie, Tom Fleming, Margaret Robinson, Blake Thomson, Nicholas Graetz, Christopher Margono, Erin C. Mullany, et al. "Global, Regional, and National Prevalence of Overweight and Obesity in Children and Adults During 1980–2013: A Systematic Analysis for the Global Burden of Disease Study 2013." *Lancet* 384, no. 9945 (2014): 766–81.

Ng, Shu Wen, and Barry M. Popkin. "Time Use and Physical Activity: A Shift Away from Movement across the Globe." *Obesity Reviews* 13, no. 8 (2012): 659–80.

Nieuwenhuijsen, M., and H. Khreis. *Integrating Human Health into Urban and Transport Planning: A Framework*. Cham, Switzerland: Springer International Publishing, 2018. https://books.google.com/books?id=iAFkDwAAQBAJ.

Nimegeer, Amy, Jane Farmer, Christina West, and Margaret Currie. "Addressing the Problem of Rural Community Engagement in Healthcare Service Design." *Health and Place* 17, no. 4 (2011): 1004–06.

Nord, Mark. "Poor People on the Move: County-to-County Migration and the Spatial Concentration of Poverty." *Journal of Regional Science* 38, no. 2 (1998): 329–51.

Norman, Gregory J., Sandra K. Nutter, Sherry Ryan, James F. Sallis, Karen J. Calfas, and Kevin Patrick. "Community Design and Access to Recreational Facilities as Correlates of Adolescent Physical Activity and Body-Mass Index." *Journal of Physical Activity and Health* 3, no. s1 (2006): S118–S28.

Norman, Lee A. *2020: The State of the Health of Kansans*. Topeka: Kansas Department of Health and Environment, 2020.

Nothwehr, Faryle, and N. Andrew Peterson. "Healthy Eating and Exercise: Strategies for Weight Management in the Rural Midwest." *Health Education and Behavior* 32, no. 2 (2005): 253–63.

Nubani, Linda, and Jean Wineman. "The Role of Space Syntax in Identifying the Relationship between Space and Crime." Paper presented at the Proceedings of the 5th International Space Syntax Symposium, TU Delft, 2005.

Oakes, J. Michael. "The (Mis) Estimation of Neighborhood Effects: Causal Inference for a Practicable Social Epidemiology." *Social Science and Medicine* 58, no. 10 (2004): 1929–52.

Oakley, Peter. *Projects with People: The Practice of Participation in Rural Development*. Geneva: International Labour Organization, World Employment Program, 1991.

O'Campo, Patricia. "Invited Commentary: Advancing Theory and Methods for Multilevel Models of Residential Neighborhoods and Health." *American Journal of Epidemiology* 157, no. 1 (2003): 9–13.

Ogden, Cynthia L., Margaret D. Carroll, Brian K. Kit, and Katherine M. Flegal. "Prevalence of Childhood and Adult Obesity in the United States, 2011–2012." *Journal of the American Medical Association* 311, no. 8 (2014): 806–14.

O'Hare, W. *The Rise of Poverty in Rural America*. Washington, DC: Population Reference Bureau, 1988.

O'Hare, W. P., and K. M. Johnson. "Child Poverty in Rural America." In *Reports on America*. Washington, DC: Population Reference Bureau, 2004.

O'Neil, Kevin. "Hazelton and Beyond: Why Communities Try to Restrict Immigration." *Migration Information Source*, November 10, 2010.

OpenStreetMap. "OpenStreetMap." Accessed September 26, 2021. https://www.openstreetmap.org/.

Organization for Economic Co-operation and Development. *Strategies to Improve Rural Service Delivery*. Paris: OECD Publishing, 2010.

Oropesa, R. S., and Leif Jensen. "Dominican Immigrants and Discrimination in a New Destination: The Case of Reading, Pennsylvania." *City and Community* 9, no. 3 (2010): 274–98.

Orstad, Stephanie L., Meghan H. McDonough, Shauna Stapleton, Ceren Altincekic, and Philip J. Troped. "A Systematic Review of Agreement between Perceived and Objective Neighborhood Environment Measures and Associations with Physical Activity Outcomes." *Environment and Behavior* 49, no. 8 (2017): 904–32.

Ortega-Andeane, Patricia, Eric Jiménez-Rosas, Serafín Mercado-Doménech, and Cesáreo

Estrada-Rodríguez. "Space Syntax as a Determinant of Spatial Orientation Perception." *International Journal of Psychology* 40, no. 1 (2005): 11–18.

Osgood, D. Wayne, and Jeff M. Chambers. "Social Disorganization Outside the Metropolis: An Analysis of Rural Youth Violence." *Criminology* 38, no. 1 (2000): 81–116.

Owen, Neville. "Sedentary Behavior: Understanding and Influencing Adults' Prolonged Sitting Time." *Preventive Medicine* 55, no. 6 (2012): 535–39.

Owen, Neville, Geneviève N. Healy, Charles E. Matthews, and David W. Dunstan. "Too Much Sitting: The Population-Health Science of Sedentary Behavior." *Exercise and Sport Sciences Reviews* 38, no. 3 (2010): 105.

Owen, Neville, Jo Salmon, Mohammad Javad Koohsari, Gavin Turrell, and Billie Giles-Corti. "Sedentary Behaviour and Health: Mapping Environmental and Social Contexts to Underpin Chronic Disease Prevention." *British Journal of Sports Medicine* 48, no. 3 (2014): 174–77.

Owen, Neville, Phillip B. Sparling, Geneviève N. Healy, David W. Dunstan, and Charles E. Matthews. "Sedentary Behavior: Emerging Evidence for a New Health Risk." Paper presented at the Mayo Clinic Proceedings, 2010.

Owen, Neville, Takemi Sugiyama, Elizabeth E. Eakin, Paul A. Gardiner, Mark S. Tremblay, and James F. Sallis. "Adults' Sedentary Behavior: Determinants and Interventions." *American Journal of Preventive Medicine* 41, no. 2 (2011): 189–96.

Ozbil, Ayse, John Peponis, and Sonit Bafna. "The Effects of Street Configuration on Transit Ridership." Paper presented at the Proceedings of the 7th International Space Syntax Symposium, KTH School of Architecture and the Built Environment, Stockholm, 2009.

Paffenbarger, Ralph S., Jr., Alvin L. Wing, and Robert T. Hyde. "Physical Activity as an Index of Heart Attack Risk in College Alumni." *American Journal of Epidemiology* 108, no. 3 (1978): 161–75.

Pampel, Fred C., Patrick M. Krueger, and Justin T. Denney. "Socioeconomic Disparities in Health Behaviors." *Annual Review of Sociology* 36 (2010): 349–70.

Pan, Sai Yi, Christine Cameron, Marie DesMeules, Howard Morrison, Cora Lynn Craig, and XiaoHong Jiang. "Individual, Social, Environmental, and Physical Environmental Correlates with Physical Activity among Canadians: A Cross-Sectional Study." *BMC Public Health* 9, no. 1 (2009): 21.

Panter, Jenna Rachel, and Andy Jones. "Attitudes and the Environment as Determinants of Active Travel in Adults: What Do and Don't We Know?" *Journal of Physical Activity and Health* 7, no. 4 (2010): 551–61.

Parks, S. E., Robyn A. Housemann, and Ross C. Brownson. "Differential Correlates of Physical Activity in Urban and Rural Adults of Various Socioeconomic Backgrounds in the United States." *Journal of Epidemiology and Community Health* 57, no. 1 (2003): 29–35.

Parvin, Afroza, Arlen Min Ye, and Beisi Jia. "Multilevel Pedestrian Movement." Paper presented at the Proceedings of the 6th International Space Syntax Symposium, Istanbul Technical University, 2007.

Patterson, Paul Daniel, Charity G. Moore, Janice C. Probst, and Judith Ann Shinogle. "Obesity and Physical Inactivity in Rural America." *Journal of Rural Health* 20, no. 2 (2004): 151–59.

Patterson, Ruth E., Laura L. Frank, Alan R. Kristal, and Emily White. "A Comprehensive Examination of Health Conditions Associated with Obesity in Older Adults." *American Journal of Preventive Medicine* 27, no. 5 (2004): 385–90.

Patton, Carl V. "Rural Public Transportation: Problems and Possibilities." In *Rural and Small Town Planning*, edited by Judith Getzels and Charles Thurow, 219–50. Chicago: Planners Press, 1979.

Patz, Jonathan A., Diarmid Campbell-Lendrum, Tracey Holloway, and Jonathan A. Foley. "Impact of Regional Climate Change on Human Health." *Nature* 438, no. 7066 (2005): 310.

Patz, Jonathan A., and Douglas E. Norris. "Land Use Change and Human Health." In *Ecosystems and Land Use Change, 2004*, edited by Ruth S. Defries, Gregory P. Asner, and Richard A. Houghton, 159–67. Hoboken, NJ: Blackwell Publishing, 2004.

Paul, Abhijit. "An Integrated Approach to Modeling Vehicular Movement Networks: Trip Assignment and Space Syntax." PhD diss., Texas Tech University, 2009.

Pearson, Thomas A., and Carol Lewis. "Rural Epidemiology: Insights from a Rural Population Laboratory." *American Journal of Epidemiology* 148, no. 10 (1998): 949–57.

Pearson, Tim, Jean Russell, Michael J. Campbell, and Margo E. Barker. "Do 'Food Deserts' Influence Fruit and Vegetable Consumption? A Cross-Sectional Study." *Appetite* 45, no. 2 (2005): 195–97.

Pedersen, Carsten Bøcker, and Preben Bo Mortensen. "Family History, Place and Season of Birth as Risk Factors for Schizophrenia in Denmark: A Replication and Reanalysis." *British Journal of Psychiatry* 179, no. 1 (2001): 46–52.

Pengpid, Supa, and Karl Peltzer. "High Sedentary Behaviour and Low Physical Activity Are Associated with Anxiety and Depression in Myanmar and Vietnam." *International Journal of Environmental Research and Public Health* 16, no. 7 (2019): 1251.

Penkalla, Anna Maria, and Stefan Kohler. "Urbanicity and Mental Health in Europe: A Systematic Review." *European Journal of Mental Health* 9, no. 2 (2014): 163.

Penn, Alan. "Space Syntax and Spatial Cognition: Or Why the Axial Line?" *Environment and Behavior* 35, no. 1 (2003): 30–65.

Penn, Alan, Bill Hillier, David Banister, and Jun Xu. "Configurational Modelling of Urban Movement Networks." *Environment and Planning B: Planning and Design* 25, no. 1 (1998): 59–84.

Peponis, John, Catherine Ross, and Mahbub Rashid. "The Structure of Urban Space, Movement and Co-Presence: The Case of Atlanta." *Geoforum* 28, no. 3 (1997): 341–58.

Peponis, John, and Jean Wineman. "Spatial Structure of Environment and Behavior." In *Handbook of Environmental Psychology*, edited by Robert B. Bechtel and Azra Churchman, 271–91. New York: John Wiley and Sons, 2002.

Perkins, Douglas D., John W. Meeks, and Ralph B. Taylor. "The Physical Environment of Street Blocks and Resident Perceptions of Crime and Disorder: Implications for Theory and Measurement." *Journal of Environmental Psychology* 12, no. 1 (1992): 21–34.

Perkins, Douglas D., Abraham Wandersman, Richard C. Rich, and Ralph B. Taylor. "The Physical Environment of Street Crime: Defensible Space, Territoriality and Incivilities." *Journal of Environmental Psychology* 13, no. 1 (1993): 29–49.

Perry, C. L. "Preadolescent and Adolescent Influences on Health." In *Promoting Health: Intervention Strategies from Social and Behavioral Research*, edited by B. D. Smedley and S. L. Syme, 217–53. Washington, DC: National Academies Press, 2000.

Petrzelka, Peggy, Richard S. Krannich, and Joan M. Brehm. "Identification with Resource-Based Occupations and Desire for Tourism: Are the Two Necessarily Inconsistent?" *Society and Natural Resources* 19, no. 8 (2006): 693–707.

Pfeffer, Max J., and Pilar A. Parra. "Strong Ties, Weak Ties, and Human Capital: Latino Immigrant Employment Outside the Enclave." *Rural Sociology* 74, no. 2 (2009): 241–69.

Phillips, Charles D., and Kenneth R. McLeroy. "Health in Rural America: Remembering the Importance of Place." *American Journal of Public Health* 94, no. 10 (October 2004). https://ajph.aphapublications.org/doi/full/10.2105/AJPH.94.10.1661.

Pitts, S. B., Karamie R. Bringolf, Katherine K. Lawton, Jared T. McGuirt, Elizabeth Wall-Bassett, Jo Morgan, Melissa Nelson Laska, and Joseph R. Sharkey. "Formative Evaluation for a Healthy Corner Store Initiative in Pitt County, North Carolina: Assessing the Rural Food Environment, Part 1." *Preventing Chronic Disease* 10 (2013): E121–E21.

Pitts, Stephanie B. Jilcott, Alison Gustafson, Qiang Wu, Mariel Leah Mayo, Rachel K. Ward, Jared T. McGuirt, Ann P. Rafferty, et al. "Farmers' Market Use Is Associated with Fruit and Vegetable Consumption in Diverse Southern Rural Communities." *Nutrition Journal* 13, no. 1 (2014).

Pitts, Stephanie B. Jilcott, Qiang Wu, Jared T. McGuirt, Thomas W. Crawford, Thomas C. Keyserling, and Alice S. Ammerman. "Associations between Access to Farmers' Markets and Supermarkets, Shopping Patterns, Fruit and Vegetable Consumption and Health Indicators among Women of Reproductive Age in Eastern North Carolina, USA." *Public Health Nutrition* 16, no. 11 (2013): 1944–52.

Pohl, Janet S., Barbara B. Cochrane, Karen G. Schepp, and Nancy F. Woods. "Measuring Social Isolation in the National Health and Aging Trends Study." *Research in Gerontological Nursing* 10, no. 6 (2017): 277–87.

Popke, Jeff. "Latino Migration and Neoliberalism in the US South: Notes toward a Rural Cosmopolitanism." *Southeastern Geographer* 51, no. 2 (2011): 242–59.

Porta, Sergio, Paolo Crucitti, and Vito Latora. "Multiple Centrality Assessment in Parma: A Network Analysis of Paths and Open Spaces." *Urban Design International* 13, no. 1 (2008): 41–50.

Porta, Sergio, Paolo Crucitti, and Vito Latora. "The Network Analysis of Urban Streets: A Primal Approach." *Environment and Planning B: Planning and Design* 33, no. 5 (2006): 705–25.

Poterba, James M. "Demographic Structure and the Political Economy of Public Education." *Journal of Policy Analysis and Management* 16, no. 1 (1997): 48–66.

Pothukuchi, K. "Attracting Supermarkets to Inner-City Neighborhoods: Economic Development Outside the Box." *Economic Development Quarterly* 19, no. 3 (2000).

Pouliou, Theodora, and Susan J. Elliott. "Individual and Socio-Environmental Determinants of Overweight and Obesity in Urban Canada." *Health and Place* 16, no. 2 (2010): 389–98.

Powell, Lisa M., Frank J. Chaloupka, and Yanjun Bao. "The Availability of Fast-Food and Full-Service Restaurants in the United States: Associations with Neighborhood Characteristics." *American Journal of Preventive Medicine* 33, no. 4 (2007): S240–S45.

Prentice, Andrew M., and Susan A. Jebb. "Fast Foods, Energy Density and Obesity: A Possible Mechanistic Link." *Obesity Reviews* 4, no. 4 (2003): 187–94.

Pretty, Jules, Jo Peacock, Rachel Hine, Martha Sellens, N. South, and Murray Griffin. "Green Exercise in the UK Countryside: Effects on Health and Psychological Well-Being, and Implications for Policy and Planning." *Journal of Environmental Planning and Management* 50, no. 2 (2007): 211–31.

Probst, Janice C., Charity G. Moore, Saundra H. Glover, and Michael E. Samuels. "Person and Place: The Compounding Effects of Race/Ethnicity and Rurality on Health." *American Journal of Public Health* 94, no. 10 (2004): 1695–703.

Procter, David E. "The Rural Grocery Crisis." Daily Yonder, August 18, 2010. https://daily yonder.com/author/david_c_procter/.

Pucher, John, Jennifer Dill, and Susan Handy. "Infrastructure, Programs, and Policies to Increase Bicycling: An International Review." *Preventive Medicine* 50 (2010): S106–S25.

Putnam, R. D. *Bowling Alone: The Collapse and Revival of American Community*. New York: Touchstone, 2000.

Quillian, Lincoln. "Why Is Black-White Residential Segregation So Persistent? Evidence on Three Theories from Migration Data." *Social Science Research* 31, no. 2 (2002): 197–229.

Quiñones, Ana R., Sheila Markwardt, and Anda Botoseneanu. "Multimorbidity Combinations and Disability in Older Adults." *Journals of Gerontology Series A: Biomedical Sciences and Medical Sciences* 71, no. 6 (2016): 823–30.

Raford, Noah. "Looking Both Ways: Space Syntax for Pedestrian Exposure Forecasting and Collision Risk Analysis." Paper presented at the Proceedings to the 4th International Space Syntax Symposium, University College London, London, 2003.

Raford, Noah, Alain Chiaradia, and Jorge Gil. *Space Syntax: The Role of Urban Form in Cyclist Route Choice in Central London.* Berkeley, CA: Safe Transportation Research and Education Center, 2007. http://escholarship.org/uc/item/8qz8m4fz.

Raford, Noah, and David Ragland. "Space Syntax: Innovative Pedestrian Volume Modeling Tool for Pedestrian Safety." *Transportation Research Record: Journal of the Transportation Research Board*, no. 1878 (2004): 66–74.

Raja, Samina, Changxing Ma, and Pavan Yadav. "Beyond Food Deserts: Measuring and Mapping Racial Disparities in Neighborhood Food Environments." *Journal of Planning Education and Research* 27, no. 4 (2008): 469–82.

Raleigh, Veena Soni, and Victor A. Kiri. "Life Expectancy in England: Variations and Trends by Gender, Health Authority, and Level of Deprivation." *Journal of Epidemiology and Community Health* 51, no. 6 (1997): 649–58.

Ramirez, Laura K. Brennan, Christine M. Hoehner, Ross C. Brownson, Rebeka Cook, C. Tracy Orleans, Marla Hollander, Dianne C. Barker, et al. "Indicators of Activity-Friendly Communities: An Evidence-Based Consensus Process." *American Journal of Preventive Medicine* 31, no. 6 (2006): 515–24.

Rand, George. "Crime and Environment: A Review of the Literature and Its Implications for Urban Architecture and Planning." *Journal of Architectural and Planning Research* 1, no. 1 (1984): 3–19.

Rashid, Mahbub. *The Geometry of Urban Layouts: A Global Comparative Study.* Switzerland: Springer International Publishing, 2016. https://books.google.com/books?id=Iuh6 DAAAQBAJ.

Rashid, Mahbub. "On Space Syntax as a Configurational Theory of Architecture from a Situated Observer's Viewpoint." *Environment and Planning B: Planning and Design* 39, no. 4 (2012): 732–54.

Rashid, Mahbub. "The Question of Knowledge in Evidence-Based Design for Healthcare Facilities: Limitations and Suggestions." *HERD: Health Environments Research and Design Journal* 6, no. 4 (2013): 101–26.

Rashid, Mahbub. "Space Syntax: A Network-Based Configurational Approach for Urban Morphological Studies." In *Mathematics of Urban Morphology*, edited by L. D'Acci. Modeling and Simulation in Science, Engineering and Technology, 199–251. Basel, Switzerland: Springer Nature Series: Birkhäuser Mathematics, 2019.

Rashid, Mahbub. "Studies on the Geometry of Urban Layouts: A Review of the Literature." Chap. 3 in *The Geometry of Urban Layouts: A Global Comparative Study*, 19–45. Switzerland: Springer International Publishing, 2016.

Ratti, Carlo. "Space Syntax: Some Inconsistencies." *Environment and Planning B: Planning and Design* 31, no. 4 (2004): 487–99.

Ray, Achintya, and Soumendra N. Ghosh. "City Size and Health Outcomes: Lesson from the USA." *Economics Bulletin* 9, no. 5 (2007): 1–7.

Reed, Leslie. "Young Men Increasingly Outnumber Young Women in Rural Great Plains." Science X, May 15, 2014. https://phys.org/news/2014-05-young-men-increasingly-out number-women.html.

Reidpath, Daniel D., Cate Burns, Jan Garrard, Mary Mahoney, and Mardie Townsend. "An Ecological Study of the Relationship between Social and Environmental Determinants of Obesity." *Health and Place* 8, no. 2 (2002): 141–45.

Ricketts, Thomas C. "The Changing Nature of Rural Health Care." *Annual Review of Public Health* 21, no. 1 (2000): 639–57.

Ricketts, Thomas C. *Rural Health in the United States*. New York: Oxford University Press, 1999. https://books.google.com/books?id=kEErphxU1m4C.

Ricketts, Thomas C., Karen D. Johnson-Webb, and Patricia Taylor. *Definitions of Rural: A Handbook for Health Policy Makers and Researchers. Prepared for the Federal Office of Rural Health Policy, Health Resources and Services Administration: U.S. Department of Health and Human Services*. Chapel Hill, NC: Cecil G. Sheps Center, 1998.

Riney-Kehrberg, P., ed. *The Routledge History of Rural America*. New York: Taylor and Francis, 2016.

Robert Wood Johnson Foundation. "Finney County, Kansas." Accessed May 31, 2021. https:// www.rwjf.org/en/about-rwjf/how-we-work/learning-and-evaluation/sentinel-communities /finney-county-kansas.html.

Robinson, W. S. "Ecological Correlations and the Behavior of Individuals." *International Journal of Epidemiology* 38, no. 2 (2009): 337–41.

Rogers, David L., and Larry R. Whiting, eds. *Aspects of Planning for Public Services in Rural Areas. Monograph Composed of Papers Presented at Conference Developed by the North Central Regional Center for Rural Development (Lincoln, Nebraska)*. Ames, IA: North Central Regional Center for Rural Development, 1976.

Rogot, Eugene, Paul D. Sorlie, and Norman J. Johnson. "Life Expectancy by Employment Status, Income, and Education in the National Longitudinal Mortality Study." *Public Health Reports* 107, no. 4 (1992): 457.

Roncek, D. W. "Schools and Crime." In *Analyzing Crime Patterns: Frontiers of Practice*, edited by V. Goldsmith, P. G. McGuire, J. H. Mollenkopf, and T. A. Ross. Thousand Oaks, CA: Sage Publications, 2000.

Röösli, Martin. "Radiofrequency Electromagnetic Field Exposure and Non-Specific Symptoms of Ill Health: A Systematic Review." *Environmental Research* 107, no. 2 (2008): 277–87.

Rose, Donald, and Rickelle Richards. "Food Store Access and Household Fruit and Vegetable Use among Participants in the US Food Stamp Program." *Public Health Nutrition* 7, no. 08 (2004): 1081–88.

Rose, Geoffrey. "Sick Individuals and Sick Populations." *International Journal of Epidemiology* 14, no. 1 (1985): 32–38.

Rose, Geoffrey. "Sick Individuals and Sick Populations." *International Journal of Epidemiology* 30, no. 3 (2001): 427–32.

Ross, Catherine E., and Chia-ling Wu. "The Links between Education and Health." *American Sociological Review* (1995): 719–45.

Rott, Nathan. "3 Men Charged with Plotting Attack on Somali Immigrants in Kansas." NPR, October 14, 2016. https://www.npr.org/sections/thetwo-way/2016/10/14/498013572/three -men-charged-with-plotting-attack-on-somali-immigrants-in-kansas.

Rowles, Graham D. "What's Rural About Rural Aging? An Appalachian Perspective." *Journal of Rural Studies* 4, no. 2 (1988): 115–24.

Ruddell, Rick, and G. Larry Mays. "Rural Jails: Problematic Inmates, Overcrowded Cells, and Cash-Strapped Counties." *Journal of Criminal Justice* 35, no. 3 (2007): 251–60.

Ruff, Corrine. "Monsanto, BASF Will Pay $250 Million in Punitive Damages in First Dicamba Trial." Harvest Public Media, February 17, 2020. https://news.stlpublicradio.org/economy -innovation/2020-02-15/monsanto-basf-will-pay-250-million-in-punitive-damages-in -first-dicamba-trial.

Rundle, Andrew, Ana V. Diez-Roux, Lance M. Freeman, Douglas Miller, Kathryn M. Neckerman, and Christopher C. Weiss. "The Urban Built Environment and Obesity in New York City: A Multilevel Analysis." *American Journal of Health Promotion* 21, no. S4 (2007): 326–34.

Rundle, Andrew, Kathryn M. Neckerman, Lance Freeman, Gina S. Lovasi, Marnie Purciel, James Quinn, Catherine Richards, Neelanjan Sircar, and Christopher Weiss. "Neighborhood Food Environment and Walkability Predict Obesity in New York City." *Environmental Health Perspectives* 117, no. 3 (2009): 442–47.

Rupprecht, Erhardt O. "Private Motor Vehicles—Rural America's Pervasive Transportation Mode." Paper presented at the National Symposium on Transportation for Agriculture and Rural America, Washington, DC, 1977.

Rural Health Information Hub. "Substance Abuse in Rural Areas." Accessed August 2, 2020. https://www.ruralhealthinfo.org/topics/substance-abuse.

Rutt, Candace D., and Karen J. Coleman. "Examining the Relationships among Built Environment, Physical Activity, and Body Mass Index in El Paso, TX." *Preventive Medicine* 40, no. 6 (2005): 831–41.

Rydin, Yvonne, Ana Bleahu, Michael Davies, Julio D. Dávila, Sharon Friel, Giovanni De Grandis, Nora Groce, et al. "Shaping Cities for Health: Complexity and the Planning of Urban Environments in the 21st Century." *Lancet* 379, no. 9831 (2012): 2079–108.

Saarloos, Dick, Helman Alfonso, Billie Giles-Corti, Nick Middleton, and Osvaldo P. Almeida. "The Built Environment and Depression in Later Life: The Health in Men Study." *American Journal of Geriatric Psychiatry* 19, no. 5 (2011): 461–70.

Saelens, Brian E., and Susan L. Handy. "Built Environment Correlates of Walking: A Review." *Medicine and Science in Sports and Exercise* 40, no. S7 (2008): S550.

Saelens, Brian E., James F. Sallis, Jennifer B. Black, and Diana Chen. "Neighborhood-Based Differences in Physical Activity: An Environment Scale Evaluation." *American Journal of Public Health* 93, no. 9 (2003): 1552–58.

Saelens, Brian E., James F. Sallis, and Lawrence D. Frank. "Environmental Correlates of Walking and Cycling: Findings from the Transportation, Urban Design, and Planning Literatures." *Annals of Behavioral Medicine* 25, no. 2 (2003): 80–91.

Saha, Sukanta, David Chant, Joy Welham, and John McGrath. "A Systematic Review of the Prevalence of Schizophrenia." *PLoS Med* 2, no. 5 (2005): e141.

Salamon, S. *Newcomers to Old Towns: Suburbanization of the Heartland.* Chicago: University of Chicago Press, 2003.

Sallis, James F., Heather R. Bowles, Adrian Bauman, Barbara E. Ainsworth, Fiona C. Bull, Cora L. Craig, Michael Sjöström, et al. "Neighborhood Environments and Physical Activity among Adults in 11 Countries." *American Journal of Preventive Medicine* 36, no. 6 (2009): 484–90.

Sallis, James F., Terry L. Conway, Kelli L. Cain, Jordan A. Carlson, Lawrence D. Frank, Jacqueline Kerr, Karen Glanz, James E. Chapman, and Brian E. Saelens. "Neighborhood Built Environment and Socioeconomic Status in Relation to Physical Activity, Sedentary Behavior, and Weight Status of Adolescents." *Preventive Medicine* 110 (2018): 47–54.

Sallis, James F., and Karen Glanz. "Physical Activity and Food Environments: Solutions to the Obesity Epidemic." *Milbank Quarterly* 87, no. 1 (2009): 123–54.

Sallis, James F., and Karen Glanz. "The Role of Built Environments in Physical Activity, Eating, and Obesity in Childhood." *Future of Children* (2006): 89–108.

Sallis, James F., Melbourne F. Hovell, C. Richard Hofstetter, John P. Elder, Mimi Hackley, Carl J. Caspersen, and Kenneth E. Powell. "Distance between Homes and Exercise Facilities Related to Frequency of Exercise among San Diego Residents." *Public Health Reports* 105, no. 2 (1990): 179–85.

Sallis, James F., and Brian E. Saelens. "Assessment of Physical Activity by Self-Report: Status, Limitations, and Future Directions." *Research Quarterly for Exercise and Sport* 71, no. S2 (2000): 1–14.

Salmon, Jo, Louisa Salmon, David A. Crawford, Clare Hume, and Anna Timperio. "Associations among Individual, Social, and Environmental Barriers and Children's Walking or Cycling to School." *American Journal of Health Promotion* 22, no. 2 (2007): 107–13.

Samet, Jonathan. "Community Design and Air Quality." In *Making Healthy Places: Designing and Building for Health, Wellbeing, and Sustainability,* edited by Andrew L. Dannenberg, Howard Frumkin, and Richard J. Jackson, 63–76. Washington, DC: Island Press, 2011.

Samet, Jonathan, and Daniel Krewski. "Health Effects Associated with Exposure to Ambient Air Pollution." *Journal of Toxicology and Environmental Health, Part A* 70, no. 3–4 (2007): 227–42.

Sampson, Robert J., Jeffrey D. Morenoff, and Thomas Gannon-Rowley. "Assessing 'Neighborhood Effects': Social Processes and New Directions in Research." *Annual Review of Sociology* 28, no. 1 (2002): 443–78.

Sampson, Robert J., and Stephen W. Raudenbush. "Systematic Social Observation of Public Spaces: A New Look at Disorder in Urban Neighborhoods." *American Journal of Sociology* 105, no. 3 (1999): 603–51.

Sampson, Robert J., Stephen W. Raudenbush, and Felton Earls. "Neighborhoods and Violent Crime: A Multilevel Study of Collective Efficacy." *Science* 277, no. 5328 (1997): 918–24.

Sandel, Megan, and Rosalind J. Wright. "When Home Is Where the Stress Is: Expanding the Dimensions of Housing That Influence Asthma Morbidity." *Archives of Disease in Childhood* 91, no. 11 (2006): 942–48.

Sanderson, Bonnie, MaryAnn Littleton, and Lea Vonne Pulley. "Environmental, Policy, and Cultural Factors Related to Physical Activity among Rural, African American Women." *Women and Health* 36, no. 2 (2002): 73–88.

Sarkar, Chinmoy, John Gallacher, and Chris Webster. "Urban Built Environment Configuration and Psychological Distress in Older Men: Results from the Caerphilly Study." *BMC Public Health* 13. (30 July 2013).

Sarkar, Chinmoy, Chris Webster, and John Gallacher. *Healthy Cities: Public Health through Urban Planning.* Cheltenham, UK: Edward Elgar, 2014. https://books.google.com/books?id=xuBnAwAAQBAJ.

Sarnat, Jeremy A., Joel Schwartz, and Helen H. Suh. "Fine Particulate Air Pollution and Mortality in 20 US Cities." *New England Journal of Medicine* 344, no. 16 (2001): 1253–54.

Saunderson, Thomas, Robin Haynes, and Ian H. Langford. "Urban-Rural Variations in Suicides and Undetermined Deaths in England and Wales." *Journal of Public Health* 20, no. 3 (1998): 261–67.

Saville, G., and G. Cleveland. "Second-Generation CPTED: The Rise and Fall of Opportunity Theory." Chap. 7 in *21st Century Security and CPTED: Designing for Critical Infrastructure Protection and Crime Prevention,* edited by R. Atlas, 79–90. Boca Raton, FL: CRC Press, 2008.

Scerri, Andy, and Paul James. "Communities of Citizens and 'Indicators' of Sustainability." *Community Development Journal* 45, no. 2 (2010): 219–36.

Schafft, Kai A., Eric B. Jensen, and C. Clare Hinrichs. "Food Deserts and Overweight Schoolchildren: Evidence from Pennsylvania." *Rural Sociology* 74, no. 2 (2009): 153–77.

Schelin, Else Marie, P. Munk-Jørensen, Anne Vingaard Olesen, and Jes Gerlach. "Regional Differences in Schizophrenia Incidence in Denmark." *Acta Psychiatrica Scandinavica* 101, no. 4 (2000): 293–99.

Schläpfer, Markus, Luís M. A. Bettencourt, Sébastien Grauwin, Mathias Raschke, Rob Claxton, Zbigniew Smoreda, Geoffrey B. West, and Carlo Ratti. "The Scaling of Human Interactions with City Size." *Journal of the Royal Society Interface* 11, no. 98 (2014): 20130789.

Schoenborn, Charlotte A., Patricia F. Adams, and Jennifer A. Peregoy. "Health Behaviors of Adults: United States, 2008–2010." *Vital and Health Statistics. Series 10, Data from the National Health Survey,* no. 257 (2013): 1–184.

Schoeni, Robert F., Vicki A. Freedman, and Robert B. Wallace. "Persistent, Consistent, Widespread, and Robust? Another Look at Recent Trends in Old-Age Disability." *Journals of Gerontology Series B: Psychological Sciences and Social Sciences* 56, no. 4 (2001): S206–S18.

Schoeni, Robert F., Linda G. Martin, Patricia M. Andreski, and Vicki A. Freedman. "Persistent and Growing Socioeconomic Disparities in Disability among the Elderly: 1982–2002." *American Journal of Public Health* 95, no. 11 (2005): 2065–70.

Schreiner, Dean F. "A Planning Framework for Rural Public Sector Analysis." In *Aspects of Planning for Public Services in Rural Areas. Monograph Composed of Papers Presented at Conference Developed by the North Central Regional Center for Rural Development (Lincoln, Nebraska)*, edited by David L. Rogers and Larry R. Whiting. Ames, IA: North Central Regional Center for Rural Development, 1976.

Schüle, Steffen Andreas, and Gabriele Bolte. "Interactive and Independent Associations between the Socioeconomic and Objective Built Environment on the Neighbourhood Level and Individual Health: A Systematic Review of Multilevel Studies." *PLoS One* 10, no. 4 (2015): e0123456.

Schulz, Jochen, Inga Ruddat, Jörg Hartung, Gerd Hamscher, Nicole Kemper, and Christa Ewers. "Antimicrobial-Resistant Escherichia Coli Survived in Dust Samples for More Than 20 Years." *Frontiers in Microbiology* 7 (2016): 866.

Schumaker, Erin, and Mark Nichols. "An American Tragedy: Inside the Towns Hardest Hit by Coronavirus." ABC News, November 19, 2020, https://abcnews.go.com/Health/small-towns-face-covid-19-pandemic-us-passes/story?id=74271392.

Schwanen, Tim. "Urban Form and Commuting Behaviour: A Cross-European Perspective." *Tijdschrift voor economische en sociale geografie* 93, no. 3 (2002): 336–43.

Schwasinger-Schmidt, Tiffany E., Jon P. Schrage, Justin B. Moore, and Betty M. Drees. "The State of Diabetes in Kansas: A Community Centered Approach to the Treatment of Diverse Populations." *Kansas Journal of Medicine* 10, no. 4 (2017): 96.

Scoppa, Martin, Steven French, and John Peponis. "The Effects of Street Connectivity Upon the Distribution of Local Vehicular Traffic in Metropolitan Atlanta." Paper presented at the Proceedings of the 7th International Space Syntax Symposium, KTH School of Architecture and the Built Environment, Stockholm, 2009.

Seiler, Anthony. "Farmers Struggle with Health Care." *Ark Valley (KS) News*, February 21, 2019. http://www.arkvalleynews.com/web/isite.dll?1550782592720~health.

Seligman, Hilary K., Barbara A. Laraia, and Margot B. Kushel. "Food Insecurity Is Associated with Chronic Disease among Low-Income Nhanes Participants." *Journal of Nutrition* 140, no. 2 (2010): 304–10.

Selvin, Hanan C. "Durkheim's Suicide and Problems of Empirical Research." *American Journal of Sociology* 63, no. 6 (1958): 607–19.

Sesso, Howard D., I-Min Lee, and Ralph S. Paffenbarger. "Physical Activity and Breast Cancer Risk in the College Alumni Health Study (United States)." *Cancer Causes and Control* 9, no. 4 (1998): 433–39.

Sesso, Howard D., Ralph S. Paffenbarger, Tina Ha, and I-Min Lee. "Physical Activity and Cardiovascular Disease Risk in Middle-Aged and Older Women." *American Journal of Epidemiology* 150, no. 4 (1999): 408–16.

Sesso, Howard D., Ralph S. Paffenbarger Jr., and I-Min Lee. "Physical Activity and Coronary Heart Disease in Men: The Harvard Alumni Health Study." *Circulation* 102, no. 9 (2000): 975–80.

Shah, Anoop S. V., Jeremy P. Langrish, Harish Nair, David A. McAllister, Amanda L. Hunter, Ken Donaldson, David E. Newby, and Nicholas L. Mills. "Global Association of Air Pollution and Heart Failure: A Systematic Review and Meta-Analysis." *Lancet* 382, no. 9897 (2013): 1039–48.

Shaper, A. Gerald, S. Goya Wannamethee, and Mary Walker. "Body Weight: Implications for the Prevention of Coronary Heart Disease, Stroke, and Diabetes Mellitus in a Cohort Study of Middle Aged Men." *BMJ* 314, no. 7090 (1997): 1311.

Sharp, Richard. "Land Giveaway Helps Keep Marquette Vibrant." KSHB, June 9, 2016. https:// www.kshb.com/news/state/kansas/small-kansas-town-gives-away-land-for-new-homes -to-attract-new-residents.

Shaw, C. R., and H. D. McKay. *Juvenile Delinquency and Urban Areas.* Chicago: University of Chicago Press, 1942.

Sheard, M. *Report on Burglary Patterns: The Impact of Cul-de-Sacs.* Delta, British Columbia: Delta Police Department, 1991.

Shephard, Roy J. "Is Active Commuting the Answer to Population Health?" *Sports Medicine* 38, no. 9 (September 2008): 751–58. https://doi.org/10.2165/00007256-200838090-00004.

Shiels, Meredith S., Pavel Chernyavskiy, William F. Anderson, Ana F. Best, Emily A. Haozous, Patricia Hartge, Philip S. Rosenberg, et al. "Trends in Premature Mortality in the USA by Sex, Race, and Ethnicity from 1999 to 2014: An Analysis of Death Certificate Data." *Lancet* 389, no. 10073 (2017): 1043–54.

Shouls, Susanna, Peter Congdon, and Sarah Curtis. "Modelling Inequality in Reported Long Term Illness in the UK: Combining Individual and Area Characteristics." *Journal of Epidemiology and Community Health* 50, no. 3 (1996): 366–76.

Shoup, Lilly, and Becca Homa. *Principles for Improving Transportation Options in Rural and Small Town Communities.* Washington, DC: Transportation for America, 2010.

Shriver, Thomas E., and Gary R. Webb. "Rethinking the Scope of Environmental Injustice: Perceptions of Health Hazards in a Rural Native American Community Exposed to Carbon Black." *Rural Sociology* 74, no. 2 (2009): 270–92.

Shultis, Wendy, Robert Graff, Chara Chamie, Cherish Hart, Palina Louangketh, Mike Mc-Namara, Nick Okon, and David Tirschwell. "Striking Rural-Urban Disparities Observed in Acute Stroke Care Capacity and Services in the Pacific Northwest: Implications and Recommendations." *Stroke* 41, no. 10 (2010): 2278–82.

Singh, Gopal K. "Rural-Urban Trends and Patterns in Cervical Cancer Mortality, Incidence, Stage, and Survival in the United States, 1950–2008." *Journal of Community Health* 37, no. 1 (2012): 217–23.

Singh, Gopal K., and Mohammad Siahpush. "Increasing Rural-Urban Gradients in US Suicide Mortality, 1970–1997." *American Journal of Public Health* 92, no. 7 (2002): 1161–67.

Singh, Gopal K., and Mohammad Siahpush. "Widening Rural-Urban Disparities in All-Cause Mortality and Mortality from Major Causes of Death in the USA, 1969–2009." *Journal of Urban Health* 91, no. 2 (2014): 272–92.

Singh, Gopal K., and Mohammad Siahpush. "Widening Rural-Urban Disparities in Life Expectancy, US, 1969–2009." *American Journal of Preventive Medicine* 46, no. 2 (2014): e19–e29.

Skinner, Asheley Cockrell, and Rebecca T. Slifkin. "Rural/Urban Differences in Barriers to and Burden of Care for Children with Special Health Care Needs." *Journal of Rural Health* 23, no. 2 (2007): 150–57.

Slack, Tim, Joachim Singelmann, Kayla Fontenot, Dudley L. Poston Jr., Rogelio Saenz, and Carlos Siordia. "Poverty in the Texas Borderland and Lower Mississippi Delta: A Comparative Analysis of Differences by Family Type." *Demographic Research* 20 (2009): 353–76.

Sloggett, Andrew, and Heather Joshi. "Deprivation Indicators as Predictors of Life Events 1981–1992 Based on the UK ONS Longitudinal Study." *Journal of Epidemiology and Community Health* 52, no. 4 (1998): 228–33.

Sloggett, Andrew, and Heather Joshi. "Higher Mortality in Deprived Areas: Community or Personal Disadvantage?" *BMJ* 309, no. 6967 (1994): 1470–74.

Smalley, K. Bryant, and Jacob C. Warren, eds. *Rural Public Health: Best Practices and Preventive Models*. N.p.: Springer Publishing Company, 2014.

Smalley, K. Bryant, Jacob C. Warren, and J. P. Rainer. *Rural Mental Health: Issues, Policies, and Best Practices*. New York: Springer Publishing Company, 2012. https://books.google.com/books?id=ia6bpsTT62AC.

Smith, Chery, and Lois W. Morton. "Rural Food Deserts: Low-Income Perspectives on Food Access in Minnesota and Iowa." *Journal of Nutrition Education and Behavior* 41, no. 3 (2009): 176–87.

Smith, G. Davey, Carole Hart, Graham Watt, David Hole, and Victor Hawthorne. "Individual Social Class, Area-Based Deprivation, Cardiovascular Disease Risk Factors, and Mortality: The Renfrew and Paisley Study." *Journal of Epidemiology and Community Health* 52, no. 6 (1998): 399–405.

Smith, G. Davey, M. Shipley, D. Hole, C. Hart, G. Watt, C. Gillis, M. G. Marmot, and V. Hawthorne. "Explaining Male Mortality Differentials between the West of Scotland and the South of England." *Journal of Epidemiology and Community Health* 49 (1995): 541.

Smith, Judith M. "Portraits of Loneliness: Emerging Themes among Community-Dwelling Older Adults." *Journal of Psychosocial Nursing and Mental Health Services* 50, no. 4 (2012): 34–39.

Smith, Michael D., and Richard S. Krannich. "'Culture Clash' Revisited: Newcomer and Longer-Term Residents' Attitudes toward Land Use, Development, and Environmental Issues in Rural Communities in the Rocky Mountain West." *Rural Sociology* 65, no. 3 (2000): 396–421.

Smithies, Jan, and Lee Adams. "Walking the Tightrope: Issues in Evaluation and Community Participation for Health for All." Chap. 5 in *Healthy Cities: Research and Practice*, edited by John K. Davies and Michael Kelly, 55–70. New York: Routledge, 1993.

Sorlie, Paul D., Eric Backlund, and Jacob B. Keller. "US Mortality by Economic, Demographic, and Social Characteristics: The National Longitudinal Mortality Study." *American Journal of Public Health* 85, no. 7 (1995): 949–56.

Sorokin, Pitirim Aleksandrovich, and Carle Clark Zimmerman. *Principles of Rural-Urban Sociology*. New York: Henry Holt, 1929.

Spauwen, Janneke, Lydia Krabbendam, Roselind Lieb, Hans-Ulrich Wittchen, and Jim van Os. "Does Urbanicity Shift the Population Expression of Psychosis?" *Journal of Psychiatric Research* 38, no. 6 (2004): 613–18.

Stafford, M., T. Chandola, and M. Marmot. "Association between Fear of Crime and Mental Health and Physical Functioning." *American Journal of Public Health* 97, no. 2076–81 (2007).

Stamm, B. Hudnall, ed. *Rural Behavioral Health Care: An Interdisciplinary Guide*. Washington, DC: American Psychological Association, 2003.

Stansfeld, Stephen, Mary Haines, and Bernadette Brown. "Noise and Health in the Urban Environment." *Reviews on Environmental Health* 15, no. 1–2 (2000): 43–82.

Stansfeld, Stephen A., and Mark P. Matheson. "Noise Pollution: Non-Auditory Effects on Health." *British Medical Bulletin* 68, no. 1 (2003): 243–57.

Stanton, Mark W. "The High Concentration of U.S. Health Care Expenditures." In *Research in Action Issue 19. AHRQ Pub. No. 06-0060*. Rockville, MD: Agency for Healthcare Research and Quality, 2005. http://www.ahrq.gov/research/findings/factsheets/costs/expriach/index.html.

Stark, Rodney. "Deviant Places: A Theory of the Ecology of Crime." *Criminology* 25, no. 4 (1987): 893–910.

State of Kansas. "Constitution of the State of Kansas." Accessed September 14, 2021. https://www.kssos.org/other/pubs/KS_Constitution.pdf.

Stedman, Richard C., Stephan J. Goetz, and Benjamin Weagraff. "Does Second Home Development Adversely Affect Rural Life?" In *Population Change and Rural Society*, 277–92. N.p.: Springer, 2006.

Steinberger, Julia, D. R. Jacobs, S. Raatz, Antoinette Moran, C. P. Hong, and Alan R. Sinaiko. "Comparison of Body Fatness Measurements by BMI and Skinfolds vs Dual Energy X-Ray Absorptiometry and Their Relation to Cardiovascular Risk Factors in Adolescents." *International Journal of Obesity* 29, no. 11 (2005): 1346–52.

Steiner, Phillip, Wyatt J. Beckman, Sydney McClendon, and Kari M. Bruffett. *Disrupting Disparities in Kansas: A Review of Social Isolation among Older Adults*. Topeka: Kansas Health Institute, 2020.

Stephenson, J., and A. Bauman. *The Cost of Illness Attributable to Physical Inactivity in Australia*. Canberra: CDHAC and Australian Sports Commission, 2000.

Steptoe, Andrew, Aparna Shankar, Panayotes Demakakos, and Jane Wardle. "Social Isolation, Loneliness, and All-Cause Mortality in Older Men and Women." *Proceedings of the National Academy of Sciences* 110, no. 15 (2013): 5797–801.

Stewart, Orion T., Anne Vernez Moudon, Brian E. Saelens, Chanam Lee, Bumjoon Kang, and Mark P. Doescher. "Comparing Associations between the Built Environment and Walking in Rural Small Towns and a Large Metropolitan Area." *Environment and Behavior* 48, no. 1 (2016): 13–36.

Stommes, Eileen S., and Dennis M. Brown. "Transportation in Rural America: Issues for the 21st Century." *Rural America / Rural Development Perspectives* 16, no. 4 (2002): 2–10.

Stowe, Ellen W., S. Morgan Hughey, Shirelle H. Hallum, and Andrew T. Kaczynski. "Associations between Walkability and Youth Obesity: Differences by Urbanicity." *Childhood Obesity* 15, no. 8 (2019): 555–59.

Sturm, Roland, and Deborah Cohen. "Proximity to Urban Parks and Mental Health." *Journal of Mental Health Policy and Economics* 17, no. 1 (2014): 19–24.

Suchan, Trudy A., Marc J. Perry, James D. Fitzsimmons, Anika E. Juhn, Alexander M. Tait, and Cynthia A. Brewer. "Population Distribution." Chap. 2 in *Census Atlas of the United States*. Washington DC: US Census Bureau, 2000.

Suchy, Daniel R., and K. David Newell. "Hydraulic Fracturing of Oil and Gas Wells in Kansas." In *Public Information Circular (PIC)* 32. Lawrence: Kansas Geological Survey, 2012. https://www.kgs.ku.edu/Publications/PIC/pic32.html.

Sugiyama, Takemi, Ester Cerin, Neville Owen, Adewale L. Oyeyemi, Terry L. Conway, Delfien Van Dyck, Jasper Schipperijn, et al. "Perceived Neighbourhood Environmental Attributes Associated with Adults' Recreational Walking: IPEN Adult Study in 12 Countries." *Health and Place* 28 (2014): 22–30.

Sugiyama, Takemi, Ding Ding, and Neville Owen. "Commuting by Car: Weight Gain among Physically Active Adults." *American Journal of Preventive Medicine* 44, no. 2 (2013): 169–73.

Sugiyama, Takemi, Jacinta Francis, Nicholas J. Middleton, Neville Owen, and Billie Giles-Corti. "Associations between Recreational Walking and Attractiveness, Size, and Proximity of Neighborhood Open Spaces." *American Journal of Public Health* 100, no. 9 (2010): 1752–57.

Sugiyama, Takemi, Eva Leslie, Billie Giles-Corti, and Neville Owen. "Associations of Neighborhood Greenness with Physical and Mental Health: Do Walking, Social Coherence and Local Social Interaction Explain the Relationships?" *Journal of Epidemiology and Community Health* 62, no. 5 (2008): e9–e9.

Sugiyama, Takemi, Maike Neuhaus, Rachel Cole, Billie Giles-Corti, and Neville Owen. "Destination and Route Attributes Associated with Adults' Walking: A Review." *Medicine and Science in Sports and Exercise* 44, no. 7 (2012): 1275–86.

Sugiyama, Takemi, Maike Neuhaus, and Neville Owen. "Active Transport, the Built Environment, and Human Health." In *Sustainable Environmental Design in Architecture*, edited by S. Rassia and P. Pardalos, 43–65. New York: Springer, 2012.

Sugiyama, Takemi, and Catharine Ward Thompson. "Associations between Characteristics of Neighborhood Open Space and Older People's Walking." *Urban Forestry and Urban Greening* 7, no. 1 (2008): 41–51.

Sugiyama, Takemi, Catharine Ward Thompson, and Susana Alves. "Associations between Neighborhood Open Space Attributes and Quality of Life for Older People in Britain." *Environment and Behavior* 41, no. 1 (2009): 3–21.

Sullivan, John M., and Michael J. Flannagan. "Determining the Potential Safety Benefit of Improved Lighting in Three Pedestrian Crash Scenarios." *Accident Analysis and Prevention* 39, no. 3 (2007): 638–47.

Sun, Guibo, Nicolas M. Oreskovic, and Hui Lin. "How Do Changes to the Built Environment Influence Walking Behaviors? A Longitudinal Study within a University Campus in Hong Kong." *International Journal of Health Geographics* 13, no. 28 (2014). https://doi.org/10.1186 /1476-072X-13-28.

Sun, Qi, Rob M. Van Dam, Donna Spiegelman, Steven B. Heymsfield, Walter C. Willett, and Frank B. Hu. "Comparison of Dual-Energy X-Ray Absorptiometric and Anthropometric Measures of Adiposity in Relation to Adiposity-Related Biologic Factors." *American Journal of Epidemiology* 172, no. 12 (2010): 1442–54.

Sundquist, Kristina, Marilyn Winkleby, Helena Ahlén, and Sven-Erik Johansson. "Neighborhood Socioeconomic Environment and Incidence of Coronary Heart Disease: A Follow-Up Study of 25,319 Women and Men in Sweden." *American Journal of Epidemiology* 159, no. 7 (2004): 655–62.

Susser, Mervyn. "The Logic in Ecological: I. The Logic of Analysis." *American Journal of Public Health* 84, no. 5 (1994): 825–29.

Susser, Mervyn. "The Logic in Ecological: II. The Logic of Design." *American Journal of Public Health* 84, no. 5 (1994): 830–35.

Swinburn, B. A., I. Caterson, J. C. Seidell, and W. P. T. James. "Diet, Nutrition and the Prevention of Excess Weight Gain and Obesity." *Public Health Nutrition* 7, no. 1a (2004): 123–46.

Takano, Takehito, Keiko Nakamura, and Masafumi Watanabe. "Urban Residential Environments and Senior Citizens' Longevity in Megacity Areas: The Importance of Walkable Green Spaces." *Journal of Epidemiology and Community Health* 56, no. 12 (2002): 913–18.

Tan, Jianguo, Youfei Zheng, Xu Tang, Changyi Guo, Liping Li, Guixiang Song, Xinrong Zhen, et al. "The Urban Heat Island and Its Impact on Heat Waves and Human Health in Shanghai." *International Journal of Biometeorology* 54, no. 1 (2010): 75–84.

Taylor, Harry Owen. "Social Isolation's Influence on Loneliness among Older Adults." *Clinical Social Work Journal* 48, no. 1 (2020): 140–51.

Taylor, Judy, David Wilkinson, and Brian Cheers. "Is It Consumer or Community Participation? Examining the Links between 'Community' and 'Participation.'" *Health Sociology Review* 15, no. 1 (2006): 38–47.

Taylor, M., and C. Nee. "The Role of Cues in Simulated Residential Burglary." *British Journal of Criminology* 28, no. 3 (1988): 396–401.

Taylor, R. B., and A. V. Harrell. *Physical Environment and Crime*. Rockville, MD: National Institute of Justice, US Department of Justice, 1996. https://www.ncjrs.gov/App/Publications /abstract.aspx?ID=157311.

Taylor, Ralph B., Sally Ann Shumaker, and Stephen D. Gottfredson. "Neighborhood-Level Links between Physical Features and Local Sentiments: Deterioration, Fear of Crime, and Confidence." *Journal of Architectural and Planning Research* 2, no. 4 (1985): 261–75.

Taylor, Shelley E., and Teresa E. Seeman. "Psychosocial Resources and the SES-Health Relationship." *Annals-New York Academy of Sciences* 896 (1999): 210–25.

Teedon, P., T. Reid, P. Griffiths, and A. McFadyen. "Evaluating Secured by Design Door and Window Installations: Effects on Residential Crime." *Crime Prevention and Community Safety* 12, no. 4 (2010): 246–62.

ten Brink, Patrick, Konar Mutafoglu, Jean-Pierre Schweitzer, Marianne Kettunen, Clare Twigger-Ross, Jonathan Baker, Yoline Kuipers, et al. *The Health and Social Benefits of Nature and Biodiversity Protection. A Report for the European Commission (Env. B. 3/ ETU/2014/0039)*. London: Institute for European Environmental Policy, 2016.

Thomas, John K., and Frank M. Howell. "Metropolitan Proximity and US Agricultural Productivity, 1978–1997." *Rural Sociology* 68, no. 3 (2003): 366–86.

Thompson, A., A. O. Yeboah, and S. H. Evans. "Determinants of Poverty among Farm Operators in North Carolina." In *Agricultural Change*, edited by J. Molnar, 177–99. Boulder, CO: Westview Press, 1986.

Thompson, Bryan. "Coffeyville Trail Project Gets Boost from EPA Grant." Kansas Public Radio, May 29, 2014. https://kansaspublicradio.org/kpr-news/coffeyville-trail-project -gets-boost-epa-grant.

Thompson, Bryan. "Kansas Rural Hospitals Struggle to Stay Afloat." KHI News Service, April 27, 2015. https://www.kcur.org/health/2015-04-27/kansas-rural-hospitals-struggle-to-stay -afloat.

Thompson, Bryan. "Rural Drop-In Centers Aim to Address Dangers of Isolation." Kansas Public Radio, March 28, 2017. https://kansaspublicradio.org/kpr-news/rural-drop-centers -aim-address-dangers-isolation.

Thompson, Janice L., Peg Allen, Leslie Cunningham-Sabo, Dedra A. Yazzie, Michelle Curtis, and Sally M. Davis. "Environmental, Policy, and Cultural Factors Related to Physical Activity in Sedentary American Indian Women." *Women and Health* 36, no. 2 (2002): 57–72.

Thompson, Susan. "The Human Experience." In *The Routledge Handbook of Planning for Health and Well-Being: Shaping a Sustainable and Healthy Future*, edited by Hugh Barton, Susan Thompson, Sarah Burgess, and Marcus Grant, 85–88. New York: Routledge, 2015.

Thompson, Susan, and Jennifer Kent. "Connecting and Strengthening Communities in Places for Health and Well-Being." *Australian Planner* 51, no. 3 (2014): 260–71.

Thorndike, Edward L. "On the Fallacy of Imputing the Correlations Found for Groups to the Individuals or Smaller Groups Composing Them." *American Journal of Psychology* 52, no. 1 (1939): 122–24.

Thorp, Alicia A., Neville Owen, Maike Neuhaus, and David W. Dunstan. "Sedentary Behaviors and Subsequent Health Outcomes in Adults: A Systematic Review of Longitudinal Studies, 1996–2011." *American Journal of Preventive Medicine* 41, no. 2 (2011): 207–15.

Thrive Allen County. "Thrive's Innovative Approach to Rural Bike Share." September 11, 2017. http://thriveallencounty.org/news/thrive-innovative-rural-bike-share/.

Thurow, Charles. "Zoning and Development Permit Systems." In *Rural and Small Town Planning*, edited by Judith Getzels and Charles Thurow, 53–96. Chicago: Planners Press, 1979.

Tickamyer, Ann, and Janet Bokemeier. "Sex Differences in Labor Market Experiences." *Rural Sociology* 53, no. 2 (1988): 166–89.

Tickamyer, Ann R., and Cynthia L. Duncan. "Economic Activity and the Quality of Life in Eastern Kentucky." *Growth and Change* 15, no. 4 (1984): 43–51.

Tickamyer, Ann R., and Cynthia M. Duncan. "Poverty and Opportunity Structure in Rural America." *Annual Review of Sociology* 16, no. 1 (1990): 67–86.

Tickamyer, A. R., J. Sherman, and J. Warlick. *Rural Poverty in the United States*. New York: Columbia University Press, 2017. https://books.google.com/books?id=zKAvDwAAQBAJ.

Tickamyer, Ann R., and Cecil H. Tickamyer. "Gender and Poverty in Central Appalachia." *Social Science Quarterly* 69, no. 4 (1988): 874–91.

Tinsley, Howard E. A., Diane J. Tinsley, and Chelsey E. Croskeys. "Park Usage, Social Milieu, and Psychosocial Benefits of Park Use Reported by Older Urban Park Users from Four Ethnic Groups." *Leisure Sciences* 24, no. 2 (2002): 199–218.

Titze, Sylvia, Billie Giles-Corti, Matthew W. Knuiman, Terri J. Pikora, Anna Timperio, Fiona C. Bull, and Kimberly Van Niel. "Associations between Intrapersonal and Neighborhood Environmental Characteristics and Cycling for Transport and Recreation in Adults: Baseline Results from the Reside Study." *Journal of Physical Activity and Health* 7, no. 4 (2010): 423–31.

Tobías, Aurelio, Alberto Recio, Julio Díaz, and Cristina Linares. "Health Impact Assessment of Traffic Noise in Madrid (Spain)." *Environmental Research* 137 (2015): 136–40.

Toner, William. "Getting to Know the People and the Place." In *Rural and Small Town Planning*, edited by Judith Getzels and Charles Thurow, 1–26. Chicago: Planners Press, 1979.

Town, S., C. Davey, and A. Wooton. *Design against Crime: Secure Urban Environments by Design*. Salford, England: University of Salford, 2003.

Trapp, Georgina S. A., Billie Giles-Corti, Hayley E. Christian, Max Bulsara, Anna F. Timperio, Gavin R. McCormack, and Karen P. Villanueva. "Increasing Children's Physical Activity: Individual, Social, and Environmental Factors Associated with Walking to and from School." *Health Education and Behavior* 39, no. 2 (2012): 172–82.

Trapp, Georgina S. A., Billie Giles-Corti, Hayley E. Christian, Max Bulsara, Anna F. Timperio, Gavin R. McCormack, and Karen P. Villanueva. "On Your Bike! A Cross-Sectional Study of the Individual, Social and Environmental Correlates of Cycling to School." *International Journal of Behavioral Nutrition and Physical Activity* 8, no. 123 (2011). https://doi.org/https://doi.org/10.1186/1479-5868-8-123.

Trivedi, Tushar, Jihong Liu, Janice C. Probst, Anwar Merchant, Sonya Jones, and Amy Block Martin. "Obesity and Obesity-Related Behaviors among Rural and Urban Adults in the USA." *Rural and Remote Health* 15, no. 3276 (2015). www.rrh.org.au/journal/article/3267.

Troped, Philip J., Jeffrey S. Wilson, Charles E. Matthews, Ellen K. Cromley, and Steven J. Melly. "The Built Environment and Location-Based Physical Activity." *American Journal of Preventive Medicine* 38, no. 4 (2010): 429–38.

Trust for America's Health. "A Funding Crisis for Public Health and Safety: State-by-State Public Health Funding and Key Health Facts." Washington, DC: Trust for America's Health, 2018. https://www.tfah.org/report-details/a-funding-crisis-for-public-health-and-safety-state-by-state-and-federal-public-health-funding-facts-and-recommendations/.

Tsai, Yuping. "Education and Disability Trends of Older Americans, 2000–2014." *Journal of Public Health* 39, no. 3 (2017): 447–54.

Tsouros, Agis D. "City Leadership for Health and Sustainable Development: The World Health Organization European Healthy Cities Network." *Health Promotion International* 24, no. S1 (2009): i4–i10.

Tsouros, Agis D. "Healthy Cities: A Political Movement Which Empowered Local Governments to Put Health and Equity High on Their Agenda." In *Integrating Human Health into Urban and Transport Planning: A Framework*, edited by Mark Nieuwenhuijsen and Haneen Khreis, 73–88. Cham: Springer International Publishing, 2019.

Tsouros, Agis D. "Healthy Cities: A Political Project Designed to Change How Cities Understand and Deal with Health." In *Healthy Cities: The Theory, Policy, and Practice of Value-Based Urban Planning*, edited by Evelyne de Leeuw and Jean Simos, 489–504. New York: Springer, 2017.

Tsouros, Agis D. "Healthy Cities Means Community Action." *Health Promotion International* 5, no. 3 (1990): 177–78.

Tsouros, Agis D. "The WHO Healthy Cities Project: State of the Art and Future Plans." *Health Promotion International* 10, no. 2 (1995): 133–41.

Turnbull, George C., Jr., "Using Natural Resources as a Planning Guide." In *Rural and Small Town Planning*, edited by Judith Getzels and Charles Thurow, 39–52. Chicago: Planners Press, 1979.

Ulrich, Roger S. "View through a Window May Influence Recovery from Surgery." *Science* 224, no. 4647 (1984): 420–21.

Ulrich, Roger S., Robert F. Simons, Barbara D. Losito, Evelyn Fiorito, Mark A. Miles, and Michael Zelson. "Stress Recovery during Exposure to Natural and Urban Environments." *Readings in Environmental Psychology* (1995): 149–78.

Umstattd, M. Renée, Stephanie L. Baller, Erin Hennessy, David Hartley, Christina D. Economos, Raymond R. Hyatt, Anush Yousefian, and Jeffrey S. Hallam. "Development of the Rural Active Living Perceived Environmental Support Scale (RALPESS)." *Journal of Physical Activity and Health* 9, no. 5 (2012): 724–30.

United Health Foundation. "America's Health Rankings: Analysis of America's Health Rankings Composite Measure." Accessed September 18, 2021. https://www.americashealth rankings.org/explore/annual/state/KS.

United Health Foundation. *America's Health Rankings: Annual Report 2020*. Minneapolis, MN: United Health Foundation, 2020. https://www.americashealthrankings.org/explore /annual.

United Nations. *Global Environment Outlook—Geo-6: Healthy Planet, Healthy People*. Nairobi: United Nations Environment Programme, 2019. https://www.unep.org/resources/global -environment-outlook-6.

United Nations. *Preventing the Next Pandemic: Zoonotic Diseases and How to Break the Chain of Transmission*. Nairobi: United Nations Environment Programme, 2020. https://www .unep.org/resources/report/preventing-future-zoonotic-disease-outbreaksprotecting -environment-animals-and.

United Nations Commission on Human Settlements. "Report of the United Nations Conference on Human Settlements (Habitat II)." Paper presented at the United Nations Conference on Human Settlements (Habitat II), Istanbul, Turkey, 1996.

United States Census Bureau. Accessed September 26, 2021, https://www.census.gov/.

United States Census Bureau. "About the American Community Survey." Accessed August 3, 2020. https://www.census.gov/programs-surveys/acs/about.html.

United States Census Bureau. "American Community Survey (ACS)." Accessed September 26, 2021, https://www.census.gov/programs-surveys/acs/.

United States Census Bureau. "Explore Census Data." Accessed 31 July, 2020, https://data .census.gov/cedsci/.

United States Census Bureau. "Growth in Urban Population Outpaces Rest of Nation, Census Bureau Reports." March 26, 2012. https://www.census.gov/newsroom/releases/archives /2010_census/cb12-50.html.

United States Census Bureau. "Nation's Urban and Rural Populations Shift Following 2020 Census." December 29, 2022. https://www.census.gov/newsroom/press-releases/2022 /urban-rural-populations.html.

United States Congress. "Minority Health and Health Disparities Research and Education Act of 2000, United States Public Law 106–525."

United States Department of Agriculture. "Key Statistics and Graphics: Food Security Status of U.S. Households in 2020." Economic Research Service, accessed September 30, 2021, https://www.ers.usda.gov/topics/food-nutrition-assistance/food-security-in-the-us/key -statistics-graphics/.

United States Department of Agriculture. "Rural Economy and Population—Population and Migration 2014." Economic Research Service, accessed August 3, 2020. http://www.ers .usda.gov/topics/rural-economy-population/population-migration.aspx.

United States Department of Agriculture, Natural Resources Conservation Service. *Community Garden Guide: Vegetable Garden Planting and Development*. East Lansing, MI: Rose Lake Plant Materials Center, 2009.

United States Department of Health and Human Services. "Agency for Healthcare Research and Quality 2009 National Healthcare Quality and Disparities Report." Rockville, MD: Agency for Healthcare Research and Quality, 2016.

United States Environmental Protection Agency. *Hydraulic Fracturing for Oil and Gas: Impacts from the Hydraulic Fracturing Water Cycle on Drinking Water Resources in the United States (Final Report)*. Washington, DC: Environmental Protection Agency, 2016.

United States Office of Management and Budget. "2010 Standards for Delineating Metropolitan and Micropolitan Statistical Areas: Notice." *Federal Register* 75, no. 123 (2010): 37246–52.

United States Supreme Court. Village of Euclid, Ohio v. Ambler Reality Co., 272 US 365. 1926.

University of Rochester Medical Center. "Older Adults and the Importance of Social Interaction." Health Encyclopedia, accessed August 5, 2020, http://www.urmc.rochester.edu/encyclopedia/content.aspx?ContentTypeID=1&ContentID=4513.

University of Wisconsin Population Health Institute. *2020 County Health Rankings Key Findings Report*. N.p.: University of Wisconsin Population Health Institute and Robert Wood Johnson Foundation, 2021. https://www.countyhealthrankings.org/reports/2020-county-health-rankings-key-findings-report.

Usher, Kareem M. "Exploring the Effects of Formalized, Targeted Municipal Food Planning Initiatives on Access to Healthy Food." PhD diss., Florida State University, 2015.

Vallance, Jeff K., Terry Boyle, Kerry S. Courneya, and Brigid M. Lynch. "Accelerometer-Assessed Physical Activity and Sedentary Time among Colon Cancer Survivors: Associations with Psychological Health Outcomes." *Journal of Cancer Survivorship* 9, no. 3 (2015): 404–11.

Vallance, Jeff K., Elisabeth A. H. Winkler, Paul A. Gardiner, Genevieve N. Healy, Brigid M. Lynch, and Neville Owen. "Associations of Objectively-Assessed Physical Activity and Sedentary Time with Depression: NHANES (2005–2006)." *Preventive Medicine* 53, no. 4–5 (2011): 284–88.

Valverde, Rochelle. "Is Illegal Immigration a Problem in Kansas? Despite Small Numbers, Kobach Says Yes." *Lawrence (KS) Journal-World*, September 9, 2018. https://www2.ljworld.com/news/2018/sep/09/is-illegal-immigration-a-problem-in-kansas-despite-small-numbers-kobach-says-yes/.

Vandersmissen, Marie-Hélène, Paul Villeneuve, and Marius Thériault. "Analyzing Changes in Urban Form and Commuting Time." *Professional Geographer* 55, no. 4 (2003): 446–63.

Van Holle, Veerle, Benedicte Deforche, Jelle Van Cauwenberg, Liesbet Goubert, Lea Maes, Nico Van de Weghe, and Ilse De Bourdeaudhuij. "Relationship between the Physical Environment and Different Domains of Physical Activity in European Adults: A Systematic Review." *BMC Public Health* 12, no. 807 (2012).

Van Kempen, Elise E. M. M., Hanneke Kruize, Hendriek C. Boshuizen, Caroline B. Ameling, Brigit A. M. Staatsen, and Augustinus E. M. de Hollander. "The Association between Noise Exposure and Blood Pressure and Ischemic Heart Disease: A Meta-Analysis." *Environmental Health Perspectives* 110, no. 3 (2002): 307–17.

van Os, Jim, Carsten B. Pedersen, and Preben B. Mortensen. "Confirmation of Synergy between Urbanicity and Familial Liability in the Causation of Psychosis." *American Journal of Psychiatry* 161, no. 12 (2004): 2312–14.

Varoudis. "DepthmapX: Multi-Platform Spatial Network Analyses Software." Accessed September 26, 2021. https://varoudis.github.io/depthmapX/.

Veenhoven, Ruut. "Greater Happiness for a Greater Number." *Journal of Happiness Studies* 11, no. 5 (2010): 605–29.

Veitch, Jenny, Jo Salmon, and Kylie Ball. "Individual, Social and Physical Environmental Correlates of Children's Active Free-Play: A Cross-Sectional Study." *International Journal of Behavioral Nutrition and Physical Activity* 7, no. 11 (2010). https://doi.org/https://doi.org/10.1186/1479-5868-7-11.

Ver Ploeg, M., V. Breneman, T. Farrigan, K. Hamrick, D. Hopkins, P. Kaufman, B. H. Lin, et al. *Access to Affordable and Nutritious Food: Measuring and Understanding Food Deserts and Their Consequences.* Report to Congress. Washington, DC: Department of Agriculture, 2009.

Vias, Alexander C. "Bigger Stores, More Stores, or No Stores: Paths of Retail Restructuring in Rural America." *Journal of Rural Studies* 20, no. 3 (2004): 303–18.

Villanueva, Karen, Billie Giles-Corti, Max Bulsara, Gavin R. McCormack, Anna Timperio, Nick Middleton, Bridget Beesley, and Georgina Trapp. "How Far Do Children Travel from Their Homes? Exploring Children's Activity Spaces in Their Neighborhood." *Health and Place* 18, no. 2 (2012): 263–73.

Villanueva, Karen, Billie Giles-Corti, Max Bulsara, Anna Timperio, Gavin McCormack, Bridget Beesley, Georgina Trapp, and Nicholas Middleton. "Where Do Children Travel to and What Local Opportunities Are Available? The Relationship between Neighborhood Destinations and Children's Independent Mobility." *Environment and Behavior* 45, no. 6 (2013): 679–705.

Vitruvius. *Vitruvius: The Ten Books on Architecture.* Translated by Morris Hicky Morgan. Cambridge, MA: Harvard University Press, 1960. First published 1914.

Von Korff, Michael, Thomas Koepsell, Susan Curry, and Paula Diehr. "Multi-Level Analysis in Epidemiologic Research on Health Behaviors and Outcomes." *American Journal of Epidemiology* 135, no. 10 (1992): 1077–82.

Vrijheid, Martine. "Health Effects of Residence near Hazardous Waste Landfill Sites: A Review of Epidemiologic Literature." *Environmental Health Perspectives* 108, no. S1 (2000): 101–12.

Waite, Linda J., and Maggie Gallagher. *The Case for Marriage: Why Married People Are Happier, Healthier, and Better Off Financially.* New York: Crown Publishing Group, 2001.

Wallace, Amy E., Yinong Young-Xu, David Hartley, and William B. Weeks. "Racial, Socioeconomic, and Rural-Urban Disparities in Obesity-Related Bariatric Surgery." *Obesity Surgery* 20, no. 10 (2010): 1354–60.

Wandersman, Abraham, and Maury Nation. "Urban Neighborhoods and Mental Health: Psychological Contributions to Understanding Toxicity, Resilience, and Interventions." *American Psychologist* 53, no. 6 (1998): 647–56.

Wang, Fahui, Ming Wen, and Yanqing Xu. "Population-Adjusted Street Connectivity, Urbanicity and Risk of Obesity in the U.S." *Applied Geography* 41 (2013): 1–14. https://doi.org/10.1016/j.apgeog.2013.03.006.

Wang, Xiao, Yuexuan Li, and Haoliang Fan. "The Associations between Screen Time–Based Sedentary Behavior and Depression: A Systematic Review and Meta-Analysis." *BMC Public Health* 19, no. 1 (2019): 1524.

Wannamethee, S. Goya, A. Gerald Shaper, and Mary Walker. "Changes in Physical Activity, Mortality, and Incidence of Coronary Heart Disease in Older Men." *Lancet* 351, no. 9116 (1998): 1603–08.

Warren, Jacob C., and K. Bryant Smalley. "What Is Rural?" In *Rural Public Health: Best Practices and Preventive Models,* edited by K. Bryant Smalley and Jacob C. Warren, 1–9. N.p.: Springer, 2014.

Weaver, Kathryn E., Ann M. Geiger, Lingyi Lu, and L. Douglas Case. "Rural-Urban Disparities in Health Status among US Cancer Survivors." *Cancer* 119, no. 5 (2013): 1050–57.

Weaver, Kathryn E., Nynikka Palmer, Lingyi Lu, L. Douglas Case, and Ann M. Geiger. "Rural-

Urban Differences in Health Behaviors and Implications for Health Status among US Cancer Survivors." *Cancer Causes and Control* 24, no. 8 (2013): 1481–90.

Weber, B. A., A. Marre, M. Fisher, R. Gibbs, and J. Cromartie. "Education's Effect on Poverty: The Role of Migration." *Review of Agricultural Economics* 29, no. 3 (2007): 437–45.

Weber, Lauren, Laura Ungar, Michelle R. Smith, Hannah Recht, and Anna Maria Barry-Jester. "Hollowed-Out Public Health System Faces More Cuts Amid Virus." Kaiser Health News, July 1, 2020. https://khn.org/news/us-public-health-system-underfunded-under-threat -faces-more-cuts-amid-covid-pandemic/.

Wei, Ming, James B. Kampert, Carolyn E. Barlow, Milton Z. Nichaman, Larry W. Gibbons, Ralph S. Paffenbarger Jr., and Steven N. Blair. "Relationship between Low Cardiorespiratory Fitness and Mortality in Normal-Weight, Overweight, and Obese Men." *Journal of the American Medical Association* 282, no. 16 (1999): 1547–53.

Weinert, Clarann, and Robert J. Boik. "MSU Rurality Index: Development and Evaluation." *Research in Nursing and Health* 18, no. 5 (1995): 453–64.

Weinert, Clarann, and Kathleen Ann Long. "Understanding the Health Care Needs of Rural Families." *Family Relations* 36, no. 4 (1987): 450–55.

Weir, Lori A., Debra Etelson, and Donald A. Brand. "Parents' Perceptions of Neighborhood Safety and Children's Physical Activity." *Preventive Medicine* 43, no. 3 (2006): 212–17.

Weisheit, R. A., and J. F. Donnermeyer. "Change and Continuity in Crime in Rural America." In *Criminal Justice 2000. The Nature of Crime: Continuity and Change*, edited by G. LaFree, 309–57. Washington, DC: National Institute of Justice, 2000.

Weisheit, R. A., D. N. Falcone, and L. E. Wells. *Crime and Policing in Rural and Small-Town America*. 2nd ed. Prospect Heights, IL: Waveland Press, 1999.

Weisheit, R. A., and L. E. Wells. "Deadly Violence in the Heartland: Comparing Homicide Patterns in Nonmetropolitan and Metropolitan Counties." American Society of Criminology Annual Meeting, Atlanta, GA, November 2001.

Weisheit, R. A., and L. E. Wells. "Rural Crime and Justice: Implications for Theory and Research." *Crime and Delinquency* 42, no. 3 (1996): 379–97.

Wells, L. Edward, and Ralph A. Weisheit. "Patterns of Rural and Urban Crime: A County-Level Comparison." *Criminal Justice Review* 29, no. 1 (2004): 1–22.

Wells, Nancy M., and Yizhao Yang. "Neighborhood Design and Walking: A Quasi-Experimental Longitudinal Study." *American Journal of Preventive Medicine* 34, no. 4 (2008): 313–19.

Wen, Ming, Christopher R. Browning, and Kathleen A. Cagney. "Poverty, Affluence, and Income Inequality: Neighborhood Economic Structure and Its Implications for Health." *Social Science and Medicine* 57, no. 5 (2003): 843–60.

Wendel, Monica L. "Social Capital and Health: Individual Measures, Community Influences, and Persistent Questions." PhD diss., Texas A&M University System Health Science Center, 2009.

Werna, Edmundo, Trudy Harpham, Ilona Blue, and Grey Goldstein. *Healthy City Projects in Developing Countries: An International Approach to Local Problems*. New York: Routledge, 2014.

White, Eric M., Anita T. Morzillo, and Ralph J. Alig. "Past and Projected Rural Land Conversion in the US at State, Regional, and National Levels." *Landscape and Urban Planning* 89, no. 1–2 (2009): 37–48.

White, Martin. "Food Access and Obesity." *Obesity Reviews* 8 (2007): 99–107.

White, Mathew P., Ian Alcock, Benedict W. Wheeler, and Michael H. Depledge. "Would You Be Happier Living in a Greener Urban Area? A Fixed-Effects Analysis of Panel Data." *Psychological Science* 24, no. 6 (2013): 920–28.

Whitehead, M., P. Townsend, M. Whitehead, and N. Davidson, eds. *The Health Divide*.

Inequalities in Health (the Black Report and the Health Divide). New edition. London: Penguin Books, 1992.

W. K. Kellogg Foundation. *Perceptions of Rural America*. Battle Creek, MI: W. K. Kellogg Foundation, 2002.

Wilcox, Pamela, Neil Quisenberry, Debra T. Cabrera, and Shayne Jones. "Busy Places and Broken Windows? Toward Defining the Role of Physical Structure and Process in Community Crime Models." *Sociological Quarterly* 45, no. 2 (2004): 185–207.

Wilcox, Sara, Melissa Bopp, Larissa Oberrecht, Sandra K. Kammermann, and Charles T. McElmurray. "Psychosocial and Perceived Environmental Correlates of Physical Activity in Rural and Older African American and White Women." *Journals of Gerontology Series B: Psychological Sciences and Social Sciences* 58, no. 6 (2003): 329–37.

Wilcox, Sara, Cynthia Castro, Abby C. King, Robyn Housemann, and Ross C. Brownson. "Determinants of Leisure Time Physical Activity in Rural Compared with Urban Older and Ethnically Diverse Women in the United States." *Journal of Epidemiology and Community Health* 54, no. 9 (2000): 667–72.

Wilkinson, R. G., and M. Marmot. *Social Determinants of Health: The Solid Facts*. 2nd ed. Copenhagen: World Health Organization Regional Office for Europe, 2003.

Willett, Kamali, Rui Jiang, Elizabeth Lenart, Donna Spiegelman, and Walter Willett. "Comparison of Bioelectrical Impedance and BMI in Predicting Obesity-Related Medical Conditions." *Obesity* 14, no. 3 (2006): 480–90.

Willett, Walter C., William H. Dietz, and Graham A. Colditz. "Guidelines for Healthy Weight." *New England Journal of Medicine* 341, no. 6 (1999): 427–34.

Williams, D. R. "Race, Socioeconomic Status, and Health: The Added Effects of Racism and Discrimination." *Annals of the New York Academy of Sciences* 896 (1999): 173–88.

Williams, David R. "Socioeconomic Differentials in Health: A Review and Redirection." *Social Psychology Quarterly* (1990): 81–99.

Wilson, Dawn K., Karen A. Kirtland, Barbara E. Ainsworth, and Cheryl L. Addy. "Socioeconomic Status and Perceptions of Access and Safety for Physical Activity." *Annals of Behavioral Medicine* 28, no. 1 (2004): 20–28.

Wilson, Kenneth, Patricia Mottram, and Andrew Sixsmith. "Depressive Symptoms in the Very Old Living Alone: Prevalence, Incidence and Risk Factors." *International Journal of Geriatric Psychiatry: A Journal of the Psychiatry of Late Life and Allied Sciences* 22, no. 4 (2007): 361–66.

Wing, Steve, Elizabeth Barnett, Michele Casper, and H. A. Tyroler. "Geographic and Socioeconomic Variation in the Onset of Decline of Coronary Heart Disease Mortality in White Women." *American Journal of Public Health* 82, no. 2 (1992): 204–09.

Wing, Steve, Michele Casper, Carl G. Hayes, Patricia Dargent-Molina, Wilson Riggan, and H. A. Tyroler. "Changing Association between Community Occupational Structure and Ischaemic Heart Disease Mortality in the United States." *Lancet* 330, no. 8567 (1987): 1067–70.

Winkler, Elisabeth, Gavin Turrell, and Carla Patterson. "Does Living in a Disadvantaged Area Mean Fewer Opportunities to Purchase Fresh Fruit and Vegetables in the Area? Findings from the Brisbane Food Study." *Health and Place* 12, no. 3 (2006): 306–19.

Wohlfahrt-Veje, C., J. Tinggaard, K. Winther, A. Mouritsen, C. P. Hagen, M. G. Mieritz, K. T. de Renzy-Martin, et al. "Body Fat Throughout Childhood in 2647 Healthy Danish Children: Agreement of BMI, Waist Circumference, Skinfolds with Dual X-Ray Absorptiometry." *European Journal of Clinical Nutrition* 68, no. 6 (2014): 664–70.

Wolch, Jennifer, Michael Jerrett, Kim Reynolds, Rob McConnell, Roger Chang, Nicholas Dahmann, Kirby Brady, et al. "Childhood Obesity and Proximity to Urban Parks and Recreational Resources: A Longitudinal Cohort Study." *Health and Place* 17, no. 1 (2011): 207–14.

Wood, Lisa, Lawrence D. Frank, and Billie Giles-Corti. "Sense of Community and Its Relationship with Walking and Neighborhood Design." *Social Science and Medicine* 70, no. 9 (2010): 1381–90.

Woods, Michael. "Rural Geography: Blurring Boundaries and Making Connections." *Progress in Human Geography* 33, no. 6 (2009): 849–58.

World Health Organization. *Constitution of the World Health Organization*. New York: World Health Organization, 1946.

World Health Organization. *Indoor Environment: Health Aspects of Air Quality, Thermal Environment, Light and Noise*. Geneva: World Health Organization, 1990.

World Health Organization. *Nature, Biodiversity and Health: An Overview of Interconnections*. Copenhagen: WHO Regional Office for Europe, 2021.

World Health Organization. *Obesity and Overweight*. Geneva: World Health Organization, 2006.

World Health Organization. *The Ottawa Charter for Health Promotion*. Ottawa: WHO, Canadian Public Health Association, Health and Welfare Canada, 1986.

World Health Organization. *Primary Health Care: Report of the International Conference on Primary Health Care, Alma-Ata, USSR, September 6–12, 1978*. N.p.: World Health Organization, 1978.

World Health Organization. *Rural Poverty and Health Systems in the WHO European Region*. Copenhagen: WHO Regional Office for Europe, 2010.

World Health Organization. *Twenty Steps for Developing a Healthy Cities Project*. Copenhagen: World Health Organization Regional Office for Europe, 1995.

World Health Organization Commission on Social Determinants of Health. *Addressing the Social Determinants of Health: The Urban Dimension and the Role of Local Government*. Copenhagen: World Health Organization Regional Office for Europe, 2012. https://books .google.com/books?id=XYvIMQEACAAJ.

World Health Organization European Healthy Cities Network. *Phase V (2009–2013) of the WHO European Healthy Cities Network: Goals and Requirements*. Copenhagen: WHO Regional Office for Europe, 2009.

World Health Organization Regional Office for Europe. *Community Participation in Local Health and Sustainable Development: Approaches and Techniques*. Copenhagen: Centre for Urban Health, WHO Regional Office for Europe, 2002. https://apps.who.int/iris/handle /10665/107341.

World Health Organization Regional Office for Europe. *Health 21: The Health for All Policy Framework for the European Region*. Copenhagen: WHO Regional Office for Europe, 1998.

WSP and Arup. *Impacts of Land Use Planning Policy on Transport Demand and Congestion, Research Report for Department for Transport*. Cambridge: WSP Policy and Research, 2005. www.wspgroup.com/upload/documents/pdf/news%20attachments/ppg13_Final _Report.pdf.

Wuthnow, Robert. *Small-Town America: Finding Community, Shaping the Future*. Princeton, NJ: Princeton University Press, 2013. https://books.google.com/books?id=N5u-QZ _oHmUC.

Xu, Yanqing, and Fahui Wang. "Built Environment and Obesity by Urbanicity in the US." *Health and Place* 34 (2015): 19–29.

Yang, Wei, and Stanley T. Omaye. "Air Pollutants, Oxidative Stress and Human Health." *Mutation Research / Genetic Toxicology and Environmental Mutagenesis* 674, no. 1–2 (2009): 45–54.

Yang, X. *Exploring the Influence of Environmental Features on Residential Burglary Using Spatial-*

Temporal Pattern Analysis. Gainesville: University of Florida, 2006. http://etd.fcla.edu/UF /UFE0013390/yang_x.pdf.

Yannis, George, Alexandra Kondyli, and Xenia Georgopoulou. "Investigation of the Impact of Low Cost Traffic Engineering Measures on Road Safety in Urban Areas." *International Journal of Injury Control and Safety Promotion* 21, no. 2 (2014): 181–89.

Youmans, E. G. *Older Rural Americans.* Lexington: University Press of Kentucky, 2015. https:// books.google.com/books?id=nsofBgAAQBAJ.

Yousefian, Anush, Erin Hennessy, M. Renee Umstattd, Christina D. Economos, Jeffrey S. Hallam, Raymond R. Hyatt, and David Hartley. "Development of the Rural Active Living Assessment Tools: Measuring Rural Environments." *Preventive Medicine* 50 (2010): S86–S92.

Yousefian, Anush, Erika Ziller, Jon Swartz, and David Hartley. "Active Living for Rural Youth: Addressing Physical Inactivity in Rural Communities." *Journal of Public Health Management and Practice* 15, no. 3 (2009): 223–31.

Zajacova, Anna, Jennifer B. Dowd, and Allison E. Aiello. "Socioeconomic and Race/Ethnic Patterns in Persistent Infection Burden among US Adults." *Journals of Gerontology Series A: Biomedical Sciences and Medical Sciences* 64, no. 2 (2009): 272–79.

Zajacova, Anna, Robert A. Hummer, and Richard G. Rogers. "Education and Health among US Working-Age Adults: A Detailed Portrait across the Full Educational Attainment Spectrum." *Biodemography and Social Biology* 58, no. 1 (2012): 40–61.

Zajacova, Anna, and Jennifer Karas Montez. "Physical Functioning Trends among US Women and Men Age 45–64 by Education Level." *Biodemography and Social Biology* 63, no. 1 (2017): 21–30.

Zajacova, Anna, and Elizabeth M. Lawrence. "The Relationship between Education and Health: Reducing Disparities through a Contextual Approach." *Annual Review of Public Health* 39 (2018): 273–89.

Zakus, J. David L., and Catherine L. Lysack. "Revisiting Community Participation." *Health Policy and Planning* 13, no. 1 (1998): 1–12.

Zenk, Shannon N., Amy J. Schulz, Barbara A. Israel, Sherman A. James, Shuming Bao, and Mark L. Wilson. "Fruit and Vegetable Access Differs by Community Racial Composition and Socioeconomic Position in Detroit, Michigan." *Ethnicity and Disease* 16, no. 1 (2006): 275–80.

Zhang, Junfeng, and Kirk R. Smith. "Indoor Air Pollution: A Global Health Concern." *British Medical Bulletin* 68, no. 1 (2003): 209–25.

Zhang, Xingyou, James B. Holt, Hua Lu, Stephen Onufrak, Jiawen Yang, Steven P. French, and Daniel Z. Sui. "Neighborhood Commuting Environment and Obesity in the United States: An Urban-Rural Stratified Multilevel Analysis." *Preventive Medicine* 59 (2014): 31–36.

Zhou, Bin, Diego Rybski, and Jürgen P. Kropp. "The Role of City Size and Urban Form in the Surface Urban Heat Island." *Scientific Reports* 7, no. 1 (2017): 4791. https://doi.org/10.1038 /s41598-017-04242-2.

Zhu, X., and C. Lee. "Ethnic Disparity in the Multi-Level Walkability and Safety of Public Elementary School's Attendance Areas." *American Journal of Preventive Medicine* 34, no. 4 (2008): 282–90.

Ziegler, Laura. "Atchison, Kansas, Residents Find Themselves in the Crosshairs of Economic Change." KMUW, April 13, 2017. https://www.kmuw.org/post/atchison-kansas-residents -find-themselves-crosshairs-economic-change.

Ziersch, Anna Marie, and F. E. Baum. "Involvement in Civil Society Groups: Is It Good for Your Health?" *Journal of Epidemiology and Community Health* 58, no. 6 (2004): 493–500.

Ziglio, E., S. Hagard, and J. Griffiths. "Health Promotion Development in Europe: Achievements and Challenges." *Health Promotion International* 15, no. 2 (2000): 143–54.

Zipf, George Kingsley. *Human Behavior and the Principle of Least Effort*. Oxford: Addison-Wesley Press, 1949.

Zurek, Ludek, and Anuradha Ghosh. "Insects Represent a Link between Food Animal Farms and the Urban Environment for Antibiotic Resistance Traits." *Applied and Environmental Microbiology* 80, no. 12 (2014): 3562–67.

Figures and tables are indicated by "f" and "t" following page numbers.

active commuting (AC), 197–99

Affordable Care Act of 2010, 79, 107

African Americans, 12–13, 38–39, 53, 64–66, 96–97, 105, 143, 178

aging in place, 52, 66

Agnew, Robert, 269

agriculture: corporate, 56, 60; employment in, 51, 55, 64, 78, 112; farm bill (2002), 46; in flood lands, 329–30; livestock operations, 79, 88–89, 92; monocrop, 113, 139; pollution from, 79, 87; safeguarding land for, 301; in small Kansas cities, xii, 77–79; subsidy programs, 77; trade and, 49, 55

air quality, 7–9, 14, 16, 17, 86–88, 90

alcohol use. *See* substance use and abuse

Amazon, 80

American Community Survey (ACS), 155–58, 205

American Diabetes Association, 143

American Hospital Association, 106–7

American Indians. *See* Native Americans

American Public Health Association, 94

America's Health Rankings, 94–95, 102

Antonovsky, Aaron, 26

anxiety, 12, 16, 80, 95, 99–100, 113, 140, 145, 211, 234, 241

any mental illness (AMI), 262

Appalachia, 14, 38, 51, 58

aquifers, 87, 330

Arnstein, S., 341

arthritis, 96, 105, 144

Asian populations, 12, 13, 53

Association of American Indian Physicians, 106

asthma, 7, 15, 96, 99, 105, 112, 336

attention-deficit/hyperactivity disorder (ADHD), 234

axial maps, 134–36, 160

Bader, Michael D. M., 205

Barton, Hugh, 5

behavioral health, 94, 100

Behavioral Risk Factor Surveillance System (BRFSS), 96, 99, 105, 157, 235, 259

bicycling, 138, 141, 162, 174–75, 180–81, 187–88, 197, 214–17, 300

birth rates, 50–51, 55, 62, 66

Black Americans. *See* African Americans

Black Belt, 38–39

body mass index (BMI), 96, 138, 143–44, 206, 213, 234, 236, 239, 242–45, 259–61

Boehmer, Tegan K., 234

Boer, R., 181, 184

Briggs, Ronald, 123

Britton, M., 123

Brown, Barbara B., 239, 243

built environments: active commuting and, 198–99; density, 49–50, 128–29; disability accommodations in, 142; mental health and, 99–100; natural elements within, 8; pathways of influence in, 126, 304; physical activity and, 95, 100, 212, 304; in socio-ecological model, 5, 6f, 9–11, 120–22, 286–87. *See also* spatial design and planning

Burgoine, T., 236, 243

Campoli, J., 175

cancer, 10, 106, 130, 137, 139–44, 211, 258

capital improvement programs (CIPs), 322–23, 345

cardiovascular disease, 7, 10, 16, 22, 97, 125, 130, 140, 144, 197, 211

carpooling, 138, 162, 179, 187, 190, 197, 200–202

Carr-Hill, Roy, 125

census block density, 129, 158, 176, 189, 233

census tracts, 40, 42–44, 156, 197, 204–5, 235, 243, 258

Centers for Disease Control and Prevention (CDC), 102, 106, 137, 140, 157, 158

Centers for Medicare and Medicaid Services, 144

Cerin, Ester, 182, 240

Cervero, Robert, 182

Chang, Virginia W., 235–36

Chen, Juan, 230

Cheung, Monit, 230

children: health, 51, 111; mental disorders, 3; nutrition assistance, 105; obesity, 140, 234, 235; physical activity, 177, 185, 199, 212; poverty, 65; walking to school, 185, 199

chronic diseases, 4, 12–17, 94, 96, 99–101, 106, 139. *See also specific conditions*

city size, 128, 172–74, 188, 230–32, 246

Coleman, Karen J., 242–43

Commonwealth Fund Commission on the Elderly Living Alone, 146

Community Care Network of Kansas, 157

community empowerment, 24–26, 28, 308, 340–44, 349

community participation: challenges in, 350–51; defined, 340; in food consumption experience, 303–4; "health in all policies" and, 347–48; in health promotion projects, 24–26, 28; intersectoral planning, 316; participation fatigue, 351; population density and, 232; as protection from social isolation, 98; in rural America, 344–45; in social activities, 309. *See also* participatory spatial design and planning

community planning and development, 104, 309, 322, 328

commute time: eating and food shopping, 209–10, 221; health and, 261, 266, 274; mortality/morbidity and, 256; physical and sedentary activities, 217, 221; work-related travel behaviors, 62, 147, 198, 202, 221

comorbid conditions, xiii, 96, 105, 144–45

concentrated animal feeding operations (CAFOs), 88–89

constitutional home rule, 75, 76

convenience stores, 80, 130–31, 179–80, 235, 237–38, 302

Corn Belt, 51

coronary heart disease, 99, 123, 125, 234, 236, 256, 258

counties: in fringe areas, 61–63; as geographical units of analysis, 40; as local government administrative units, 40; rural-urban classification schemes, 43–44, 46

COVID-19 pandemic, xiii–xv, 107

crime: built environments and, 11; city size and, 231–32; data sources on, 156; density and, 232; land use mix and, 240–42, 247; in neighborhoods, 16–17; prevention, 3, 145, 308; reduction, 4, 166, 309, 343; in rural America, 37, 67, 268–69, 290–91; in small Kansas cities, 102–3, 163, 164*t*, 166; street properties and, 243; substance use and, 100; in urban America, 103, 268–69, 290–91; violent, 86, 102–3, 145–46, 156, 231–32, 238, 242, 245, 268. *See also* property crime

Crime Prevention through Environmental Design (CPTED), 308, 309

critical access hospitals, xiv, 82, 107–8

cultural diversity. *See* race and ethnicity

Dahlgren, Göran, 5

Davidson, Scott, 341

daytime population change: eating and food shopping, 208, 220; health and, 260–61, 265, 272–73; mortality/morbidity and, 255; physical and sedentary activities and, 215–16, 220; work-related travel behaviors and, 147, 201, 220

demographics: data sources, 155–56; in rural America, 38–40, 52–54, 66–67; rural poverty, 52–53, 64–65, 67; in small Kansas cities, 83–86; sociodemographics, 9, 99, 204–5, 304, 311; urban poverty, 64–65

Dengel, Donald R., 235

density: of built environments, 49–50, 128–29; census block, 129, 158, 176, 189, 233; health and, 232–33, 246; of housing, 129, 158, 175, 176, 233; lifestyle and, 174–76, 189; of streets, 133, 184, 242–43. *See also* population density

dental care, 62, 94, 111, 112, 252

depression: comorbid conditions, 144; food insecurity and, 139; global burden of disease and, 3; major depressive episodes, 262–63; physical activity and, 106, 211; risk factors, 4, 95, 140, 234, 240, 269–70; in small Kansas cities, 99; unemployment and, 80, 113, 241

Depthmap, 157, 163

design. *See* spatial design and planning; urban design and planning

determinants of health: in area-level studies, 123, 124; assessment methods, 27; economic, 25, 345, 350; environmental, 25, 345; health promotion and, 316, 347; key destinations and facility availability, 129; social, 5, 11–14, 25, 108–9, 147, 345, 350

diabetes mellitus: active commuting and, 197; city size and, 231; economic costs, 97, 143; food insecurity and, 139; physical activity and, 106, 139, 178, 211; prevalence, 142–43; racial/ethnic differences, 97; risk factors, 95–97, 112, 140, 211, 237, 256–58; street properties and, 244; treatment, 97–98; type 2, 22, 130, 137, 141, 144, 211

Diehr, P., 125

Diez-Roux, A. V., 125, 177

disabilities, 11, 13, 57, 96, 99–100, 106, 142, 244

disability-adjusted life years (DALYs), 10

discrimination, 12–13, 17, 54, 65, 86, 349

disease: dense housing and, 15; global burden, 3, 7; prevention efforts, 111; treatment, 88–89. *See also* chronic diseases; *specific conditions*

distal factors, 5, 6

diversity. *See* race and ethnicity

domestic violence, 67, 112, 270

Donnermeyer, J. F., 268

Douglass, H. Paul, 44

driving to work, 108, 113, 138, 162, 179, 187, 197, 200–202

drug use. *See* substance use and abuse

Dutko, Paula, 204–5

Eames, Margaret, 123

earthquakes, 81, 90–91

eating behaviors: city size and, 174; commute time and, 209–10, 221; daytime population change and, 208, 220; distance to nearest city and, 208–9, 221; as health risk factors, 139; key destinations and facility availability and, 180; land use types and, 182–83, 190; overeating, 16; population density and, 207–8, 219–20; population size and, 207, 219; rurality and spatial associations, 203–11, 210*t*; in small Kansas cities, 103,

113, 161*t*, 162, 165, 207–11; spatial design/planning for, 301–4; street properties and, 186–87, 190

economic health, 39, 49

Economic Research Service, 41–42

economic well-being, 64, 137, 301

economy: city size and, 172–73; data sources on, 155–56; global, 54, 60, 77, 85; health and, 13–14; in Healthy Cities and Communities, 25; recessions, 57, 80–81; in rural America, 39, 49, 57–60, 67; in small Kansas cities, 77–83; in urban America, 57

education level: diabetes and, 97; employment and, 20; food desert tracts and, 204–5; health outcomes and, 13; of immigrants, 54, 86; mental disorders and, 3; obesity and, 96; as pathway of influence, 20–21; physical activity and, 21, 105, 178; in rural America, 52, 67; substance use and, 100–101

elderly populations. *See* older adults

Elliott, Susan J., 239–40

employment: agricultural, 51, 55, 64, 78, 112; education level and, 20; health hazards in, 16; for immigrants, 77, 84, 91; in manufacturing, 56–57, 64, 67, 80; workers' compensation, 105. *See also* unemployment; work-related travel behaviors

environmental health, 49, 60, 323, 330

environmental issues: air quality, 7–9, 14, 16, 17, 86–88, 90; anthropogenic activities and, 7–10; greenhouse effects, 8, 21, 22, 88. *See also* pollution

environmental justice, 63–64, 67, 172

Environmental Protection Agency (EPA), 90

ethnicity. *See* race and ethnicity

Evans, Robert G., 4

Ewing, Reid, 181

Fan, Jessie X., 197–98, 211–12

farmers' markets, 111, 206, 302–3, 310, 316, 343

fast food restaurants, 80, 130, 235–36

Federal Bureau of Investigation (FBI), 102, 145, 156

Feeding America, 104

Ferré, Céline, 230

flood lands, 329–30

floor area ratio, 236

food: access to, 4, 6, 16, 104, 111, 204; anthropogenic activities affecting, 7, 10; farmers' markets, 111, 206, 302–3, 310, 316, 343; health promotion and, 315–16; meat industry, 53, 56, 63–64, 77, 81, 84, 91, 325; processing plants, 39, 53, 63–64, 67, 120;

food (*cont.*)

    safety concerns, 56; in small Kansas cities, 103–5, 113; SNAP and, 104, 105, 303. *See also* eating behaviors

Food Access Research Atlas, 104

Food and Drug Administration, 88

food deserts, 12, 37, 56, 95, 104, 113, 204–5, 290

food insecurity, 56, 94, 103–4, 139, 186, 204

food shopping: city size and, 174, 188; commute time and, 209–10, 221; daytime population change and, 208, 220; distance to nearest city and, 208–9, 221; as health risk factors, 139; key destinations and facility availability and, 179–80; land use types and, 182–83, 190; population density and, 207–8, 219–20; population size and, 207, 219; rurality and spatial associations, 203–11, 210*t*; in small Kansas cities, 161*t*, 162, 165, 207–11; spatial design/planning for, 301–4; street properties and, 186–87, 190. *See also* grocery stores

Forsyth, A., 184

Fox, Anthony John, 123

fracking, 60, 81, 90–91

Frank, Lawrence D., 181, 239, 242

fringe areas, 61–63

frontier communities, 44, 49, 101

geographical units of analysis, 40

geographic information system (GIS), 155, 157

geographic isolation, 37, 43, 96, 152, 258, 285, 334

Ghosh, Soumendra N., 230

Giles-Corti, Billie, 21, 234

global burden of disease, 3, 7

Goldblatt, P. O., 123

Gomez, L. F., 183–84

Google Maps, 157

Government Accountability Office (GAO), 107

Grant, Marcus, 5

Great Lakes region, 51, 53, 58

Great Plains, 38, 39, 51, 53, 83

greenhouse effects, 8, 21, 22, 88

green spaces. *See* parks and green spaces

grocery stores: availability, 130, 176, 179–80, 205, 235, 237–38, 302; closure, 80, 104; local, 13, 56, 78, 83, 84, 104–5

Haan, M., 124–25

Hancock, Trevor, 5

Handy, Susan L., 128, 181, 184–85

Hansen, Anush Yousefian, 258

Hanson, Julienne, 133

health: behavioral, 94, 100; of children, 51, 111; data sources on, 156–57; defined, 1–4, 285; economic, 39, 49; environmental, 49, 60, 323, 330; income and, 12, 109, 125; mandala of, 5; maternal, 51, 111; positive model, 5, 24, 26; spatial design/planning for, 307–9. *See also* determinants of health; mental health; physical health; population health; public health; social health; spatial associations of health

health behaviors, 18–19, 28, 51, 123, 269. *See also* *specific behaviors*

health care: access to, 13, 21, 43, 65–66, 86, 107, 111, 130, 237–38; dental, 62, 94, 111, 112, 252; expenditures related to, 5, 52, 143; rural, 14, 43, 52, 65–66, 106–8, 290; skilled nursing care, 107; urban, 14–16, 65–66

health disparities: green space access and, 237; in natural environments, 8; racial/ethnic, 13, 86; in small Kansas cities, 99–100, 108–9, 109–10*t*; in social environments, 11; urban-rural, 119, 195, 198, 258–59, 262–64, 289–91

Health for All, 5, 24, 316, 340–41

"health in all policies," 347–48

health indicators: fringe area residents and, 62–63; limitations, 288; mental health, 144–45; physical health, 142–44; for population health monitoring, 95, 99; racial/ethnic, 13, 86; rankings of rural America, 51; rurality and spatial associations for, 276–77, 278*t*; social health, 145–46

health inequities, 5, 7–8, 21, 24, 27–28, 51, 344

health insurance, 62, 86, 107, 108, 111

health outcomes: in area-level studies, 123–26; education level and, 13; health rankings, 94; quality of life, 22, 111–12; rurality and spatial associations, 276–77, 278*t*; segregation and, 12; spatial design/planning and, 21–22, 23*f*; spatial factors and, 14; urban design and, 1

health promotion: community empowerment and, 24, 28; community participation in, 24–26, 28; defined, 4, 24; individual interventions, 19; intersectoral approach, 315–16; Ottawa Charter for Health Promotion, 4, 24, 25; of population health, 3, 5, 24–27, 113, 301, 306, 311; public policies, 5, 24–25, 347–48; spatial design/planning and, 113–14, 309–11, 335–40, 345–52

health rankings, 51, 94–95, 102, 108, 109–10*t*
Health Resources and Services Administration (HRSA), 43
health risk factors: in area-level studies, 123, 125; eating behaviors as, 139; food shopping and, 139; health rankings on, 94; in households, 15–16; in natural environments, 8; obesity, 21, 95–96, 256–57; sedentary activity and, 21, 140–41; in small Kansas cities, 95; spatial design/planning and, 21–22, 23*f*
health status, 27, 52, 86, 98, 141–42, 234
Healthy Cities and Communities, 24–27, 316, 344
Healthy Kansans 2020 initiative, 109
heart disease, 99, 123, 125, 139, 143–44, 234, 236, 239, 256, 258
Heinrich, Katie M., 199
High Plains aquifer, 87
Hillier, Bill, 133
Hispanic people, 12, 39, 53–54, 66, 84, 97, 105, 143
home rule, 75, 76
hospitals, xiv, 66, 68, 79, 82, 107–8, 113
housing. affordable, 6, 41, 111; data sources, 155–56; density, 129, 158, 175, 176, 233; discrimination, 86; poverty and, 15–16; in rural America, 41, 51, 58–59; second homes, 58–59; in small Kansas cities, 81–82; spatial factors, 15–16; urban health and, 14–15. *See also* neighborhoods
Humphreys, Keith, 125
hydraulic fracturing, 60, 81, 90–91
hyperlipidemia, 139, 211, 257
hypertension, 10, 97, 138–40, 144, 211, 256–58, 270

immigrants, 3, 39, 53–54, 67–68, 77, 84–86, 91–92
inactivity. *See* sedentary activity
income level: anxiety and, 99; diabetes and, 97; food desert tracts and, 204–5; health and, 12, 109, 125; obesity and, 96; physical activity and, 105, 178; restaurant availability and, 236; in rural America, 51, 57, 67
industrial land use, 181–83, 190, 241–42, 293, 300, 337
infant mortality, 12, 123, 308
infrastructure: civic, 84; food-related, 104; pedestrian, 199; for physical activity, 177; for rural health care, 106; strains on, 51. *See also* transportation infrastructure
insurance. *See* health insurance
intensive care units (ICUs), xiv

ischemic heart disease, 123, 143
isolation. *See* geographic isolation; social isolation

Jiao, Junfeng, 204
Joshi, Heather, 125
Julian, David A., 240

Kaczynski, Andrew T., 239
KanCare, 97
Kansas Association of Local Health Departments, 157
Kansas Bureau of Investigation (KBI), 156, 157
Kansas Care Planning Council, 99
Kansas Corporation Commission (KCC), 90–91
Kansas Department of Health and Environment (KDHE), xiii, 101, 105–6, 109, 156, 157
Kansas Foundation for Medical Care, 157
Kansas Health Foundation, 157
Kansas Health Institute, 157
Kansas Health Matters, 156–57
Kansas Hospital Association, 100, 157
Kansas Partnership for Improving Community Health, 156–57
Kansas Sampler Foundation, 105
Kansas State University, 105
Kansas Violent Death Reporting System, 101
Keller, Suzanne, 45, 46
key destinations and facility availability: businesses, 131, 176–77, 180, 236–38; computation methods, 129–30; convenience stores, 80, 130–31, 179–80, 235, 237–38, 302; health and, 130, 233–39, 246; lifestyle and, 176–81, 189; restaurants, 131, 179–80, 235–38, 302. *See also* grocery stores; parks and green spaces
Kim, Hyung Jin, 199
Kindig, David, 4
Kiri, Victor A., 123
Kockelman, K., 182
Kohler, Stefan, 263–64

land use mix (LUM): crime rates and, 103; defined, 131; density and, 174; health and, 239–42, 247; lifestyle and, 181–83, 189–90; at macro-spatial scale, 17; mixed-use, 103, 131, 181, 232, 240–41; quantification, 132; spatial design/planning and, 300, 305
land use types, 63, 131, 181–83, 189–90, 239–42, 247. *See also* industrial land use

Latinos/Latinas. *See* Hispanic people

Lawrence-Douglas County Health Department, 111–12

Leonard, William A., IV, 123

Leslie, Eva, 240

Li, Fuzhong, 184, 236, 239

life expectancy, 12, 13, 109, 130, 211

lifestyle: active, 37, 106, 130, 132, 199, 211, 258; behaviors selected for study, 288; in Healthy Cities and Communities, 25; pathways of health influence and, 126; in small Kansas cities, 160–62, 161*t*, 165; spatial design/planning for, 21–22, 23*f*, 106, 299–307. *See also* spatial associations of lifestyle

linear map analysis, 133–37

livestock operations, 79, 88–89, 92

local governments, 24–27, 40, 59, 75–76, 341, 344, 347–48

local health departments, xiv, 157

locally undesirable land use (LULU), 63

loneliness, 4, 98, 234, 269–70, 290, 308, 335–36. *See also* social isolation

Lower Mississippi Delta, 39

Lund, Hollie, 240

Mackenbach, Joreintje D., 239

macro-spatial scale, 5, 6*f*, 17, 19–20, 20*f*, 286–87, 299

major depressive episodes (MDEs), 262–63

manufacturing, 7, 39, 56–57, 64, 67, 80, 91, 120, 140

Map the Meal Gap, 104

McKenzie, Brian S., 205

Medicaid, 79, 107, 111, 113

Medicare, 52, 97, 107, 111, 113

Mehta, Neil K., 235–36

mental disorders: older adults, 3, 144; risk factors, 3, 4, 99; suicide rates, 101, 113; unemployment and, 3, 80, 113, 241; unwillingness to reveal, 43; urban-rural disparities, 262–64. *See also specific conditions*

mental health: city size and, 230, 231; commute time and, 266; daytime population change and, 265; defined, 2; density and, 232, 246; distance to nearest city and, 266; food insecurity and, 139; in fringe areas, 62; as global concern, 3; indicators, 144–45; integration with physical and social health, 5; key destinations and facility availability and, 238; land use mix and, 240–42, 247;

microenvironments and, 15–16; noise exposure, 10; parks / green spaces and, 233–34; physical activity and, 100; population density and, 265; population size and, 264; rurality and spatial associations, 262–66, 267*t*; in small Kansas cities, 99–100, 163, 164*t*, 166, 264–66; in small-town America, 37, 69; social isolation and, 4, 43, 100; spatial design/planning and, 22; street properties and, 243–45, 247; substance use and, 100

mental well-being, 2–4, 8, 10, 26–27, 100, 232, 241, 262, 285, 345

meso-spatial scale, 5, 6*f*, 16–17, 19–20, 20*f*, 286–87, 299

metabolic syndrome (METS), 130, 235

metropolitan areas: defined, 41–42; employment, 57; migration patterns, 51; proximity to, 43, 46; small towns and cities within, 39; urban cores, 37, 50, 62, 63, 241, 293. *See also* urban America

micropolitan areas, 46, 259, 262

micro-spatial scale, 5, 6*f*, 14–16, 19–20, 20*f*, 286–87, 299

Midwest: agriculture, 51, 87, 103; Great Lakes region, 51, 53, 58; Great Plains, 38, 39, 51, 53, 83. *See also* small Kansas cities

migration: age-selective, 14, 51–52; of farm families, 55–56; in-migration, 39, 50, 52, 58–59, 66; out-migration, 14, 39, 50–52, 55, 67–69, 91; quality of life and, 67; white flight, 54. *See also* immigrants

mining, 37, 51, 55, 57, 64–65, 89–92

Mobley, Lee R., 234, 236, 239

moderate to vigorous physical activity (MVPA), 177–78, 181, 184–85, 187, 199

Morland, Kimberly B., 235

Morris, J. N., 123

mortality and morbidity: air pollution and, 7; anxiety and, 99; cardiovascular disease and, 7, 125; city size and, 231; commute time and, 256; death rate, 142, 163, 254–56; depression and, 99; diabetes and, 97; disabilities and, 142; distance to nearest city and, 255–56; in fringe areas, 62; indicators, 96, 141–42; infant mortality, 12, 123, 308; population density and, 254–55; population size and, 254; rurality and spatial associations, 252–56, 257*t*; in small Kansas cities, 163, 164*t*, 237, 254–56; in small-town America, 38, 51; social isolation and, 98; street properties and, 244; suicide and, 142, 253

MRSA (methicillin-resistant Staphylococcus aureus), 89

Murray, Christopher J. L., 14

Nasar, Jack L., 240

National Center for Health Statistics (NCHS), 46

National Comorbidity Survey, 144

National Health and Nutrition Examination Survey (NHANES), 211

National Health Interview Survey (NHIS), 46, 230, 258

National Institute on Drug Abuse, 145

National Vital Statistics System (NVSS), 46

Native Americans, 3, 39, 53, 106, 178

natural environments, 5–10, 6*f*, 286–87. *See also* parks and green spaces

natural resources, 6, 57–60, 317, 325, 328–31

neighborhoods: crime and violence, 16–17; inner-city, 54, 65, 185; land use mix, 181, 240; property abandonment, 14; safety, 6, 11–12, 16–17, 241; segregation, 12, 65; walkability, 213. *See also* housing

Nelson, Melissa C., 185

noise, 9–17, 37, 197, 241

nonmetropolitan areas, 42, 51, 53–54. *See also* rural America

Norman, Gregory J., 177–78, 185, 239

North American Free Trade Agreement (NAFTA), 77

North Carolina Rural Health Research Program, 107

Oakley, Peter, 346

obesity and overweight: children, 140, 234, 235; city size and, 231; comorbid conditions, 96; food deserts and, 56; as health risk factor, 21, 95–96, 256–57; land use mix and, 239; older adults, 257–58; physical activity and, 105–6, 139, 211, 234–35; prevalence, 143–44, 203; quality of life, 143; racial/ethnic differences, 13, 96; restaurant availability and, 235–36; risk factors, 22, 95–96, 106, 140, 259; in rural America, 37, 96, 103, 138; sedentary activity and, 22; social isolation and, 11; street properties and, 244, 245; work-related travel behaviors and, 197, 198

Office of Management and Budget (OMB), 41–42, 44–46, 155

oil industry, 79–82, 90–91

older adults: aging in place, 52, 66; chronic diseases, 14; COVID-19 pandemic, xiii, xiv; Medicare, 52, 97, 107, 111, 113; mental disorders, 3, 144; obesity, 257–58; physical activity, 105; poverty, xiv, 52–53, 65, 67; in rural America, 52–53, 58–59, 66–67; as second-home owners, 58–59; social isolation, 98, 146, 163, 166, 238; transportation services, 41, 98

OpenStreetMap, 157

Ottawa Charter for Health Promotion, 4, 24, 25

Ozarks region, 51, 58

Pan, Sai Yi, 178

parks and green spaces: availability, 130, 177, 233–35, 238; health benefits, 233–35, 237, 246; land use mix, 239; at meso-spatial scale, 16; scarcity, 12; in small-town America, 37, 91, 106, 189; spatial design/planning and, 299–300, 305–6

participatory spatial design and planning, 340–52; advantages, 342–44; health promotion and, 345–52; levels of participation, 340–41; limitations, 341–42; traditional approach versus, 316–17

pathways of health influence: in built environments, 126, 304; education level as, 20–21; interpersonal networks as, 18; lifestyle and, 126; in natural environments, 8; in social environments, 11; spatial design/planning and, 6, 21, 23*f*, 28, 126–28, 127*f*

Penkalla, Anna Maria, 263–64

physical activity: built environments and, 95, 100, 212, 304; CDC guidelines, 137, 140; city size and, 174; commute time and, 217, 221; daytime population change and, 215–16, 220; defined, 139; density and, 175; distance to nearest city and, 216–17, 221; education level and, 21, 105, 178; health benefits, 130, 137, 139–40, 211, 234; key destinations and facility availability and, 176–80; land use types and, 181, 183, 190; moderate to vigorous, 177–78, 181, 184–85, 187, 199; in natural environments, 7, 8; neighborhood safety and, 11–12, 16–17; park access and, 177, 234–35; population density and, 215, 220; population size and, 214–15, 219; race/ethnicity and, 105, 178; rurality and spatial associations, 211–17, 218*t*; in small Kansas cities, 105–6, 112, 161*t*, 162, 165, 214–17;

physical activity (*cont.*)
  spatial design/planning for, 304–7; street
  properties and, 184–88, 190; urban-rural
  disparities, 212–14, 289–90. *See also* bicycling;
  walking
physical health: city size and, 231; commute time
  and, 261; daytime population change and,
  260–61; defined, 2; density and, 232, 246; distance to nearest city and, 261; in fringe areas, 62;
  indicators, 142–44; integration with mental and
  social health, 5; key destinations and facility
  availability and, 237–38; land use mix and, 241,
  242, 247; microenvironments and, 15–16; noise
  exposure and, 10; parks / green spaces and,
  233–34; physical activity and, 100; population
  density and, 260; population size and, 259–60;
  rurality and spatial associations, 256–61, 262*t*;
  in small Kansas cities, 163–65, 164*t*, 259–61; in
  small-town America, 69; social isolation and, 4,
  43; spatial design/planning for, 22, 307–8; street
  properties and, 243–45, 247; substance use and,
  100; urban-rural disparities, 258–59, 290
physical well-being, 2, 4, 26–27, 100, 232, 241, 285,
  345
Pivo, G., 181
place based approach, 120, 148, 288, 336 37
placemaking, 335–36
planning. *See* spatial design and planning; urban
  design and planning
Planning Walkable Places Program, 106
political environments, 25, 85, 317
pollution: agricultural, 79, 87; air, 7–10, 12, 17, 37,
  89–90, 197, 232; chemical, 87–88, 92; as health
  risk factor, 21, 92; industrial, 7–8; from livestock
  operations, 88–89, 92; from mining and oilfields,
  89–92; noise, 12, 17, 197; water, 10, 17, 56, 64,
  87–90, 327
population density: active commuting and, 198;
  census tracts and, 40, 44; crime rates and,
  103; eating and food shopping, 207–8, 219–20;
  health and, 260, 265, 271–72; measurement, 147;
  mortality/morbidity and, 254–55; physical and
  sedentary activities, 215, 220; in rural-urban
  classification schemes, 43–44; in small-town
  America, 49, 98; in urban America, 119, 232, 269;
  work-related travel behaviors and, 200–201, 219
population health: area-level studies, 122–26, 148;
  286; contexts, 5–14, 6*f*; defined, 4; health rank-

ings, 94–95; individual-level studies, 120–24, 148;
  pollution and, 92; principles, 5; promotion, 3, 5,
  24–27, 113, 301, 306, 311; in small Kansas cities,
  95–108, 112–13, 162–66, 164*t*; in small-town
  America, 37–38, 51, 69, 120. *See also* socio-
  ecological model of population health
population size: city classifications based on,
  75–76; eating and food shopping, 207, 219;
  health and, 259–60, 264, 271; in metropolitan-
  nonmetropolitan definitions, 42; mortality/
  morbidity and, 254; physical and sedentary
  activities and, 214–15, 219; of rural America,
  37, 45, 50–51, 55; in rural-urban classification
  schemes, 43, 45–46; of urban America, 45, 50;
  work-related travel behaviors and, 200, 219
Pouliou, Theodora, 239–40
poverty: air pollution and, 7, 12; city size and, 174,
  230–31; COVID-19 pandemic and, xiii–xiv; food
  deserts and, 12, 56, 205; food insecurity and, 139;
  generational, 109; health effects, 3, 12, 112; housing and, 15–16; industrial land use and, 182, 183,
  242; rural, 28, 51–53, 64–65, 67; in small Kansas
  cities, 77, 81, 111; SNAP threshold for, 104; substance use and, 100; urban, 64–65
property crime, 102, 145–46, 156, 232, 238, 242, 245,
  268
proximal factors, 5, 6
public health: data sources on, 157; defined, 5;
  federal and state allocations for, 111; as field of
  study, 119, 126, 148; in fringe areas, 62; funding
  for, 94; improvements in, 1, 186; spatial design/
  planning partnerships, 339
public policy and administration, 5, 24–25, 347–48
public services, 319, 334–35
public transportation, 138, 197–98, 213, 289–90,
  300, 331–34

quality of life, 10–11, 22, 67, 98–99, 111–12, 143–44,
  253

race and ethnicity: diabetes and, 97, 143; health
  disparities and, 13, 86; obesity and, 13, 96;
  physical activity and, 105, 178; in rural America,
  38–40, 53–54; segregation based on, 12, 17, 54,
  65; transportation access and, 98. *See also* immigrants; *specific racial and ethnic groups*
Raleigh, Veena Soni, 123
Ramirez, Laura K., 239

randomized controlled trials (RCTs), 338

Ray, Achintya, 230

restaurants, 80, 130–31, 179–80, 212, 235–38, 302

Robert Wood Johnson Foundation, 111

Rundle, Andrew, 239, 243

rural America: active commuting in, 197–99; agriculture in, 49, 51, 55–57, 60; birth rates in, 50–51, 55, 66; challenges for, 41, 49; changing trends in, 50–69; community participation in, 344–45; consumption in, 57–60; crime in, 37, 67, 268–69, 290–91; diversity in, 38–40, 53–54; economy in, 39, 49, 57–60, 67; employment in, 51, 55–57, 64; food deserts in, 12, 37, 56, 95, 104, 113, 204–5, 290; fringe areas, 61–63; frontier communities, 44, 49, 101; geography, 38–39; health care in, 14, 43, 52, 65–66, 106–8, 290; health indicator rankings in, 51; housing in, 41, 51, 58–59; immigrants in, 39, 53, 54, 67–68; in-migration to, 39, 50, 52, 58–59, 66; interdependency with urban America, 60–61, 67; obesity in, 37, 96, 103, 138; older adults in, 52–53, 58–59, 66–67; out-migration from, 14, 39, 50–52, 55, 67–69, 91; population size, 37, 45, 50–51, 55; poverty in, 28, 51–53, 64–65, 67; social and environmental justice issues in, 63–64, 67, 172; social determinants of health in, 14. *See also* nonmetropolitan areas; small-town America; *specific regions*

rurality: crime rates and, 102; defined, 40–45, 47, 195; eating behaviors and, 203–11, 210*t*; factors of, 146–47, 195; food shopping and, 203–11, 210*t*; geographic isolation and, 37, 43, 96, 152, 258, 285, 334; measurement, 42–44, 46, 129; mental health and, 262–66, 267*t*; mortality/morbidity and, 252–56, 257*t*; physical activity and, 211–17, 218*t*; physical health and, 256–61, 262*t*; sedentary activity and, 211–17, 218*t*; social health and, 266, 268–74, 275*t*; spatial associations of health and, 251–78, 257*t*, 262*t*, 267*t*, 275*t*, 278*t*, 296–99; spatial associations of lifestyle and, 195–222, 203*t*, 210*t*, 218*t*, 222*t*, 296–99; work-related travel behaviors and, 196–203, 203*t*

Rural-Urban Community Areas (RUCAs), 43

Rural-Urban Continuum Codes (RUCCs), 43

Rutt, Candace D., 242–43

Saarloos, Dick, 240

safety: city size and, 174; neighborhood, 6, 11–12,

16–17, 241; sense of, 3, 175, 188; spatial design/planning and, 232–33; street properties and, 185; walking and, 212–13

salutogens, 8, 26–27

SARS-CoV-2 global pandemic, xiii–xv, 107

scale-based approach, 120, 148, 288

second homes, 58–59

sedentary activity: city size and, 174; commute time and, 217, 221; daytime population change and, 216, 220; diabetes and, 95, 97, 140, 211; distance to nearest city and, 216–17, 221; driving to work and, 138; as health risk factor, 21, 140–41; key destinations and facility availability and, 180; land use types and, 183, 190; obesity and, 22, 95, 106, 140; population density and, 215, 220; population size and, 214–15, 219; rurality and spatial associations, 211–17, 218*t*; in small Kansas cities, 161*t*, 162, 165, 214–17; in small-town America, 37; spatial design/planning for, 304–7; street properties and, 187, 188

segment maps, 134–37, 160

segregation, 12, 17, 54, 65

Selvin, Hanan C., 124

serious mental illness (SMI), 262

serious psychological distress (SPD), 263

settlement health maps, 5

Shouls, Susanna, 123

single-occupancy vehicles (SOVs), 174, 181

skilled nursing care, 107

Sloggett, Andrew, 125

small Kansas cities: classifications for, 75–76; data sources on, 152, 155–58; demographic challenges in, 83–86; initiatives to identify health priorities, 109, 111–12; in study sample, 152, 153*t*, 154*f*, 285, 288–89

small-town America: challenges in, 37, 67–69; defined, 44–47, 152, 287–88; geographically isolated cities in, 37, 96, 152, 285, 334; population health in, 37–38, 51, 69, 120. *See also* rural America; small Kansas cities

Smith, G. Davey, 125

smoking, 11–13, 16–17, 21, 99, 125, 211, 257, 263

social environments, 5, 6*f*, 11–14, 98, 142, 286–87

social goods, 4, 62–63

social health: challenges, 49; city size and, 231–32; commute time and, 274; daytime population change and, 272–73; defined, 2–3; density and, 246; distance to nearest city and, 273–74;

social health (*cont.*)
  in fringe areas, 62; indicators, 145–46; individual versus collective dimensions, 3–4; integration with physical and mental health, 5; key destinations and facility availability and, 238; land use mix and, 240–42, 247; population density and, 271–72; population size and, 271; rurality and spatial associations, 266, 268–74, 275*t*; self-assessment, 290; in small Kansas cities, 164*t*, 271–74; in small-town America, 69; spatial design/planning and, 22; street properties and, 243–45, 247; substance use and, 100
social interactions, 2, 16, 306, 309, 314
social isolation: health effects, 4, 11, 22, 43, 96, 100, 269–70; older adults, 98, 146, 163, 166, 238; quality of place, 95; rural poverty, 65; in small-town America, 13, 37, 98–99. *See also* loneliness
social justice, 3, 11, 37, 63–64, 172
social realities, 3, 122
social support, 2–3, 11–13, 16, 21, 146, 233–34, 238, 308
social well-being, 2–4, 26–27, 241, 285, 345
sociocultural considerations, 9, 66, 311
sociodemographics, 9, 99, 204–5, 304, 311
socio-ecological model of population health, 5–29; built environments in, 5, 6*f*, 9 11, 120 22, 286–87; contexts of health in, 5–14, 6*f*; in Healthy Cities and Communities, 24–27; limitations, 286–87; natural environments in, 5–9, 6*f*, 286–87; organizational levels in, 5, 6*f*, 17–20, 20*f*, 27–29, 285–87; pathways of influence in, 6, 20–24, 28; placemaking and, 335–36; social environments in, 5, 6*f*, 11–14, 286–87; spatial scales in, 5, 6*f*, 14–17, 19–20, 20*f*, 27–28, 285–87
socioeconomic status (SES), 11, 18, 22, 121, 123–24, 177, 236. *See also* poverty
sociological units, 287
socio-spatial disparities, 205
soil composition, 330
space syntax, 133–37, 157, 185–86, 243
spatial associations of health, 229–78; city size and, 230–32, 246; density and, 232–33, 246; implications of findings, 294–99; key destinations and facility availability and, 233–39, 246; land use and, 239–42, 247; limitations, 289; mental health, 262–66, 267*t*; methodology for study, 229–30; mortality/morbidity and, 252–56, 257*t*; physical health, 256–61, 262*t*; rurality and, 251–78, 257*t*,

262*t*, 267*t*, 275*t*, 278*t*, 296–99; social health, 266, 268–74, 275*t*; street properties and, 242–45, 247
spatial associations of lifestyle, 171–222; city size and, 172–74, 188; density and, 174–76, 189; eating and food shopping, 203–11, 210*t*; implications of findings, 292–94, 296–99; key destinations and facility availability and, 176–81, 189; land use and, 181–83, 189–90; limitations, 289; methodology for study, 171–72; physical and sedentary activities and, 211–17, 218*t*; rurality and, 195–222, 203*t*, 210*t*, 218*t*, 222*t*, 296–99; street properties and, 183–88, 190; work-related travel behaviors and, 196–203, 203*t*
spatial data, 155, 157, 163, 291–92
spatial design and planning: for health, 307–9; health promotion and, 113–14, 309–11, 335–40, 345–52; for lifestyle, 21–22, 23*f*, 106, 299–307; pathways of influence and, 6, 21, 23*f*, 28, 126–28, 127*f*; for rural poverty, 28; safety and, 232–33; salutogenic effects, 27. *See also* participatory spatial design and planning; traditional spatial design and planning
spatial factors: city size, 128, 172–74, 188, 230–32, 246; health outcomes and, 14; housing and, 15–16; limitations, 288; segregation and, 17; in small Kansas cities, 158 60, 159 60*t*, 163, 165. *See also* density; key destinations and facility availability; land use mix; land use types; street properties
spatial scales, 5, 6*f*, 14–17, 19–20, 20*f*, 27–28, 184–85, 285–87
Stewart, Orion T., 199–200, 212
Stoddart, George L., 4
stormwater management, 327
Stowe, Ellen W., 213
street properties: active commuting and, 198–99; data sources on, 157; health and, 242–45, 247; lifestyle and, 183–88, 190; metric variables, 133; route accessibility, 133, 242–43; in small Kansas cities, 160, 186–88, 244–45; space syntax and, 133–37, 157, 185–86, 243; spatial design/planning and, 306–7; in suburban areas, 132–33, 185; urbanicity and, 132, 133
stroke, 97, 99, 143, 144, 211, 256, 258
subdivision regulations, 310, 319, 322–23, 325–28
substance use and abuse, 3, 13, 17, 21, 37, 67, 95, 100–102, 111, 125, 145
suburban areas, 57, 132–33, 181, 185, 318

suicide rates, 3–4, 38, 95, 101–2, 113, 142, 241, 253
Sundquist, Kristina, 125
Sunflower Foundation, 106
supermarkets. *See* grocery stores
Supplemental Nutrition Assistance Program
(SNAP), 104, 105, 303

3Ds (density, diversity, design), 182
topography, 328–29
traditional spatial design and planning, 317–40;
approaches, 320–22; contextual factors, 317–19;
health promotion and, 335–40; implementation
techniques, 322–28; legal and other provisions,
319–20; natural resources, 328–31; participatory
approach versus, 316–17; public services, 334–35;
public transportation, 331–34; sectoral view, 315
transportation infrastructure: access to, 6, 98, 112;
bridges, 37, 41; older adults, 41, 98; public, 138,
197–98, 213, 289–90, 300, 331–34; roads, 37, 63,
81; in small-town America, 50
Trivedi, Tushar, 211
Troped, Philip J., 181, 184
Trust for America's Health, 111
Tyson, 81

unemployment, 3, 57, 67, 80–81, 100, 113, 139, 205,
241
Uniform Crime Reporting (UCR) Program, 102
United Health Foundation, 94, 102
United Nations Human Settlement Program
(UN-Habitat), 15
units of analysis, 40, 122, 148, 287
University of Wisconsin Population Health Institute, 108, 109–10*t*
urban America: active commuting in, 197–99;
air pollution in, 7–8, 37; crime in, 103, 268–69,
290–91; economy in, 57; fringe areas, 61–63;
health care in, 14–16, 65–66; in-migration from,
39, 50, 52, 58–59, 66; interdependency with rural
America, 60–61, 67; mixed-use environments,
103, 131, 181, 232, 240–41; out-migration to, 14, 39,
50–52, 55, 67–69, 91; population density, 119, 232,
269; population size, 45, 50; poverty in, 64–65;
social determinants of health in, 14. *See also*
metropolitan areas
urban clusters (UCs), 42, 45–46, 152, 287
urban design and planning, 1, 212, 317
urban heat islands (UHIs), 17, 21, 37, 230

urbanicity: defined, 41–43, 45, 195; mental health
and, 262–64; physical activity and, 212–14,
289–90; physical health and, 258–59, 290; street
properties and, 132, 133
Urban-Rural Classification Scheme for Counties, 46
urban-rural divide, 123
US Census Bureau, 38, 41–43, 45, 155–58
US Department of Agriculture (USDA), 41–42, 46,
78, 82, 104, 139, 204
US Geological Survey, 87, 90
US-Mexico-Canada Agreement (USMCA), 77

vehicles. *See* driving to work
violence: built environments and, 11; crime and,
86, 102–3, 145–46, 156, 231–32, 238, 242, 245, 268;
domestic, 67, 112, 270; health effects, 11; immigrants and, 85; mental disorders and, 3; neighborhood, 16–17; reduction, 4; substance use and,
100
volatile organic compounds (VOCs), 90

walking: city size and, 174; density and, 174, 175,
189, 215; health benefits, 141; land use mix and,
181; park availability, 177; population size and,
214; safety concerns, 212–13; to school, 185,
199; street properties and, 184–85, 187–88, 300;
utilitarian, 199–200, 300; to work, 137–38, 162,
180, 197, 217
Walk Score, 213
Wang, Fahui, 259
water resources, 87, 90, 329–30
weight. *See* obesity and overweight
Weisheit, R. A., 268, 269
well-being: economic, 64, 137, 301; mental, 2–4, 8,
10, 26–27, 100, 232, 241, 262, 285, 345; physical, 2,
4, 26–27, 100, 232, 241, 285, 345; in rural America, 57, 60; social, 2–4, 26–27, 241, 285, 345
Wells, L. Edward, 269
Wells, Nancy M., 183
western Kansas, 78, 81–82
Whitehead, Margaret, 5
Wing, Steve, 123
Wood, Lisa, 240, 243
workers' compensation, 105
work-related travel behaviors: active commuting,
197–99; bicycling, 138, 162, 180, 197; carpooling,
138, 162, 179, 187, 190, 197, 200–202; city size and,
173; commute time and, 62, 147, 198, 202, 221;

work-related travel behaviors (*cont.*)
  daytime population change and, 147, 201, 220;
  distance to nearest city and, 201–2, 221; driving
  alone, 108, 113, 138, 162, 179, 187, 197, 200–202;
  key destinations and facility availability and, 179,
  299–300; land use and, 182, 190, 300; population
  density and, 200–201, 219; population size and,
  200, 219; public transportation and, 138, 197–98,
  300; rurality and spatial associations, 196–203,
  203*t*; in small Kansas cities, 161*t*, 162, 165,
  200–203; spatial design/planning for, 299–301;
  street properties and, 186–87, 190, 300; walking,
  137–38, 162, 180, 197, 217
World Health Organization (WHO), 5, 8, 197,
  340; European Healthy Cities Network, 314–15;

European Regional Office, 12, 24; health as
  defined by, 2–4, 285; Health for All and, 5, 24,
  316, 340–41; Healthy Cities projects, 24, 316,
  344; Ottawa Charter for Health Promotion, 4,
  24, 25
Wuthnow, Robert, 44–45

Xu, Yanqing, 259

Yang, Yizhao, 183
years of potential life lost (YPLL), 101, 253

Zhang, Xingyou, 198, 258–59
Zhou, Bin, 230
zoning ordinances, 309–10, 319–25, 327